THE
BEAUTY
BIBLE

THE

SARAH STACEY

BEAUTY

JOSEPHINE FAIRLEY

BIBLE

KYLE CATHIE LIMITED

To Clive and Craig,
who never saw us while we wrote this book,
but were always there

First published in Great Britain in 1996 by
Kyle Cathie Limited
20 Vauxhall Bridge Road, London SW1V 2SA
Reprinted 1996
ISBN 1 85626 225 1

A Cataloguing in Publication record for this title is available
from the British Library

Designed by the Senate
Printed and bound in Italy
by Editoriale Johnson

The publishers wish to thank Simon Alderton at Twentieth Century Design,
274 Upper Street, London N1 for the loan of his warehouse and props.

CONTENTS

ACKNOWLEDGEMENTS

This book couldn't have been published without the unstintingly generous help of the following people:

OUR EXPERTS: Tania Alexander, Beryl Barnard, Bobbi Brown, Dr Karen Burke, Kay Cooper, Paul Edmonds, Johanna Faber, Eva Fraser, John Frieda, Stephen Glass, Gillian Hamer, Jo Hansford, Susan Harmsworth, Patrick Holford, Dr Susan Horsewood-Lee, Maggie Hunt, Stanley Kay, Eve Lom, Kathryn Marsden, Denise McAdam, Lorna McKnight, Orlando Pita, Leigh Richmond, Dr Hugh Rushton, Magdy Saad, Gloria Thomas, Dr Luca Turin, Jacki Wadeson.

OUR TESTERS who included: Amanda Acland, Lynne Allen, Becky Bain, Maureen Barrymore, Emma Bittleston, Nicole Boyd, Cluny Brown, Joanna Brown, Olivia Brown, Alison Bullivant, Liz Calvert, Alexandra Campbell, Stephanie Cargill, Annette Clark, Penny Clay, Caroline Clegg, Sally-Anne Clifton, Penny Cobham, Barbara Coles, Heidi Crawford, Louise Crook, Alison Day, Valerie Day, Alex Douglas-Home, Marian Draper, Helen Fairley, Nicky Fairley, Suzy Fitzgerald, Adele Fletcher, Phillippa Fox, Helen Galbraith, Liz Galbraith, Felicity Geidt, Jayne Gibbons, Joy Goodman, Lily Ann Green, Gillian Greenwood, Suzanne Guyler, Annie Hanson, Anya Harris, Tessa Hatts, Joanne Hillestad, Val Holmes, Beryl Hope, Susan Hope, Kashmira Irani, Carole Justice, Sophie Kelly, Simone Klass, Jill Koops, Carolynda MacDonald, Sybil MacDonald, Jane Magnus, Jessica Mangold, Karen Mason, Clare Mastrandreas, Caitlin Maxwell, Susan Maxwell, Emma McGrath, Amanda McKee, I. Muddell, Kaye Murphy, Linda Muse, Diana Mustafa, Penny Neu, Susan Newbould, Latifa Noubiat, Sally Pardo, Claire Parker, Kathryn Parkinson, Tracey Patterson, Wendy Payne, Sue Peart, Beatrice Petty, Joanna Petty, Jane Phillimore, Ruth Pinder, Maren Price, Fiona Rowntree, Emma Ryley, Jean Ryley, Margaret Sams, Christina Sesay, Annie Shellard, Sarah Shepherd-Walwyn, Dianne Stacey, Pat Sutherland, Simone Sutherland, Sarah Tolson, Cheryl Travis, Barbara Tremble, Sara-Jane Vere Nicoll, Sally Waddell, Juliet Walker, Sophia Wallace-Turner, Rebecca Weathers, Anne Webb, Clare Willson, Francesca Yorke.

OUR 'FOREIGN CORRESPONDENTS' who included: Maggie Alderson, Bruna Bellino Weyler, Felicity Bosanquet, Pilar Boxford, Catherine Fairweather, Nicola Furey, Fiona Giannoulis, Janine di Giovanni, Angela Godfrey, Meg Guilford, Barbara Huber, Poppy King, Alison Mazzola, Karen Moline, Princess Béatrice d'Orléans, Sally Patterson, Gloria Pujol, Ruth Soh, Domenica Spencer, Bharti Vyas, Kate Williams.

AND ESPECIAL GRATITUDE to our editor Candida Hall, designer David Eldridge, illustrator David Downton, picture researcher Natalie Bray, photographer Laura Hodgson, all-round-helper Cluny Brown and researcher Sally Pardo. Also to Michael Cole and to Meg Gilmore, and all the many beauty PRs who gave us their help.

LASTLY we would like to thank our agent Laura Morris, publisher Kyle Cathie, and Dee Nolan, the Editor of YOU magazine, who backed us to the hilt.

INTRODUCTION

We wrote this book to answer the endless stream of questions lobbed at us by friends, friends of friends, readers and even perfect strangers, who have shown an insatiable appetite for information about health and beauty.

We don't just write about these subjects. Between us, we've been avid consumers for more than five decades (Sarah b. 1949, Jo b. 1956). In *The Beauty Bible* we have pooled everything we know and asked experts worldwide to add their knowledge and experience.

We love make-up, skincare and fragrance and we believe their effects are not only cosmetic: well-chosen products can lift a woman's spirits as well as offer an instant boost to her appearance. But looking and feeling great requires a long-term philosophy beyond the quick fix of a new lipstick. So we have set out what we are convinced is the ultimate two-way approach to beauty, where what goes into your body and your mind matters just as much as what goes on your eyes, skin, nails and hair.

When it came to deciding which products to recommend, we realised we needed the experience of as many women as possible – as well as a team of experts. Most magazine 'tried and testeds' are carried out by one tester alone. With this book, we hope to have done what no one else has: to discover which products, out of the bewildering array on the market, really are effective.

We recruited a panel of about one hundred women, of all ages, varying lifestyles and different colourings, and asked groups of them to test a total of around 1,000 different products, both brand leaders and lesser known names, in all price ranges. Each product went to at least six women, so that we could compile average scores as well as recording individual comments. The results are categorised as *Top Treats* and *Best Budget Buys* and, where possible, we give a *Natural Choice*. With this unique guide, we hope you can now save time and money finding the best buys for you.

We had a wonderful time writing *The Beauty Bible*. We hope you enjoy reading it.

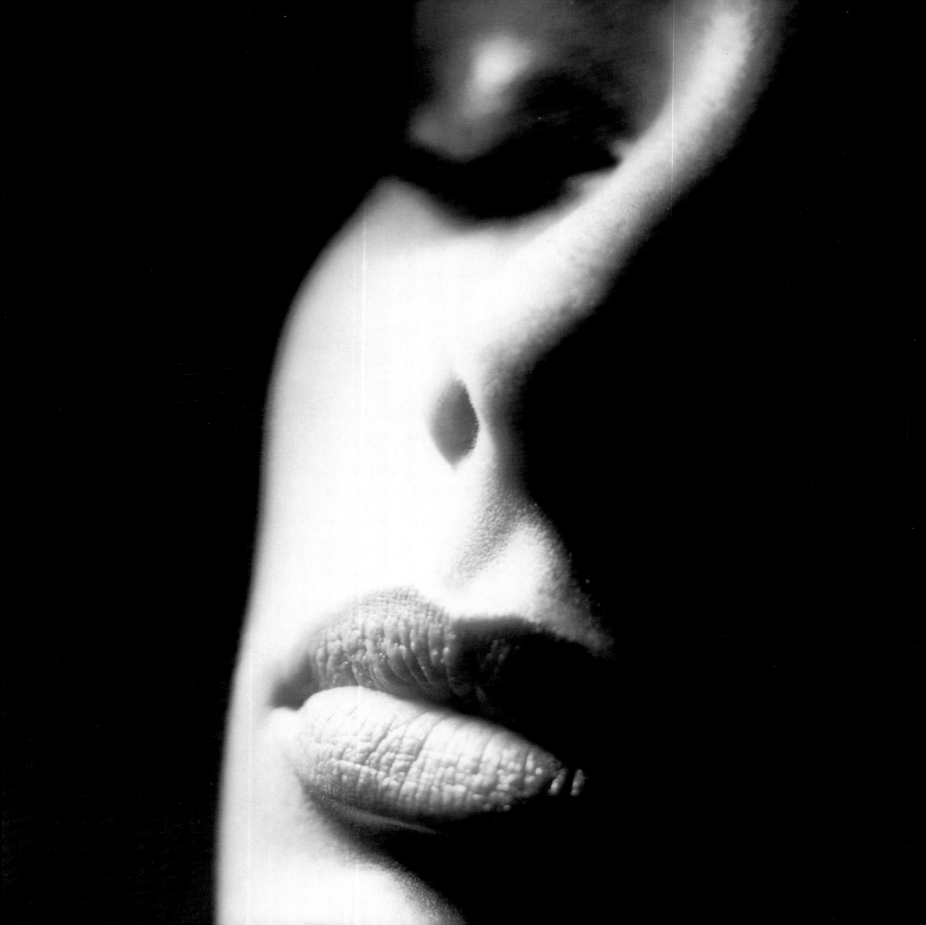

1 Face First

The right make-up won't dramatically change the way you look –

you should continue to look yourself, only lovelier. (And the

psychological boost it gives you isn't imaginary. Japanese scientists

have been able to link a stepping up of the immune system to the

application of cosmetics.) **But the secret every**

woman *really* wants to know is how to

apply perfect make-up, every time. Here is the

low-down from the world's top professionals and the world's most

attractive women, as well as reports on hundreds of make-up

products, tried and tested, to save you from wasting time. This

chapter contains the only make-up advice you'll ever need...

BOBBI BROWN
MAKE-UP MASTERCLASS

THE ONLY TEN MAKE-UP STEPS YOU'LL EVER NEED

Since she launched her bestselling signature line of cosmetics six years ago, Bobbi Brown has become the world's most famous make-up artist. Her philosophy is in tune with every busy woman's lifestyle: a pared-down regime of make-up that enhances a woman's natural beauty in the absolute minimum of time. No woman, she insists, needs more than ten make-up steps to look fabulous. 'Most days, less than that,' she adds.

Bobbi advises drawing up a list based on her steps (opposite) of the ten – or fewer – products you use most often, from the times when you rush out to walk the dog, right through to black-tie dinners. 'Decide what's the most crucial. Make that your everyday, going-to-the-shops/hanging-out-at-home regime. It really shouldn't take more than a couple of minutes. For work – or for lunch – pick the six or so steps that make the most difference. And leave the whole works for evenings only.'

Bobbi suggests choosing from her list those steps which you really can't face the world without. For day, for instance, brunettes often need concealer, but they needn't always do brows and lashes. Blondes always need to define brows and eyes, but may not need blusher because they often have a pink complexion. Redheads probably want lip pencil, even if it's a nude shade, because they often have little colour in their lips. And black women usually have to wear lipstick. A younger woman can often simply go out with foundation, lipstick and a well-groomed brow, she says. 'But anyone over 30 will probably want to add concealer to her list, since that's the age when most women start to notice under-eye circles. And every woman has positive features; if your eyes are not your best feature, play up your lips. I don't believe so much in heavily disguising flaws as drawing attention away from them to a woman's good points.'

(For our more detailed make-up steps, see page 42.)

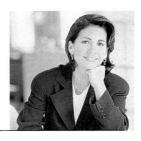

BOBBI'S TIPS

■ If you do overdo it? 'I keep a supply of cotton buds and cotton wool, and velvet powder puffs, to gently stroke it off again...'

■ 'Use shadow – not pencils – to fill in the brows, with a fine brush. It looks more natural.'

■ 'I honestly think that if you have to use an eyelash curler, there's something wrong with your mascara.'

■ Bobbi's line on evening beauty is that nobody needs much more than day make-up; the difference is in the colours. 'Maybe you wear more foundation, deeper lipstick, brighter lipstick, more shimmery lipstick – even a touch of pearl shadow on the browbone. Try darker colours on the eyes: charcoal, navy liner, slate – just darker, not heavier. The mistake most women make is to go for a complete change. The bottom line is: if the colours need blending on the skin, you're wearing the wrong make-up; it should still look very natural.'

Bobbi's step-by-step tips for perfect application

1. **Foundation**: 'I don't like to use foundation all over, just where there are imperfections: most often under the eyes, around the mouth and nose, and on any blemishes.'

2. **Concealer**: 'I like to use stick foundation because it doubles as a concealer. I blend it with my finger – especially on the bone at the inner corner of the eyes, which is where people often have grey shadows, and around the nose. Concealer is layered on top of foundation.'

3. **Powder**: 'I prefer loose powder in the morning – applied with a velour puff, then dusted off with a big fluffy brush. I put some powder in the palm of my hand and press the puff into it, then onto the face. I recommend this before you get dressed, or it goes everywhere. Then carry pressed powder for daytime touch-ups. Powder can be slightly yellow-toned, or neutral, but it shouldn't make you look pale.'

4. **Brows**: 'I use a powder, not a pencil, with a hard-edged brush – and I don't make them too dark. Just enough colour to define them.'

5. **Eyeliner**: 'I actually like to do this before eyeshadow, because for plenty of women that's all they need. I use an eyeliner brush dipped in dark shadow to line the eyes. You can use it wet or dry.'

6. **Eyeshadow**: 'On days when more impact's needed than just eyeliner, I first like to sweep a neutral highlighter shade – like bone – all over the brow and the eyelid, which doubles as a base to help shadow stay put. The more tired you are, the more you need eyeshadow. But my tip is never to use a dark shade on the eyelid – not even at the edges. I prefer a medium shade, like taupe, charcoal or heather, to shade the socket and the edges of the eyes. Darker shadows need a lot of blending and only make-up artists are really great at that.'

7. **Blusher**: 'Blush is my favourite thing in the world: if you have the right blush, you look younger, fresher, prettier. Older women should definitely add a tawny blush – which looks more natural than coral or red – to their list of basics; it becomes more important as you mature, as the skin cells don't turn over as quickly and skin doesn't look as fresh. I sometimes use two: a neutral shade, and then a brighter one on top. The darker your colouring, the more blush you need.'

8. **Lipstick**: 'I like to apply this straight from the tube – I never seem to have time for a brush, although lip brushes make lipstick last longer. Medium tones are easiest for most women to wear, and lip stains are a really natural-looking choice.'

9. **Lip pencil**: 'If the lips really need more definition, I apply this after lipstick, rather than before, for definition – it looks less hard-edged.'

10. **Mascara**: 'A good mascara should colour and curl your lashes with just one coat.'

BOBBI BROWN essentials

MAKE-UP BAGS

THE SECRETS OF THE STARS' MAKE UP BAGS

Elle Macpherson: 'If I'm feeling under the weather, I put on Guerlain's Terracotta Bronzing Powder. I can't get away with not doing my eyebrows, so I use a dark brown Shiseido pencil on them. Otherwise, I just curl my lashes, apply mascara and wear Max Factor lip gloss instead of ordinary lipstick.'

Novelist **Jackie Collins**: 'I'm a make-up fiend. I wear Estée Lauder powder, M.A.C. foundation, and Revlon mascara. Bobbi Brown lipsticks are the absolute best. My shade is No. 4 Lip Shimmer.'

Yasmin Le Bon: 'M.A.C. Satin Foundation C3, which is sheer and slightly yellow-toned, suits my skin. I like Shu Uemura loose powder, in Camel 8 – just a light dusting to stop shine. I'm not a big fan of lipsticks, but I have a collection of favourites: M.A.C. Spice Lip Pencil with Kiehl's Lip Balm on top to add gloss. M.A.C. Chilli, Paramount or Veruschka lipsticks are great worn with a coat of The Body Shop Colourings Lip Tint on top.'

Carla Bruni: 'When I wear make-up, I try to use it very lightly. I put almost nothing on the eyes, and I do my lips so it looks like me naturally, but better. But I wouldn't leave the house without my M.A.C. compact (Studiofix Powder Plus Foundation). It makes your face up in half a second. And I use Clinique CityBlock as a base. It's more like an "environment cream", good not only for the sun but to keep dust and pollution away from the skin.'

'So long as I have concealer and a hair slide, I can make myself look decent,' says supermodel **Stephanie Seymour**. But she loves lipstick, too. Favourites are Clinique's Almost Lipstick in Black Honey, M.A.C.'s X-Pose and Molton Brown's Lipcolour in Nearly Nude.

Actress **Tori Spelling**, from *Beverly Hills 90210*, knows what she likes: she was spotted at the M.A.C. make-up counter buying up 12 tubes of Del Rio lipstick, a satiny pink-brown colour.

What you'll find in our make-up bags

SARAH:
Bobbi Brown *Nude* Lipstick
Givenchy Eyeshadow Prism in *Topaz* (also works on brows)
Givenchy Beauté No. 5 Lip Pencil and Brush
Estée Lauder Dark Grey Eyeliner Pencil
Guerlain Mascara
Christian Dior Fascination Free-style Enhancing Mascara
Kiehl's Lip Balm
Tweezers and Natural Nail Company Emery Board
Yves Saint Laurent Touche Éclat Concealer
Estée Lauder Doublewear Stay-in-Place Makeup
Chanel Perfecting Bronze Powder and Powder Blush Soleil Doré

JO:
Chanel Double Perfection Makeup
Chanel Powder Blush
Aveda Cacao Definitive Eye Pencil
Bobbi Brown Black Kohl Pencil
Bobbi Brown *Taupe* Eyeshadow (for my brows)
Bobbi Brown *Sable* Eyeshadow
Bobbi Brown *Ruby Stain* Lipstick/Gloss
L'Oréal Voluminous Mascara

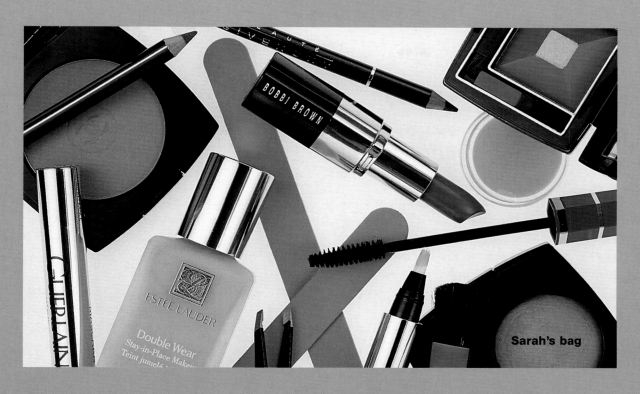

Sarah's bag

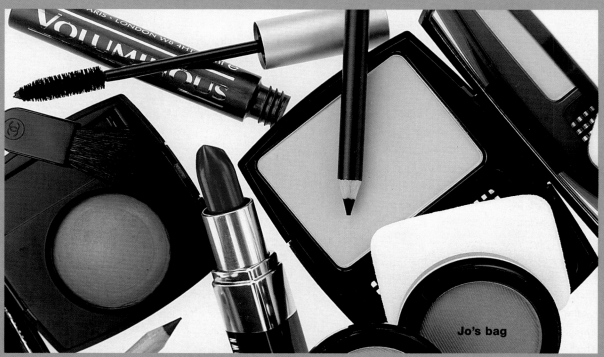

Jo's bag

FOUNDATIONS

The search for the elusive, perfect foundation is beauty's Holy Grail. In the UK 23 per cent of the money we lavish on cosmetics goes on foundation. And since finding your fabulous foundation match is so tough, you can bet that plenty of those tubes, bottles and jars wind up unworn and unwanted in the back of the bathroom cabinet.

Forty per cent of women don't even try – call it 'fear of foundation failure'. Yet applying foundation is an art that really is worth mastering. With great-looking skin, courtesy of Mother Nature or a cosmetics company, you can get away with a lot less of everything else.

MEETING YOUR MATCH

The biggest mistake most women make is choosing a foundation that's too pink. Skin isn't actually pink; it has a lot of yellow in it, so putting on pink foundation creates an unnatural flushed look and an obvious tide-mark against the neck. (There are better ways to 'perk up' skin than adding too pink a foundation. That's what blusher's designed for.) Fortunately, many cosmetic houses have recently introduced 'yellow pigments' into their foundation formulations. These don't make skin look sallow, just give natural results, instead.

■ Test foundation on the inside of the forearm – skin tone is closest to neck colour there, because it's protected from UV damage. According to US make-up artist Kevyn Aucoin, 'Make-up should blend with the skin colour of the neck, not the face.'

■ If in doubt, Bobbi Brown advises buying one shade lighter than your facial skin tone. (Going darker looks unnatural.)

■ Don't make up your mind instantly. Christian Dior's in-house make-up guru Eliane Gouriou points out: 'It takes about a minute for colour to dry and interact with the chemicals in your skin. The red pigments develop first, so it will appear pinkest at the beginning.'

■ Then go to the nearest source of natural light. (Even the most flatteringly uplit cosmetics hall tends to have colour-distorting fluorescent lighting.) If you have chosen the right colour, it will disappear into your skin.

■ Don't be shy about asking for advice; that's what beauty consultants are there for.

TIPS FROM THE PROS

■ Bobbi Brown always likes to put on make-up facing a window, if possible: 'Daylight is the truest light, and you won't get any nasty surprises.'

■ Kevyn Aucoin: 'Priming the skin before foundation is essential. To do that, cover your face with a light layer of moisturiser and let it sit for about ten minutes; less for oily complexions. Then blot off. I've found that this not only provides better coverage, but it also keeps the foundation from changing tone and looking mottled during the course of the day.'

■ Top session make-up artist Mary Greenwell (who also works with **Diana, Princess of Wales**) says: 'Forget sponges. I always prefer to apply make-up with my (clean) fingers; it enables you to reach places that sponges never can, and avoids streaking – sometimes a problem with sponged-on make-up. It also warms the foundation slightly on the skin, which allows for smoother application.' Once foundation is on the skin, the key is to blend, blend, blend – especially around the nose, hairline and jaw, which are most often the tell-tale giveaway areas.

■ Mary Greenwell, along with many other top professionals, believes in stroking foundation, powder and blusher downwards, otherwise you are pushing pigment up into pores, so highlighting them. 'And never put too much foundation under the outer eyes,' she adds, 'because it emphasises lines.'

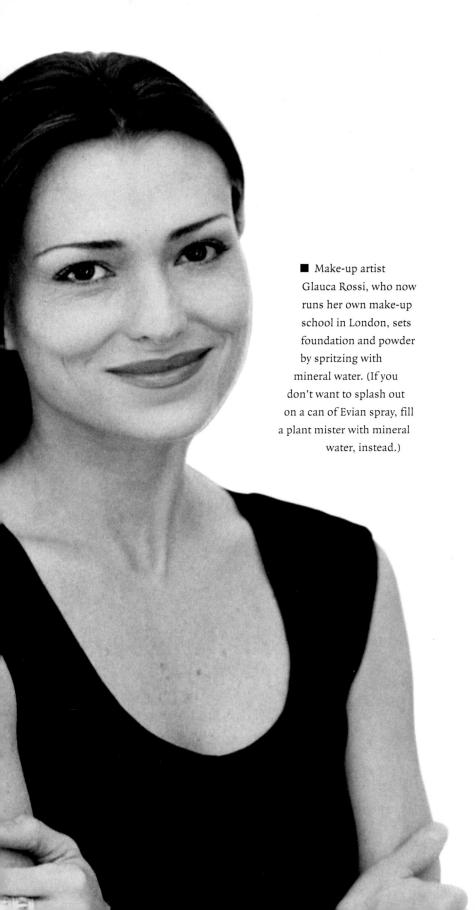

■ Make-up artist Glauca Rossi, who now runs her own make-up school in London, sets foundation and powder by spritzing with mineral water. (If you don't want to splash out on a can of Evian spray, fill a plant mister with mineral water, instead.)

■ Manhattan make-up pro Fulvia Farolfi believes in fixing foundation with an Evian spray, too. She then blots cheeks and forehead with a tissue to absorb any excess moisture.

■ Your foundation disappears? Vanishing make-up can be the result of either very dry or very oily skin, according to New York make-up artist Lynne Geller. Dry skin is so thirsty for moisture that it literally soaks up cosmetics. To combat the problem, Geller recommends choosing make-up formulations with creamy textures. Misting your face regularly with an Evian spray or a plant mister can help, too. With oily skin, enlarged pores allow make-up to seep right into your skin. Excess oils can tamper with the texture, making it rub off easily every time you touch your face. Skip the moisturiser and look for an oil-free formula – or consider all-in-one make-up/powder formulations, which are less likely to be absorbed into the skin (see *Make-Up on the Go*, page 23).

■ Christian Dior's in-house make-up artist, Eliane Gouriou, recommends applying base and powder, then (if you've time) waiting five full minutes before you add colour to the face. 'It allows make-up to "set" better, so it will last much longer.'

TIP Many companies offer free foundation samples and encourage customers to try them. Test-drive for a few days. That way, you won't get a rude awakening after you've parted with your money.

CONCEALER SECRETS

■ Mary Greenwell's concealer rules: first, match your skin tone – test on the inside of your forearm. Finding the perfect match may be harder than with foundations because there are fewer shades created. Second, don't overdo it.

■ Mary advises choosing a slightly creamy product for under-eye circles; matte concealers can cake on dry skin around the eyes. However, a product that's too slippery or liquid will 'pool' into tiny lines.

■ Which should go on first, concealer or foundation? Kevyn Aucoin believes in foundation first, concealer second. If you do it the other way round, you'll rub off the concealer when you put on your foundation. After applying concealer, he sets it by pressing firmly with a lightly dusted powder puff, 'which works powder into concealer, concealer into base, and base into skin.'

■ Joan Price, who has, since the sixties, schooled generations of women in make-up techniques at her Face Place in London, agrees that concealer should be applied after, not before, the base itself; she uses a square, stiff 2cm (3/4in) artist's brush. To get a good skin match she always mixes concealer with a dab of foundation (on the back of the hand), recommending this 'custom-blended' concealer to cover frown lines, red veins, under-eye circles and blemishes.

■ US make-up artist Trish McEvoy prefers to use an oil-free foundation rather than actual concealer to disguise blemishes: 'I dab oil-free make-up on a Q-Tip, place it on the blemish, let it dry and then "puff out" the edges with the end of the Q-Tip.'

TRIED & TESTED

CONCEALERS

With a good concealer (i.e. one which matches your skin tone) covering any small imperfections – thread veins, tiny scars, dark circles, open pores – you may well not need foundation. From an initial few – which had a sticking-plaster tint and heavy coverage – there is now a wide range of excellent products for every skin type. Remember the secret is less is more.

Top Treats

Christian Dior Anti-Cernes Perfecteur
This achieved outstanding marks from our panellists.
COMMENTS: 'looked especially natural', 'very good for eye area', 'you only need a tiny amount'.

Kanebo Exclusive Bio Concealer
A compact-style product with mirror from the internationally respected Japanese cosmetics line, which our testers reported was particularly easy to apply.
COMMENTS: 'it stayed on perfectly', 'really hid spots and even large freckles', 'filled in open pores very well'.

François Nars Concealer
This concealer was created by one of the world's top celebrity make-up artists, who has to know a thing or two about covering up blemishes!
COMMENTS: 'the texture was good', 'scored highly for thread veins and dark circles', 'good on its own for a natural look at weekends'.

Best Budget Buys

No. 7 Blemish Concealer
This product scored highest of all the products tried in any price category.
COMMENTS: 'covered dark circles very well', 'good packaging – easy to use', 'natural even without make-up – no orange tones'.

L'Oréal Perfection Magic Concealer
Shaped like a felt tip pen, the sponge applicator delivers concealer dab by dab and was praised by all our testers.
COMMENTS: 'I was surprised by how easy the applicator was to use', 'looked very natural, even without foundation'.

Natural Choice

Aveda Protective Cream Concealer
This compact-style concealer is from a pioneering 'New Age' beauty company which leads the way in providing cosmetics with no petro-chemicals and the minimum of synthetic ingredients.
COMMENTS: 'lovely compact', 'looked natural', 'I found it excellent for covering up blackheads'.

POWDER PERFECTION

❑ Which is best to set make-up – loose powder, or the pressed version? Bobbi Brown likes both (see her *Masterclass*, page 12): loose powder for first thing, then pressed powder during the day. 'The advantage of pressed powder is that it doesn't spill,' she explains. 'But if you don't use a light touch, it can sometimes appear to sit on the surface. Press it, never rub, onto the surface.'

❑ Maggie Hunt, who has made up everyone from **Paul McCartney** to **Diana, Princess of Wales**, still prefers to apply loose powder with a slim cosmetic sponge (washed regularly with warm water and a squirt of washing-up liquid or shampoo): 'I don't like big, fluffy brushes. They might look nice, but they don't get in the corners around eyes and nostrils, and they pick up grease from foundation.'

❑ French make-up artist Stéphane Marais likes lightweight, 'light-reflecting' powders – now available from many companies (such as Estée Lauder, Yves Saint Laurent and Chanel): 'So many powders are too heavy. I hate matte. It kills the light of the skin.' He also believes that perfecting the technique of applying foundation and powder matters more than any other make-up skill. With make-up the skin should be the most important focus: 'You can have not very good technique on eyes and lips – yet still look good,

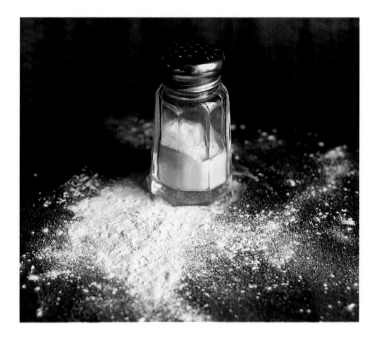

❑ If you keep loose powder in its box, it can scatter everywhere. Lesli Fader, make-up artist for America's Fox cable network show, *Breakfast Time*, decants it into glass pepper shakers. That way, you can shake out precisely how much you want – and 'custom-blend' two or more colours together.

PERFECT CAMOUFLAGE

Cosmetic camouflage creams which conceal blemishes on face and body are now extremely effective. But how you apply cosmetic camouflage is all-important. A thick layer will look obvious and – as for most forms of make-up – less is definitely more. Stephen Glass, a make-up artist who specialises in camouflage, recommends: 'Put your foundation on first, then put some camouflage make-up on your ring finger. Remove most of it with a plastic cosmetic spatula, then lightly pat a thin layer onto your face. Repeat, building up as many thin layers as you need. Do the same on your body, but first test it without foundation to see the result.'

The British Red Cross runs a cosmetic camouflage programme, available on referral from your doctor only, to help people with severe burns, scars, birthmarks or vitiligo (uneven pigmentation). Consultations with specially trained volunteers, all experienced

therapists, are free and most of the special creams (which are waterproof and contain a sunscreen) are available on prescription. Further information is available from the Beauty Care Officer at local Red Cross branches in the UK.

Advice is also available from the British Association of Skin Camouflage (BASC). The BASC will supply the name of your nearest member, who, for a modest fee, will discuss individual requirements and recommend products from the Dermablend, Dermacolour, Covermark, Veil and Keromask ranges. These are available on prescription and over-the-counter at branches of Boots.

Stephen Glass also highly rates the Doreen Savage Trust in Fife, Scotland; Doreen herself has a port wine stain down the side of her face and provides information and help for people with birthmarks. (See DIRECTORY.)

■ Estée Lauder's lightweight Maximum Cover, which Stephen Glass recommends, was voted 'absolutely brilliant' by one woman who tried it on the black scabs of shingles. It is waterproof, long-lasting and easily applied. In green and yellow colour correctors, to alter skin shade, plus four shades of foundation, Maximum Cover (available worldwide) will cover scars, bruises, broken capillaries, sunspots and pock-marks. Manufacturers say it will also hide patches of vitiligo.

■ Clinique's Continuous Coverage, in five different shades, also gives a good, natural (although slightly heavier) coverage, according to Stephen Glass; it's also available worldwide. Boots No. 7 range offers an effective allergy-screened, non-drying cover-up stick called Shade Away, which conceals small blemishes such as spots and broken veins.

DECIPHERING FOUNDATION-SPEAK

Labels can be so confusing that you can end up buying the wrong product for your skin – or not buying anything at all. Here's the lowdown.

Cream-to-powder (All-in-one or Powder/gel): Formulations that go on like a cream but rapidly dry, eliminating need to set with powder.

Demi-matte (Semi-matte, Satin): Offers the most natural look. The most wearable of all the finishes, demi-matte has the flawless coverage of matte (no imperfections show through) without its powdery texture, and allows the skin to have a healthy sheen.

Dewy: Almost a wet-look, shiny, glistening finish. Anyone can wear this, but it's sheer and won't mask imperfections. Women with oily skin (who have spent their life fighting this look) generally won't like it.

Foundation stick: Looks like a giant concealer stick, but softer to the touch; a great timesaver as it can be applied quickly, then blended.

Light-diffusing: Featuring special pigments that reflect light, this gives the optical illusion of a younger skin. Available in different strengths of cover – from medium to heavy – and in both pressed and loose powder.

Line-minimising: See *light-diffusing*.

Matte: Flat, powdery, won't reflect light, but can sap tone from skin if you don't use blusher. Good for oily skins. At its best, gives a shine-free appearance, but it can look overdone if applied heavy-handedly.

Maximum cover (Total cover): Opaque coverage, best for less-than-perfect complexions, disguising minor imperfections and even some birthmarks and moles. (See *Perfect Camouflage*, page 19.)

Microsphere: A term for tiny, microscopic particles of ingredient (which seems specially designed to blind the consumer with science).

Nanosphere: See *microsphere*.

Non-comedogenic: Won't clog pores. (Clogged pores lead to blackheads and whiteheads.) Good for oily/blemish-prone skin.

Oil-free: Special water-based formulation for oily skins, often using easy-glide silicone particles in place of moisturising elements.

Pore-minimising: A liquid foundation (shake well to mix) which deflects light from imperfections and controls oil production. Great for acne sufferers and oily skin types with large pores.

Sheer: The minimal coverage available, more a moisturiser than foundation, but just enough to even out skin tone. Best for clear skin; it won't cover freckles, blemishes or dark skin around the eyes.

Two-in-one: Versatile formulations which can be used dry – as a lightly-covering powder – or with a wetted sponge, for greater cover. (See *wet/dry*.)

UV filters: Will protect against the harmful effects of the sun's rays. (See *Weather-Beating Beauty*, page 98.) However, assume that unless it states the SPF number, only minimal protection is offered. Dermatologists consider that anything under SPF15 isn't really enough, so if you're concerned about sun damage, try switching from a regular under-foundation moisturiser to one with a SPF15 or a lightweight SPF15 sun product instead.

Velvet: A rich, not-too-matte texture, giving good cover. Perfect for evenings.

Wet/Dry: Allows you to experiment because you get two looks out of one palette. Apply dry for a lighter, silky finish, wet for more cover.

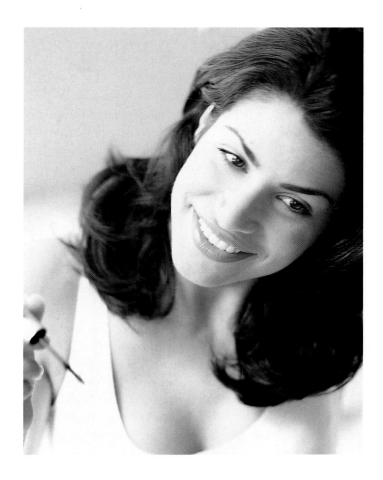

TIPS FROM THE TOP

Actress **Molly Ringwald**: 'I like Shiseido translucent powder, because it's soft and the right colour for me.'
 Singer **Chynna Phillips**: 'Clinique has a great foundation called Almost Make-up; it's so light that you can't tell that you're wearing make-up at all. It covers all the blemishes – like that little bit of acne that pops up now and again.'

MULTICULTURAL MAKE-UP

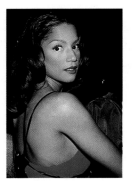

Women of colour are often frustrated by a lack of make-up choice. Flori Roberts and Fashion Fair cosmetics are specifically designed for dark skins, and offer the wide choice every woman should be able to expect at a make-up counter. Marks & Spencer Classics and Avon have now launched ranges for darker skins, too. Prescriptives offer a 'custom-blending' foundation service for every colour of skin from fairest to darkest, while Japan-based Shiseido and Shu Uemura (see DIRECTORY) have good selections for Asian and Oriental skin tones.

A HINT OF A TINT

In summer, many women swap foundation for tinted moisturiser, which gives a hint of colour and evens out skin tones. This allows freckles to show through (which is why redheads such as actress **Molly Ringwald** are fans), and avoids a foundation-and-powder look which can seem unnatural on a hot day. Stephen Glass recommends a compromise between the sheerness of tinted moisturiser and the coverage of foundation: mix the two in the palm of your hand and apply. Experiment until you achieve the texture and effect you like.

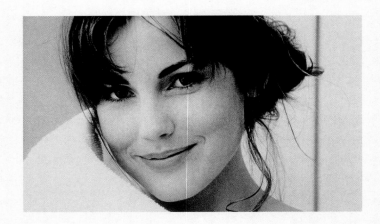

TRIED & TESTED

TINTED MOISTURISERS

These products can help you make the transition between winter-white skin and summer bronze without having to put your face in the sun. Some do contain a sun screen but rarely, if ever, at the SPF15+ level which dermatologists recommend for year-round protection. So put on your SPF first, then wait a few minutes for it to be absorbed before putting on a tinted moisturiser. These products should go on smoothly and enhance your natural skin tone rather than being a 'face dye' which will create an obvious tide-mark. If the colour is a bit strong, mix it with a dab of your usual moisturiser or, for extra cover, with a spot of foundation or concealer.

Top Treats

Shiseido Vital Perfection Tinted Moisturiser

This was a convincing winner in its category for its even application and moisture power. It's worth pointing out that tinted moisturisers rarely offer much in the way of blemish coverage, and this is no exception.
COMMENTS: 'easy to blend', 'very light, smooth and creamy', 'overall, really good – I definitely looked more healthy'.

Lancôme Imanance

This product justifiably sells like hot cakes at Lancôme beauty counters – perhaps partly because it offers a little extra coverage to conceal thread veins, open pores and small blemishes.
COMMENTS: 'light and smooth', 'packaging is easy to hold and work with, with a good lid', 'excellent blendability'.

Christian Dior Reflêt du Teint

This light-textured product was very popular, with top marks for its feel-good factor.
COMMENTS: 'I felt it gave good coverage but still looked light and fresh on my skin', 'I have an allergy to some skin products but had no problem with this one', 'very light and natural looking'.

Juvena Juvenance Soin Eclat Teintée

This was much liked by some testers, but didn't suit everyone.
COMMENTS: 'looked natural and lasted all day', 'smooth, light and creamy'.

Best Budget Buy

No. 7 Light-Diffusing Tinted Moisturiser

This contains special high-tech, light-reflecting pigments which are designed to create a 'soft focus' effect, minimising the appearance of flaws and fine lines. It scored exceptionally highly with our panel.
COMMENTS: 'instantly absorbed and lightweight', 'a great summer alternative to foundation', 'it gave me a healthy look without being greasy'.

Special Mentions

Rochas Moisturising Bronzing Gel
COMMENTS: 'gives a lovely radiance and very natural appearance'.

Vichy Lumineuse
COMMENTS: 'a pleasant, natural, matte finish', 'appeared even and soft after a while, but didn't cover blemishes'.

MAKE-UP ON THE GO

For daytime touch-ups or time-saving ease, you can't beat a mess-free, all-in-one foundation and powder (which can often be used wet or dry) – although the results may never be quite as immaculate as foundation plus loose powder.

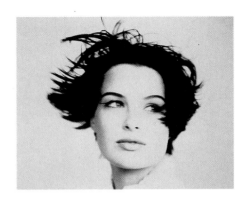

TRIED & TESTED

ALL-IN-ONE MAKE-UP

These new powder/gel formulations, which glide on wet and then rapidly dry to a lightly powdered but natural-looking finish, are one of the great contemporary beauty breakthroughs. They are a real time-saver and make light work of touch-ups.

Top Treats

Clarins Le Teint Velours Compact Foundation

Clarins again scored highly for the product and for its presentation.
COMMENTS: 'applied at 6.30 a.m., it only needed light touching up at lunch and for supper', 'beautifully presented', 'brilliant'.

Lancôme Maquilumine

This product, which was also a favourite with testers, contains light-reflecting pigments to soften the appearance of fine lines.
COMMENTS: 'nice and light and natural', 'great packaging, and I approved of the sponge', 'good for shine prevention'.

Kanebo Exclusive Bio Total Finish

All but one of our testers said that they would buy this product again, as it combined ease of application with good coverage.
COMMENTS: 'covered well but didn't clog pores', 'not at all dry-feeling on the skin', 'looked remarkably natural'.

Chanel Double Perfection Makeup

This product scored particularly highly for smoothness of application and finish, and for the compact, with its generous mirror.
COMMENTS: 'lovely and matte', 'covers with one time-saving swipe'.

Best Budget Buys

Almay SPF15 Cream Powder Make-up

We applaud the built-in sun protection in this product, which is targeted at sensitive skins.
COMMENTS: 'covered very well', 'I liked the absence of fragrance', 'the sponge made it easy to apply'.

Max Factor Sheer Genius Complete Make-up

Max Factor was the first make-up artist to have his own brand. The company still produces some of the bestselling foundations worldwide.
COMMENTS: 'very good cover', 'didn't need touching up at all during the day'.

Natural Choice

Aveda Dual Performance Cream Powder

This was far and away the top-scoring product. In addition, this compact is available with refills – a waste not, want not policy we respect.
COMMENTS: 'generally I'm not passionate about all-in-one make-ups but I loved this one – it wasn't drying and felt very comfortable', 'good yellow tone – not pink, which is sometimes a problem for me', 'hardly needed touching up; a great multi-purpose make-up'.

Special Mention

Shiseido Compact Foundation

This had some very high marks for ease of application and coverage.

THE PERFECT POUT

For most women, lipstick is the cosmetics equivalent of shoes: an instant mood-booster that's much better than buying new clothes because you don't have to get undressed to try it on. Plenty of women have told us they actually feel naked without lipstick.

Applying lipstick is the ultimate feminine gesture – but most of us have to do it more often than we'd like because it wears off so quickly. So we set out to discover the secrets of successful lipstick shopping – and of making lipstick stick.

COLOUR SAVVY

The worst reason to buy a lipstick is just because you love the colour. Understanding your skin tone is essential for error-proof lipstick shopping, believes make-up artist Brigitte Reiss-Anderson (who creates make-up for Italian designer Valentino's catwalk shows, among others), and then being able to identify which colours work best with it. 'The wrong hue can make you look sick, but the right one makes you look gorgeous.' So, here are Brigitte's guidelines:

OLIVE SKINS look good in light brown or raisin shades, with warm undertones that will light up your face. For a deeper colour, go for the browner reds (like blackberry or wine).

FAIR-COMPLEXIONED women should seek out brown-beiges with complexion-warming pink or peach undertones. For more dramatic colour, try blue-based or cherry tones with a hint of brown.

Women with really PALE SKIN and really BLACK HAIR (think of Angelica Huston and Paloma Picasso) are luckiest of all: 'They can use anything so long as it's a real contrast, including fuchsia, bright red and day-glo orange.'

DARK SKIN can carry off the deepest (but not the brightest) reds of all: those with dark blue or purplish undertones. Deep browns with wine, purple or bluish tones can look stunning, too.

Brigitte Reiss-Anderson warns the very fair- or very dark-skinned to steer clear of wishy-washy colours. 'If those women try to put on a pale rose, pale beige or a pale orange, they'll look like they're ill.'

We asked make-up artist Ariane Poole to come up with 12 lipsticks to suit all skin types, These suit everyone from Tessa Sanderson to Darryl Hannah.

Lancôme *Rose Nu*
Christian Dior *Bonbon* (lipgloss) – 'everyone I've put it on has gone out and bought it – even models'
Christian Dior *Indian Red* – 'unlike most reds, this is good with lots of different skin colourings'
Christian Dior *Figue*
Estée Lauder *Burning Rose* – 'this alters on everyone's mouth to a shade that suits them'
Estée Lauder *Copper Moon*
Bobbi Brown *Mocha Stain*
Boots No. 7 *Gay Geranium*
Clarins *Sheer Fig 104*
Clarins *Red Azalea*
Elizabeth Arden *Mauve Dream*
Guerlain Kiss Kiss *Brun Praliné* (sheer gloss)

TIP

One make-up artist told us that her pet theory is that any two lipstick colours mixed together give a great new colour. (It's certainly fun to try out.) Or copy make-up professionals and invest in a basic palette from an art supplies store, and use it to mix and match lipsticks and glosses. But keep brushes dry – water will inhibit blending, as most lipsticks are oil-based.

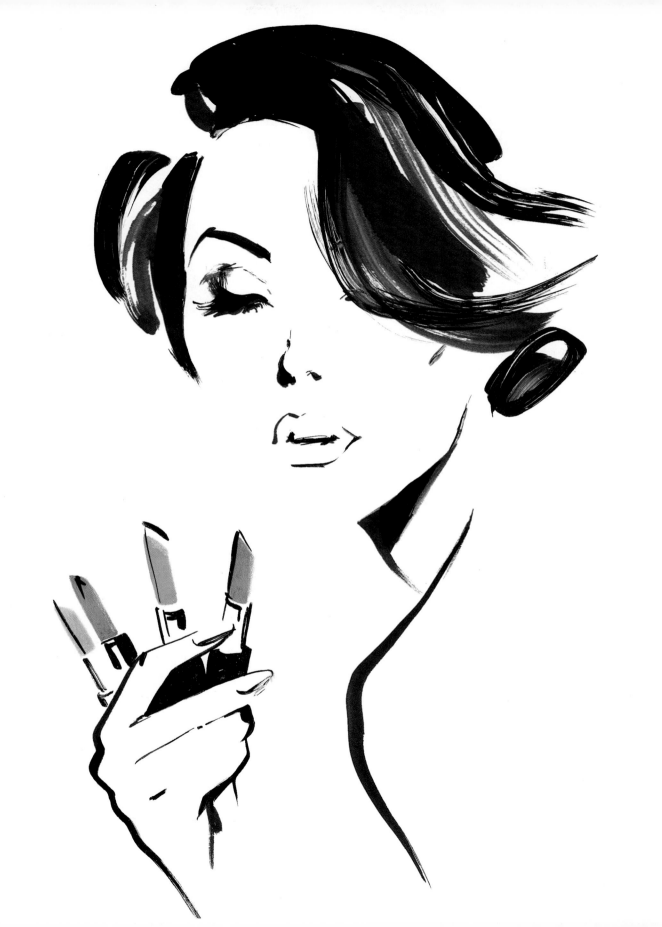

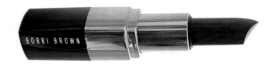

HOW TO FIND A LIPSTICK YOU'LL LOVE

Can you remember when lipstick was just lipstick? Today, lip colours come in so many different formulations – glossy, sheer, matte, creamy – that finding the one you want is harder than ever. But if you know the effect you like – barely-there colour or full, filmstar glamour – here are some clues to tracking down the perfect lipstick.

Look	Coverage	a.k.a.	Extra Features
GLOSSY	Very sheer, giving shine	Lip shine/lip sheen/lip polish	Has added moisturising ingredients, which can help dry skin. You can wear it with lip pencil or over a matte lipstick to alter their texture.
SHEER	Ultra-light, with a little shine	Semi-sheer/lip treat/stain/transparent	Moisturises, and won't wear off as quickly as gloss. Because these are usually summer shades, there's often an SPF added.
CREAMY	Opaque coverage, with little shine	Moisturising lipstick/lipmake rouge/velvet lipstick/hydrating	Features conditioners, so lips feel smooth; colour usually wears evenly. Offers the widest choice of shades.
MATTE	Extremely opaque, flat colour, with the most coverage	Demi-matte/semi-matte	The maximum amount of pigment, so giving longer wear. Often leaves a flattering, temporary stain after it's worn off.

QUICK CHANGE ACT

Today's clever lipstick 'accessories' can give your best-loved lipstick a wardrobe of different effects, adding a sweep of gloss to make it shine, a hint of shimmering gold or silver, or intensifying the colour. Try Lancaster Personal Choice Lipsticks, BeneFit Cosmetics Depth Charge and Light Switch, or surf the cosmetics counters for the many other options avabailable.

Otherwise, resurrect old favourites in your make-up bag:

For shimmer... apply lipstick lightly, then cover with a sweep of an old pearlised lipstick, or a gold colour.

For sheer cover... outline the lips with the edge of the lipstick, then cover the entire lip with colourless gloss (or lipsalve), and gently rub the lips together.

For high gloss... put on lipstick as usual and coat with clear gloss.

LIPSLICKING GOOD

■ If chapped lips are a problem, make-up artist Kevyn Aucoin suggests: 'Apply Vaseline and then buff with a baby's toothbrush to get rid of dry skin.'

■ How can you achieve lip colour that goes the distance? Bobbi Brown says it's all in the preparation: 'Apply a good lip balm and let it absorb thoroughly before applying lipstick – if your lips are dry *or* coated with waxy lip balm, your lipstick won't perform well. Build up a depth of colour by applying lipstick, then blotting it with a tissue to leave a stain on your lips. Repeating these steps before applying a final coat should give you a deeper, longer-lasting result.'

■ Women with tiny lines round the mouth will find lip liner particularly helpful, because it helps stop lipstick from bleeding. Alternatively, Colourings No Wander is a clever wax-based invisible pencil which you apply outside the lip line to stop bleeding.

■ 'Lip liner gives the mouth definition and helps lipstick stay on longer,' says Mary Greenwell. 'You can correct lips and make them bigger with a lip pencil. You don't need a different colour for each lipstick; just use a basic neutral colour a few tones darker than your natural lip colour.' On black women's lips, Mary sometimes uses a brown eye pencil as lip liner.

■ Veteran make-up artist Wayne Massarelli (who lends his skills to movies, TV and still photography) has another technique to help lipstick stay put: 'Smooth foundation over the edges of your lips, especially if you intend to accentuate the fullness of your lips with your lip liner. Then use whatever translucent powder you ordinarily use to set your foundation; take a small brush and apply a little of the powder to your lips to set the line. This stops bleeding and

feathering.' Alternatively, BeneFit Cosmetics Lip Plump acts like foundation for lips, helping lipstick stay put and actually giving the appearance of fuller, softer lips.

■ Make-up artist Jeanine Lobell, creator of her own range of cosmetics, Stila, creates a bee-sting pout by applying a rosy-brown lipstick, then dabbing a bit of concealer in the middle of the bottom lip. 'It lights the lipstick one shade in the centre, and makes lips look bigger.'

■ Scared of dark lip shades? Look for transparents, sheers or stains, recommends Mary Greenwell: 'The sheer formula allows darker colours to be worn by women who usually feel they are too strong, and it also makes for quick and easy application.'

■ Lis Williams, Revlon's in-house make-up expert, advises: 'Dark colours make lips look smaller; a light colour will expand the mouth.'

■ Frosted lipsticks – which drift in and out of fashion – only look great on very young lips. On anyone over 25, they can be instantly ageing, because they highlight lip wrinkles.

■ This is every model's technique to avoid the embarrassment of lipstick on her teeth: once lipstick has been applied, stick your index finger in your mouth, close your lips around it and pull your finger out. Any lipstick which was inside your lips will now have been transferred to your finger.

■ Any kind of oil will dissolve even long-lasting lipstick on contact. So a well-dressed salad is likely to remove all lip colour – and probably some foundation, too.

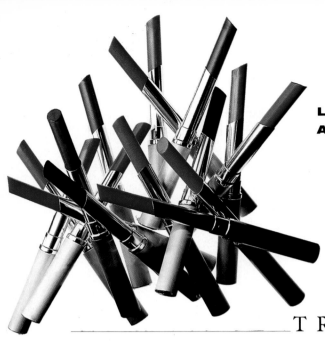

LIPSTICKS THAT KEEP ON GOING, AND GOING, AND GOING...

TRIED & TESTED

LONG-LASTING LIPSTICKS

To every woman's delight, we can report that the search for a product which stays on your lips – not on someone else's cheek or collar – may be over. The new generation of longlasting lipsticks, available in an increasingly wide and desirable choice of colours, don't dry out your lips – unlike their predecessors – and really do stay put through the day. These are the tops from our testers.

Top Treats

Prescriptives Extraordinary Lipstick

A notably rich and moisturising formulation, all our testers reported.
COMMENTS: 'this stayed put over two meals and 12 hours', 'the nicest lipstick I've ever tried – not sticky, no taste, lasts very well and looks natural', 'my dry lips improved when using it'.

Chanel Rouge Extrême Lipstick

Our testers were consistently impressed by its overall performance and the exquisite range of intense colours.
COMMENTS: 'smelt nice and was by far the best lipstick I've ever tried', 'I very much liked the slim packaging', 'colourwise this product really was long-lasting'.

Lancôme Rouge Magique

Our testers were pleased with this product, which comes in a wide range of colours, and which lasted almost as long as the packaging claimed.
COMMENTS: 'superb shade – looked good and felt good', 'there was still a stain left when I went to bed', 'a creamy feel'.

Origins Matte Stick

This is really convenient to apply as it's designed like a stubby pencil (although it needs regular sharpening, with its own sharpener).
COMMENTS: 'stayed on very well', 'gave a really good, definite outline', 'I received compliments on this lipstick'.

Best Budget Buys

Max Factor Lasting Colour Lipstick

This was the outright winner in this category, which is especially impressive considering its very reasonable price tag.
COMMENTS: 'nice and creamy', 'top marks for staying power', 'even needed eye make-up remover to get the final traces off'.

Oil of Ulay Colour Moist

This is from the new colour cosmetics collection by the company that brought you the world's top-selling moisturiser.
COMMENTS: 'I liked the colour and texture – and it was easy to apply', 'stayed fast after a couple of drinks', 'moisturising but not greasy'.

Natural Choice

Annemarie Börlind Lip Colour

This product, which is based on natural waxes makes no special claims for endurance but really goes the distance according to our testers.
COMMENTS: 'very moisturising, feels lovely', 'nice colour, nice taste', 'lasted through three drinks and lunch'.

GETTING YOUR EYES RIGHT

No physical feature expresses your individuality more than your eyes, and there are literally thousands of products out there designed to play them up.

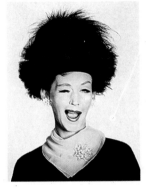

Every season, new colours in eye make-up sweep in and out of vogue on the beauty pages of magazines. Although experimenting with blues, greens and purples can be fun, the experts say that what suits most women is a basic palette of neutral shades. Like having navy, black, taupe and white as the basics of your wardrobe, which work reliably for you year after year.

Bobbi Brown (see her *Masterclass*, page 12) believes every woman needs to invest in just two basic powder eyeshadow colours. First, a light colour for sweeping over the lid (bone, ivory or the palest shell pink, depending on skin tone; for example, shell pink doesn't work well on olive skins). This also works as a base to help eye make-up stay put. Then, a medium colour – she likes taupe, charcoal or a plummy heather – for the socket and underneath the eye, if you like to wear shadow there. This might not sound dramatic, but it looks marvellous. Darker colours, Bobbi says, need more expert blending than most women can achieve.

The key to perfect application, Bobbi believes, is having the right brushes: a rounded eyeshadow brush for lids – preferably two, one for each shade – and a finer, blunt-ended brush for underneath the eyes. 'It's the best eye make-up investment you can make. Those fiddly little applicators that you get with most make-up palettes don't give enough control.' Just about any make-up artist you can name instantly throws out the manufacturer's own brushes when stocking their kits, and substitutes brushes by names like Shu Uemura, Maggie Hunt, Screenface – or Bobbi Brown's own. The Body Shop also has a wonderful, inexpensive range; Colourings.

EYE MAKE-UP SECRETS FROM THE PROS

■ More advice from Mary Greenwell: 'Grey-brown eyeshadows suit all skin types, from the very light to the very dark.'

■ Laura Geller advises women to turbo-charge the impact of a daytime eyeshadow for night by moistening the sponge applicator. This makes the colour go on darker, deeper and bolder.

■ We've all spoiled our make-up with stray specks of eyeshadow that get smeared onto cheeks. Make-up artists always liberally dot loose powder over the cheeks, so that fallen specks can be swept away, without ruining your foundation.

■ Kevyn Aucoin says: 'Depending on how you use it, eyeliner [liquid or pencil] can make the eyes appear larger or smaller. It's not always necessary to line top and bottom lashes – in fact, I rarely do, unless I'm doing a very dramatic evening look. Lining just the top lashes opens up the whole eye area and the eyes, and the eye make-up gets more definition. Another way to open up the eyes is to line the lower rims with white eyeliner.' (Yves Saint Laurent make one.)

■ Like kissing, using liquid eyeliner is an art nobody ever teaches you. If you avoid liquid eyeliner simply because your hands aren't steady, Chanel's make-up maestro has the secret of shake-free eyelining: put your mirror on the table and bend over it. Now rest your arm on the table and draw, as close to the lashes as possible and as thickly or thinly as you prefer. No more shaky lines or squinting.

■ Make-up artists use 'layering' techniques to stop cosmetics from sliding off the face and disappearing. For eyes, that means fixing pencil liner with a line of powder shadow over it. 'Really work an eye pencil into the roots of lashes,' encourages Mary Greenwell. 'It gives the optical illusion of longer lashes.' Adds Kevyn Aucoin: 'There's nothing worse than seeing white space between the lashes and liner.'

■ As the weather heats up, put your eye (and lip) pencils in the freezer for a few minutes, before sharpening them. In cold weather, pencils get too hard – and can drag. Max Factor's movie make-up artist Bob Mills advises: 'So that eyeliner pencil glides on smoothly, soften the point before use with a blast of warm air from a hairdryer.'

■ If you find eye make-up seems to fade, crease or rub off, you might like to look around for a special eyelid foundation – Estée Lauder make a great one – which fixes eye make-up.

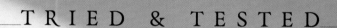

TRIED & TESTED

LASH-BUILDING MASCARAS

We asked testers not only to mark the products for lash-plumping qualities, but to note down those which looked natural and lustrous, and didn't clump, smudge, flake or crumble.

Top Treats

Lancôme Intencils

This product confirmed Lancôme's reputation for excellence in mascaras. (Beauty business insiders put this down, in particular, to the design and quality of the brushes.)

COMMENTS: 'I like thick-looking lashes – this was the best!', 'top marks for lengthening and for thickening lashes without clumpiness'.

Bobbi Brown Essentials Thickening Mascara

This mascara, from the world's No. 1 make-up artist-turned-cosmetics-producer, scored particularly highly for naturalness and non-clumpiness.

COMMENTS: 'great – but needed a lot of coats', 'excellent brush', 'all the lashes were completely separated'.

Estée Lauder More Than Mascara

Our testers were impressed by how this resisted smudging and flaking even after a long day.

COMMENTS: 'I love this – I'd buy it because it's soft and real-looking', 'went on evenly – very natural'.

Helena Rubinstein Spectacular Lash-Lengthener

Another firm favourite with testers, with good marks for the sleek gold packaging.

COMMENTS: 'looked natural and lustrous', 'easy to apply', 'a brilliant brush'.

Best Budget Buys

Oil of Ulay Lash-Building Mascara

With the exception of one tester, this inexpensive product scored the highest mark overall, in all price brackets.

COMMENTS: 'easy to use – stayed fresh all day', 'lustrous-looking but quite matte', 'nice, smooth texture – not too heavy'.

L'Oréal Voluminous

Insider info: many make-up artists use this instead of Maybelline Great Lash Mascara, which is unavailable in Europe, but a great favourite in the USA.

COMMENTS: 'I have very thin blonde lashes but this really looks natural and covers well – it's easy to get to the roots.

MORE SECRETS FROM THE PROS
– Mascaras

■ Mary Greenwell warns blondes off black mascara (and liner): 'They create Barbie-doll type lashes. Use brown, especially for day.'

■ Barbara Daly, creator of the Colourings range for The Body Shop, advises: 'To apply mascara to your upper lashes, keep your head straight but hold the mirror at chin level. This means you'll be looking down into the mirror, so that when you start to sweep the brush from root to tip, you'll be able to see the whole length of the lashes. It also prevents the smudging that can happen if you open your eyes while the mascara is wet.'

■ If mascara is too runny, don't waste money by throwing it out. Mary Greenwell advises leaving it open overnight, to dry out a bit.

■ If mascara smuts often end up on your cheeks, try applying it to top lashes only, and use a soft brown/charcoal/grey pencil underneath your eyes.

TIPS FROM THE TOP

Superbeauty **Stephanie Seymour** knows how to make the most of her lashes: 'I apply three coats of mascara. It's a trick my mom taught me. You put on one coat, wipe the brush with a tissue, dip it in the mascara again, do another coat – then repeat.'

Country and Western singer **Emmylou Harris**: 'I have to put on Lancôme mascara, even if I'm not going out. I just like the way it feels, and I really like the brush.'

Choreographer and singer **Paula Abdul** agrees with the pros that the right tools are a must. 'My Shu Uemura blending brush is essential to the process. Without it, eyeshadow would be a nightmare.'

Believe it or not, **Claudia Schiffer** insists: 'I've got really blonde lashes and if I don't wear mascara, my eyes disappear completely and look piggy. So even when I'm on holiday, it's the one make-up item that I always wear. My favourite mascara is Revlon's Water Tight Mascara, in black, which doesn't come off even when you're swimming, windsurfing or waterskiing.'

TRIED & TESTED

WATERPROOF MASCARAS

We're pleased to report that since we compiled the first edition of *The Beauty Bible*, waterproof mascara technology really has advanced. We asked our testers to try these in the rain, in the shower/steamy bathroom and in a swimming pool. The top-scorers in both categories really did stay put and the results show that this is an area where you don't have to splash out on an expensive name.

Top Treats
Kanebo 38° Silk Performance Mascara
The truly extraordinary thing about this mascara is that it won't come off with remover but needs to be taken off with hot water.
COMMENTS: 'a very good natural-looking mascara which lasted all day', 'my skin is sensitive but I had no reaction to this product', 'looked glossy, lustrous and not cake-y'.

Chanel Cils Magique Waterproof Mascara
COMMENTS: 'waterproof in the shower but OK to remove – though I did have smudges under the eyes the following morning', 'quite natural and glossy-looking'.
Guerlain Supercils
COMMENTS: 'unfailingly waterproof', 'easy to remove with oil'.

Best Budget Buys
Yardley Active Lash Mascara
COMMENTS: 'very, very natural and glossy-looking', 'didn't flake, crumble or smudge'.
L'Oréal Lash Out Lengthening Mascara
COMMENTS: 'excellent waterproofing – I've used it often for swimming', 'good marks for non-clumpiness', 'dried quickly'.

TRIED & TESTED

EYELINER PENCILS

Bobbi Brown feels eyeliner is all the eye make-up some women need and many devotees echo this. But the texture, in particular smudgeability (controlled by you) and ease of application are crucial. The more expensive brands consistently scored much higher with our testers and tended to include useful extras such as built-in sponges to smudge the line and sharpeners. Remember, the softer the pencil the more quickly it wears down, so if a sharpener doesn't come with your chosen product invest in a good one – hacking at your eyeliner pencil with a kitchen knife can be a frustrating (and risky) occupation.

Top Treats

Guerlain Eye Pencil

COMMENTS: 'the pencil worked effectively without me having to press hard', 'good strong colour and attractive design', 'didn't drag and had great smudgeability'.

Yves Saint Laurent Kohl Eyeliner Pencil

COMMENTS: 'great pencil, great colour, soft and easy to use'.

Nutri-Metics Eye Defining Pencil

COMMENTS: 'easy to use and pleasant to hold', 'the sponge tip was very useful for blending'.

Best Budget Buys

Avon Soft Definition Eye Pencil

COMMENTS: 'it went where I wanted it to go – and stayed there!', 'I'm definitely changing brands to this one'.

Max Factor Natural Eyes Eyeliner

COMMENTS: 'I have sensitive eyes but had no problem with this product', 'I would have like a built-in sponge to smudge the line'.

Natural Choice

Annemarie Börlind Kohl pour les yeux

COMMENTS: 'excellent', 'easy to use', 'smooth to apply'.

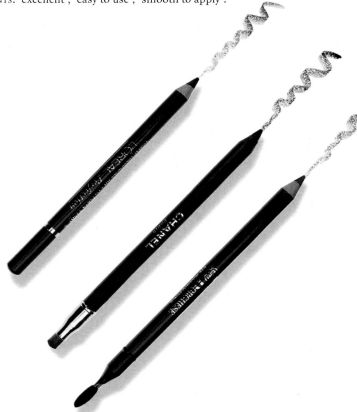

EYES TO DYE FOR

Eyelash dyeing is the perfect alternative to mascara for a beach holiday – or year-round for blondes and redheads. D-I-Y eyelash dyes contain full instructions.

A popular brand is Louis Marcel, which actress **Katie Rabett** uses on her lashes. Her tip is to apply it with a mascara brush: 'It's much less fiddly, and stops it dripping in your eyes and stinging.'

If you don't feel confident doing it at home, you can have your lashes tinted at most beauty salons. Some salons also offer brow tints. You need to re-dye lashes about every five to six weeks.

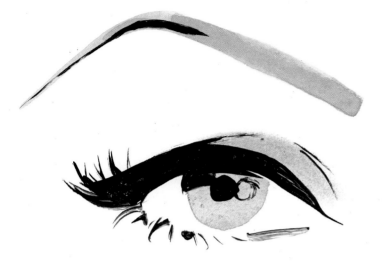

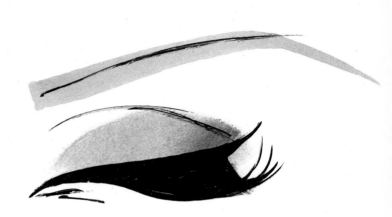

THE SECRETS OF EYELASH CURLERS

Some models and make-up artists (unlike Bobbi Brown) wouldn't be without them – but eyelash curlers can be infernal contraptions until you get the hang of them. Used properly, however, they can make your lashes look twice as long.

■ Do buy good curlers. It's worth the investment; cheap metal ones can actually cut your lashes. Tweezerman's is one of the new high-tech curlers and the rave fave of those in the know. It has non-stick silicone pads which gently curl lashes rather than 'crimping' them.

■ Don't use curlers after you've applied your mascara; mascara can stick to the curlers and the lashes get tugged out when you release it.

■ Do clean curlers, especially the pad, with a cotton wool square and alcohol. Replace the curlers as soon as the rubber starts to crack.

■ Don't pull with the curlers clamped down; you'll yank lashes out.

■ Do try the double-squeeze method: place the open curlers near the upper lash roots, and arrange your lashes between the two rims. Squeeze gently for five seconds. Release the curlers, and move them slightly towards the mid-lash area, then repeat the process. The effect is a beautifully rounded curl.

FAKING IT

False eyelashes as daywear have had their day. (For now at least.) But some women still like to wear them at night, for high drama. You can buy them either in strips, or as little clusters, packaged with their own, cement-like rubber glue that ensures painless removal (with a little tugging).

International make-up artist Chris Colbeck first applies glue from the tube to the tip of a lash cluster. Then, with tweezers, he nestles only one small cluster of false lashes into the real eyelashes just at the outside corner of the eye. 'Often, that's all a woman needs.' For a fuller effect, he places clusters closely together, along the natural lash line.

Strip lashes can be trickier, and should first be cut to fit. Then glue the band; place the strip on the lid just above the real lashes, anchoring it first in the middle, then at the edges. Applying mascara to natural and false lashes 'fuses' them for a more natural result. 'And eyeliner can fill any gap between the two,' adds Chris.

BLUSHING BEAUTY

Blusher has a reputation for being difficult to apply but, once you know what you're doing, it can make you look your best in seconds.

THE RIGHT BLUSHER FOR YOU

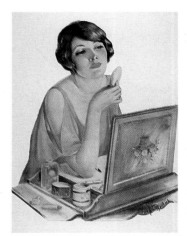

Powder blusher is easier to control and blend, which is why it's the most popular choice of all. You'll also find the widest choice of shades comes in powder form. It should be applied over foundation – and under face powder – not on bare skin; applying powder blush to clean, fresh skin gives you too bright a flash of colour. At the very least, you should wear a veil of translucent powder underneath. It will also stay put longest if 'sandwiched' between foundation and powder. Make-up artists always use powder blusher.

Cream blusher is good for dry or sun-damaged skin; it slides easily over the surface and won't settle in wrinkles. To avoid a clown effect, always put cream or liquid blusher into the palm of your hand first, then apply it to your cheek. It should be tapped on lightly with the finger and blended immediately.

Gel blusher offers the sheerest form of colour, and is great for giving a natural-looking glow to bare skin on outdoorsy weekends. Because gel blushers are transparent, they're perfect for summer. Gel should always be applied over moisturiser (not foundation), which makes it glide on more smoothly and avoids a 'polka-dot' effect (the stain 'takes' very fast when it hits the skin). Do always remember to wash your hands immediately after applying them, as the pigments can stain fingers.

Bronzing powder can be substituted for blush in summer. It's also great dusted around the hairline, on the nose and chin, as well as across the cheekbones, for giving you a truly healthy-looking tan.

■ Mary Greenwell: 'Blush is the one piece of make-up that you'll never have to change. Stick with a blush that adds the right healthy glow and change the colour of eyes and lips.'
■ Top American make-up artist Rex advises using a blusher brush with white bristles, to help you tell if you're overdoing the colour: 'If your brush suddenly looks too pink, your cheeks will, too.'

COLOUR CHOICES

Don't go too bright or too dark. Aim for a natural, soft, healthy glow. Bobbi Brown says: 'The right blusher for you is the same colour your cheeks are naturally when you're really healthy.'

FAIR-SKINNED women should look for beige, tawny and pink tones.

OLIVE/YELLOW-TONED SKINS will find warm brown, almond and copper shades most flattering.

DARK-SKINNED women can use plum, fuchsia, auburn and deep bronze shades.

REDHEADS look best in orange, apricot, peach and coral shades. These also look good on anyone with a tan.

TIPS FROM THE TOP

When Collier Strong makes up **Melanie Griffith**'s face for photo shoots, he brushes on *Coppertone* blush by M.A.C. if she has a tan, or *Rose Quartz* by Chanel if she doesn't, on top of foundation. 'The blush really brings her to life. She's such a beautiful woman – I love putting blush on her.'

Sharon Stone uses a M.A.C. eyeshadow – in *Soft Brown* – as a blush.

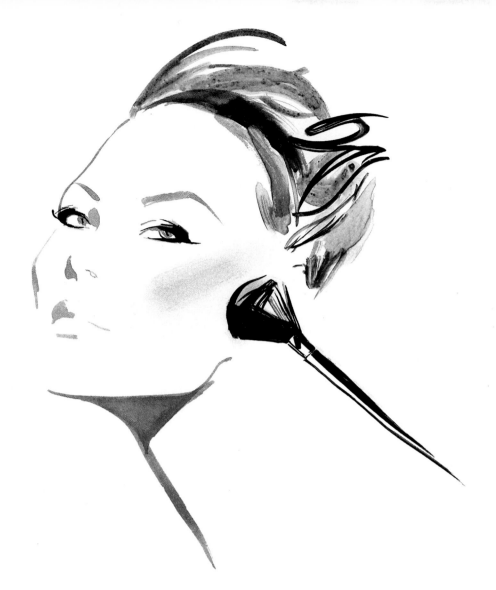

The Contour Controversy

Should you shape your face using darker powder to disguise chubby cheeks or double chins? Opinions vary. Bobbi Brown thinks it's better to play up your good points rather than try to cover up your flaws. But Maggie Hunt, who every year teaches hundreds of women how to make the most of their looks, does believe in contouring: 'I use a face shaper – a matte brown one – to help minimise double chins, chubby cheeks and high and narrow foreheads. Choose a shade of powder that's just a darker version of your own skin tone and brush it onto the heavy areas. If your forehead is too high, put a soft brown powder around the hairline.'

BLUSHER TIPS FROM THE PROS

■ 'Invest in a proper blusher brush,' advises Bobbi Brown. 'The teeny ones you find in compacts just aren't up to the job, and will give visible brush strokes.'

■ Don't use blusher to give yourself instant cheekbones. The most flattering way to apply it is on the 'apples' of the cheeks. Locate yours by drawing an imaginary line down from your pupil to the centre of your cheek. Then lightly stroke outwards, towards the top of the ear, covering the entire cheekbone area in soft, sweeping strokes.

■ Kevyn Aucoin sometimes applies blusher to the cleavage and along the hairline, too. 'It adds warmth to powder and foundation, making the whole look more realistic and healthy-looking.'

■ Carol Shaw advises applying blush when you're smiling: 'Add a little blush in that ball of your cheek and bring it back a little towards the bone.'

■ 'You want to look like the noon sun has hit you on – not under – your cheekbones,' believes Mary Greenwell.

■ Like many make-up artists, Maggie Hunt likes to 'double-blush', first applying one layer of blush, then powder, then blushing again: 'It helps the colour stay put.'

■ Shu Uemura's resident make-up artist, Andrea, says that in summer, older women should avoid powder blusher: 'It can look dusty. Instead, try rubbing some lipstick into your cheeks, which gives a much more natural result.'

■ Says Kevyn Aucoin: 'Over-blushing can always be corrected by blending in a little powder.'

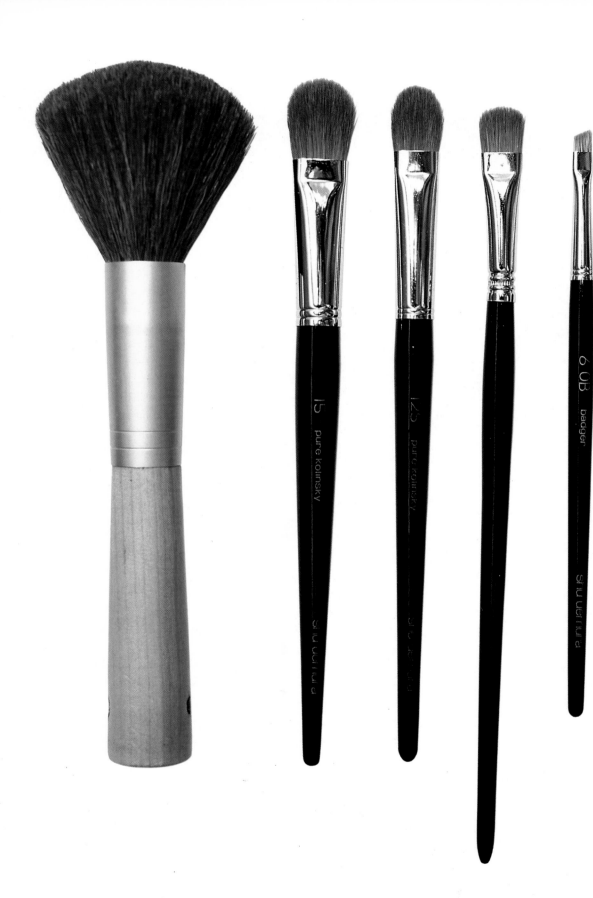

BEAUTIFUL BRUSHWORK

A make-up artist not only has skill and know-how but also the right kit. Mary Greenwell has three dozen different brushes: 'But, in fact, with just six I can do it all – and so could any woman.' Mary's box of brush tricks contains: three by Shu Uemura, in sizes 12S, 60B (both for eye defining) and 15 (blush/highlight), a Visiora lipbrush (from Christian Dior's professional range), Screenface's perfect 'blender' brush number 3/8, 'And I absolutely can't live without my cheapo-cheapo powder brush, picked up in New York.' (For mail order brushes, see DIRECTORY.) Here are the shapes – and sizes – to look for when you go brush-shopping.

GUIDELINES FOR GOLDEN GIRLS

Make-up artist Stephen Glass is a genius at enhancing older faces, from 40-somethings to 80-somethings. Clients have been known to kick up their heels and throw their first birthday party for decades after a visit to his salon (see DIRECTORY). Here are Stephen's tips to help women 'of a certain age' look wonderful.

■ **Know your skin.** Don't take it as gospel that every woman's skin dries as she gets older; women in their 60s and 70s can still have combination skin, with dry cheeks and an oily T-zone. Using too much rich nourishing cream when your skin doesn't really need it can still trigger breakouts, spots or whiteheads.

Your skin may also get so used to one product, if it's applied consistently, that it ceases to offer benefits. So get to know your skin and nourish it as and when it needs extra help. Try the alternating approach: smooth on night cream for a few evenings when your skin feels dry, then don't wear any cream at all for a night or three. If you have very dry skin, try the other alternating approach, using two creams, say collagen one night and a vitamin cream the next.

■ **Face up to your face.** Invest in the best magnifying mirror you can find and put it in the clearest (yes, that does mean cruellest) light.

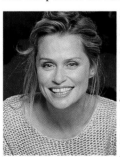

However depressing you find it initially, remember that you will end up looking infinitely better. Preparing your face like this is particularly vital for anyone who wears glasses (see *Glamour and Glasses*, page 64). There is an especially good French brand of magnifier called Beauty Look (see DIRECTORY), which has suction pads so that you can attach it to your usual mirror.

■ **Review your make-up regularly.** As your face changes, your make-up needs subtle revision, too. Don't be afraid of scrutinising the products and colours you use, and how you apply them. You may think, for instance, that your favourite foundation has changed, because it no longer looks so good on you – but the likelihood is

that your complexion has changed, just as the skin around your eyes may alter their shape, or your colouring become paler. Don't get stuck in a cosmetic rut. Take a ramble round the beauty counters and see which look you like (see *Department Store Makeovers*, page 39), then play with products, ask for advice, have a free consultation, get samples. Don't be afraid to take time; *you* make the decisions. Or go to a local make-up artist whose work you respect, or whom friends have recommended for a makeover.

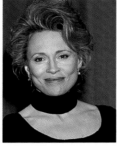

■ **Colour it natural.** Match foundation to your skin tone, however much that changes over the years. Avoid the temptation to use foundation which is tanned or darker than your own complexion. It dulls the skin, making it look lifeless and much older. Foundation should be very lightweight for older, fragile or lined skins, and always applied with a good sponge. (Best of all are Max Factor sponges, only available in America.) For skins which have grown paler, colour can be added with blusher; for those who have become more florid, concealer and foundation can work wonders.

■ Even the **drier, lined skins may need powder** as a finishing touch. The key is to drift the powder lightly over the face for a soft but flawless finish. Tip a little loose powder into the palm of your left hand (or vice versa if you're left-handed); dip your large powder brush into it, then tap the handle to shake the excess off and stroke gently across the areas which need powdering. You may want to use a tinted powder in the evening, for instance a pale mauve, if you're very sallow.

■ **Use cream or liquid blusher** rather than powder rouge on your cheeks; it looks much better on a dry or lined complexion. For cheeks with high colour or broken veins, mix a little concealer with cream rouge and pat on in thin layers.

■ **Try using lip pencil** to outline and then colour in your lips, rather than lipstick; this will avoid bleeding into any tiny lines around the mouth. Top with gloss if you wish. If your lips have grown thinner with age, never use deep, dark colours; go for soft, bright shades such as coral or apricot – Bourjois make a lovely shade called *Abricot*.

■ Every woman of every age can **get an amazing lift by using eyeliner**: use a soft pencil in charcoal, deep grey, deep blue, taupe or bronze green depending on your skin tone. Dot along the outer third to half of your upper eyelids, right up against the lashes, then smudge upwards with your little finger; you can also try a few smudges under your lower lashes, on the outer corners only. (See *Tried & Tested Eye Pencils*, page 32.)

■ **Use eye drops and** (plastic) **eyelash curlers to open and brighten eyes**, and make them look more youthful (see our tips on eyelash curlers, page 33). Then apply mascara in the direction of the lashes, rolling the wand up and away at the outer corners of the eyes, so the whole eye is drawn up. (Choose soft brown, grey or navy mascara, not black, if you have grey hair.)

■ **To minimise droopy eyes**, brush on a touch of deep brown or grey shadow on the bits which sag, usually in the creases and at the outer corners. It's important that you do this looking straight into a mirror at eye level.

■ **Check the style and shape of your eye glasses.** A different pair of specs can make a dramatic difference, and the choice today is huge. Take a trip to a good optician with a wide range of frames and sympathetic, knowledgeable staff. (Stephen's favourite is the David Clulow department in Selfridges, Oxford Street, London.)

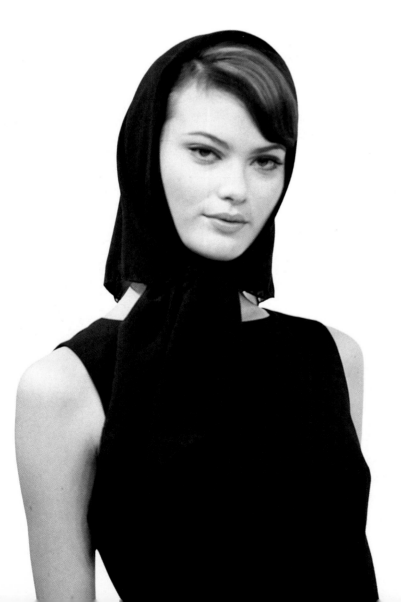

HOW MUCH MAKE-UP IS ENOUGH?

If you emphasise all your features for an everyday look – eyes, lips, cheeks – then you are going to look over-painted, although you can get away with more make-up at night. Kevyn Aucoin identifies four basic make-up combinations. Opt for the combination which enhances your good points. (If you're unsure what these are, just ask your best friend or partner, who should be relied on to give you an honest answer based on how they see you. When we look in the mirror, we tend to focus on the parts of our face that we like least.)

❶ Light eyes, light mouth – the ultra-natural look. Remember to apply a little colour to cheeks, otherwise this look can make you appear washed out.

❷ Light eyes, darker mouth – a natural-looking face, with extra emphasis on the lips.

❸ Dark eyes, light mouth – a sophisticated look, but better on younger women. Older women need some lip colour.

❹ Dark eyes, dark mouth – a dramatic look that's really only suitable for evenings and parties. (For more party looks, see page 44).

Make-up artist Shu Uemura: 'Approach make-up the way you do food. Always stop when you're 80 per cent full.'

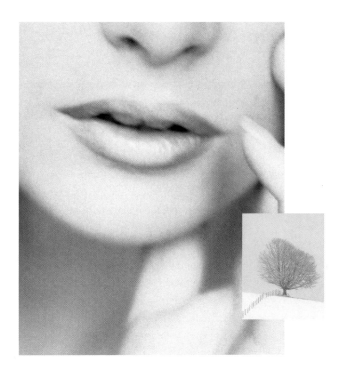

❺ Apply mascara but skip eye make-up. (You don't want to emphasise itchy, watery eyes.)

❻ Dust translucent powder or bronzer all over your face with a big, fluffy brush. A touch of glimmer or a light-reflecting powder will liven up pale skin.

❼ Sweep a rose or coral blush on the 'apples' of your cheeks.

❽ Slick on medicated lip balm and a bright lipstick, to perk up your face. But avoid brown and wine hues, which can make you look washed out.

You may not *feel* better after this. But at least you'll *look* it.

Cold Comfort Make-up

Coming down with a cold can zap good looks fast. (As can allergies such as asthma and hay fever.) Make-up pro Laura Geller, used to making up snuffly supermodels, says you can disguise the problem.

❶ Begin with non-medicated eye drops, to help soothe itchy eyes.

❷ Apply a fragrance-free moisturiser to chapped, dry zones.

❸ Use an eye gel to get rid of puffiness.

❹ Skip foundation if skin is super-dry and flaky. But dot concealer under the eyes if you need it, and over the lids, to camouflage redness and irritation. Dab a bit on both sides of your nose, to cover up any redness.

DEPARTMENT STORE MAKEOVERS – HELL OR HEAVEN?

If you can't afford a consultation with a private make-up artist, a department store makeover is a fast (and free) way to find out how your look could be updated. First, look around a department store until you see a consultant whose look you like; unless you like dragon-green eyeshadow and laminated red lips, head for a counter where the staff look fairly natural. Then, advises Bobbi Brown (who's done literally thousands of makeovers): 'Make an appointment and go to it wearing your everyday make-up so that the artist understands your style. And say exactly what you want – whether you're adapting a look from a magazine or just want to add drama to your everyday make-up.' Offer feedback: say if you like a colour, or you'd like your lips brought out more. If you're still not thrilled with the results, don't suffer in silence. 'It's often a matter of fine-tuning,' believes Bobbi. 'Try blotting your lips, rubbing in the blush and blending the eyeshadow. Talk to the artist and tell her what you'd like redone.' Never walk away until you feel comfortable.

EVENING MAKE-UP

Dressing up for the evening used to mean reaching for the scarlet lipstick and black eyeshadow. While evening make-up does demand different techniques from daytime, looking glamorous doesn't involve putting on heavy colours with a trowel.

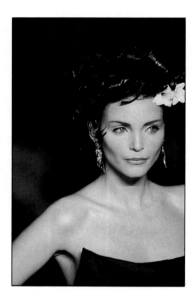

'If you vary your nighttime make-up too dramatically from day, you'll feel as uncomfortable as if you went out in someone else's dress,' says New York make-up artist Michael Criscuolo. 'If you don't look like you – if that face in the mirror seems like a stranger – you won't relax and enjoy yourself.'

These are the five most important factors to consider:

1. The occasion You wouldn't wear the same make-up to a summer picnic supper as you would to a formal prize-giving ceremony or a smoochy disco. Think through what's appropriate.

2. The time of year Summer demands lighter make-up; winter can take a more dramatic look.

3. Your choice of clothes The same make-up that works with a tuxedo-style evening suit will look overpowering with a pale satin spaghetti-strap dress.

4. The lighting That famous beauty Lady Diana Cooper was rumoured to ring hosts beforehand to check on the lighting: was it to be kind candles or sidelights, or the merciless glare of overhead beams?

5. How little time you have to get ready Think this one out ahead and – like a Girl Guide – be prepared. Have make-up and a complete outfit ready at home, or if you're going from work, pack make-up and sponge bags, evening clothes/accessories – and don't forget the spare pair of tights and scent.

TIPS FROM THE PROS ON PARTY MAKE-UP

■ Bobbi Brown: 'Think deeper, richer shades rather than just one extra-heavy application of your usual make-up.'

■ Michael Criscuolo: 'Look at what you're wearing during the day and then add in some colour that enhances that for night.'

■ Maggie Hunt: 'To avoid nasty surprises, check your make-up in several different mirrors in your house or office before going out, and don't forget to look at your neck and bosom to make sure there's no dramatic contrast with the skin of your face. Use concealer on any blemishes, then powder.'

■ Our tip: don't experiment just before a party; always have a dress and make-up rehearsal before a big evening.

However long you have, start by drinking a big glass of water to de-stress yourself; swallow a couple of algae tablets, if you like (spirulina, blue-green algae, chlorella). If you're hungry, eat something quick and energising like a banana. Then stand up straight, shoulders down, and take four slow deep breaths.

THE 5-MINUTE TIMETABLE

- brush your teeth
- turn your head upside down and brush or comb your hair; tie it back or fluff it up
- touch up lips, eyes, blusher
- spritz on scent

THE 30-MINUTE TIMETABLE

IF YOU'RE AT HOME…

- put on some upbeat music
- take off make-up
- have a 5-minute power shower. Wash hair only if it's supershort
- put on moisturiser and leave for 5 minutes while fixing hair
- do your make-up: foundation, eyes, powder, blusher, lips
- dress and spritz with scent

IF YOU'RE AT WORK…

- blot T-zone to remove shine (or whole of face if it's all shiny) with soft tissues (not loo paper – it's too hard)
- sweep face with a dry make-up sponge to remove the morning's foundation, powder and blusher
- use a cotton wool bud dipped in eye make-up remover to take off any shadow and mascara
- wipe off lipstick with a tissue and a dab of Vaseline
- if lips are flaky-dry, smooth over moisturiser and brush with a soft toothbrush
- spritz with mineral water (buy Evian spray, or use a plant mister)
- touch up foundation – compact foundations are ideal for this (see *Tried & Tested All-In-One Make-Up*, page 23)
- reapply eyeshadow, blusher, lipstick – with gloss if you wish – and a fresh coat of mascara
- spritz with scent

THE 60-MINUTE TIMETABLE

Despite the extra time, don't be tempted to dawdle or to experiment either with make-up or with clothes – it invariably leads to being late, because you're lulled into a false sense of security. Stick with the basic 30-minute strategy but add in some of these options:

- wash and style hair
- substitute long scented bath for shower
- or, if you're flagging, opt for a quick energy booster: dance around wildly to your favourite music, follow with a brisk body-brushing all over, before diving into a power shower
- smooth in body lotion so you feel silky all over
- touch up nails and give yourself a 2-minute hand and foot massage
- if your back hurts and everything aches, put on soothing music and lie flat on the floor for a few minutes, head supported by a couple of paperbacks, knees up and apart, feet flat. Let your body sink into the floor and visualise yourself in a calm, quiet, warm place. (See *Instant Stress Busters*, page 185.)

Make-up Bags for Parties	
Tweezers	Eye make-up – shadow, liner, mascara, brow pencil
Emery board	Blusher
Concealer	Lipstick
Foundation (preferably compact all-in-one)	Lipgloss
	Clear or tinted nail polish
	Scent

Sponge Bags for Parties	The above, plus:
Moisturiser	Tissues
Eye make-up remover	Deodorant/anti-perspirant
Cotton wool buds	Mineral water spray
Dry make-up sponge	Toothbrush and toothpaste

MAGGIE HUNT'S EVENING MAKE-UP

FOR THE BEAUTY BIBLE

You can adapt this comprehensive step-by-step guide to suit you individually. If, for instance, you have no blemishes, you won't need step 1. This look and these basic shades will suit most women but try varying them with different colours on eyes and lips. (See *Other Evening Faces*, page 44).

Since your evening might carry on until dawn, Maggie has designed this make-up to stay put for up to 12 hours. You don't want to find that the lights have gone up and your make-up has disappeared. As with all make-up, the secret is blending, so take time and make sure that each colour (except, of course, for your lipstick) merges imperceptibly into the next.

12 STEPS TO A PERFECT EVENING FACE:

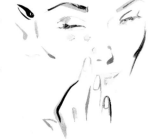

1 Paint blemishes with a small brush dipped in concealer or foundation, or pat on concealer with your ring finger; dab the blemishes gently until they have softened or, with any luck, disappeared. Do not rub.

2 To give a flawless base, look straight into a well-lit mirror and pat on a light-coloured, light-textured concealer or foundation (see *Meeting Your Match*, page 16); start from the inner corner underneath the eye and work outwards along the dark shadow. Lower eyelids and brush or pat on an even coat all over the eye zone, from lashes to brows, including the hollows on either side of the nose. Finish by thinly applying your usual foundation wherever else you need it. Put all this on lightly – you want the overall impression to be as natural as you'd look by day, especially if you are wearing a low-cut dress which shows lots of bare flesh.

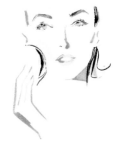

3 Before the foundation has set (and settled into any fine lines), powder lightly all over the face using translucent loose powder. Apply with a clean powder sponge, cotton wool pad or velvet puff. Whisk off any excess with a clean side of the sponge or pad, or with a big powder brush.

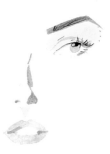

4 Now sweep an ivory semi-matte eyeshadow all over the eye area from lashes to eyebrows; this is the base for your eye make-up, whatever colours you choose, and will give 12-hour staying power. Also put the same shadow on the V above your upper lip to accentuate fullness (this is particularly effective for anyone with a thin upper lip).

5 Contour and define eyes with a semi-matte mid-brown eyeshadow (you can go for taupe/grey browns or a more golden shade). Dip your eyeshadow brush gently in the shadow and blow off any excess before applying. Put a folded tissue under lower lashes to avoid loose particles on your cheeks. Don't go up to the browbone, and avoid that little oval-shaped pad of fat on the inner corner of the eyelid. Then gently wing the shadow up and out towards the temples to lift the eyes; never take it further than the end of the eyebrows. Blend the shadow into the skin.

6 If necessary, shape face and contour cheekbones. Use slightly darker powder to slim down a broad nose, cheeks or face, disguise a double chin or bring down a high forehead. Always blend the dark powder in carefully – don't give yourself stripes. (Practise before a big evening out till you're happy with the results.)

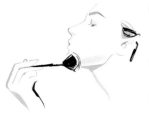

❍ for a broad nose, brush dark powder down either side of the nose.

❍ for a long nose, brush some darker powder on the tip.

❍ for round cheeks, suck in cheeks and lightly apply darker powder in hollows, blending backwards to the ear.

❍ for a heavy jaw, dust darker powder slightly under and slightly over the jawline, following the shape of the jaw.

❍ for a double chin, brush powder onto the fatty part.

❍ for a high forehead, sweep darker powder along the hairline.

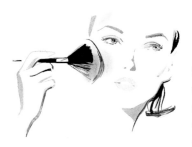

7 If you wish, brighten up your face with a bronzing powder swept across cheeks, down the nose, on the browbone, or the whole of your face. For naturalness, don't go darker than the chest and neck. Or you could try adding a bit of highlighter to upper cheekbones and browbone, to give a glow if you know the lighting will be subdued.

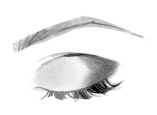

8 Now that you can judge the impact of the rest of your face, finish your eye make-up. Choose a soft golden bronze with just a touch of shine (or look at our *Other Evening Faces*, page 44) and apply across the inner two-thirds of the eyelid, up to the eye socket. Now define the outer third in a sideways V-shape, using dark brown or charcoal, smudge-blending the edges of the powder together.

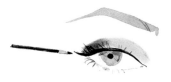

9 Define eyes in black (or a dark smokey shade) with either eyeliner pencil (for the softest finish), cake liner (medium soft) or liquid eyeliner (most dramatic).

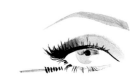

10 Apply mascara top and bottom – two coats, if you wish.

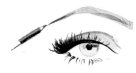

11 Define brows with powder or pencil, if necessary.

12 Define lip shape with liner, paint on lipstick, then put on gloss if you like it.

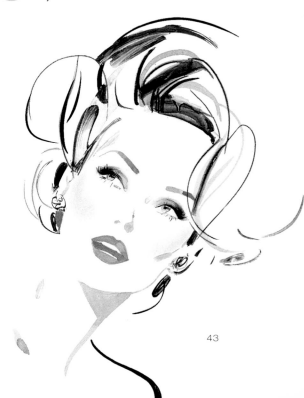

MAGGIE'S PARTY FAVOURITES

Foundation	YSL Radiant Touch, Colourings Lightening Touch
Concealer	Christian Dior Effets Blush, Lancôme Blush Subtil in Sculpture, Bourjois Hâlé moulded powder
Eyeshadow	Boots No. 7 Colour Perfect range: *Magnolia* as base, *Maple* on inner two-thirds of eye, *Calabash* on outer third. Also, Estée Lauder Compact Disc eye shadows: *Brown 1* as base, *Orange 2* for a touch of colour, *Brown 6* to shape, *Neutral 7* to define
Eye Liner	Lancome Artliner in black (liquid)
Eyebrow liner	Colourings Eyebrow Powder Pencil
Blusher	Estée Lauder Blushing Pot Pourri Passion
Lip liner	Lancôme Le Stylo Contour des Lèvres

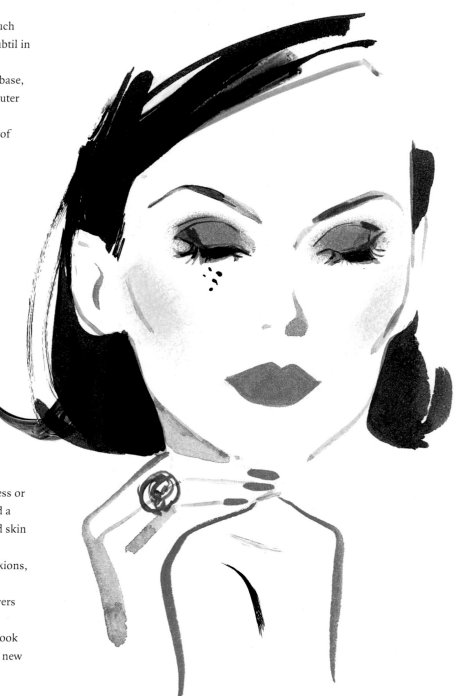

OTHER EVENING FACES

These looks will give you ideas for eyes, lips, cheeks and finishing touches, to incorporate into your party make-up.

THE PALOMA PICASSO LOOK

This is a dramatic look: try it with a tuxedo, a little black dress or any dark, rich colours. It is sensational with black velvet and a décolletage. Go for a strong accent on lips, eyes, cheeks and skin colour. Women with pale skins appear even paler and very dramatic in contrast. Medium to dark skins, or dull complexions, will take on a fresher, clearer and more vibrant tone.

✱ For a perfect canvas, you may need a foundation that covers fairly well, like Lancôme Maquilumine.

✱ Such powerful colours can be ageing, so do try out this look with products you already have before investing in an exotic new palette of colours.

✱ Scarlet nails are the finishing touch.

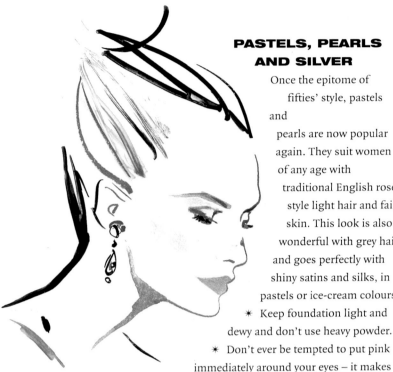

PASTELS, PEARLS AND SILVER

Once the epitome of fifties' style, pastels and pearls are now popular again. They suit women of any age with traditional English rose-style light hair and fair skin. This look is also wonderful with grey hair and goes perfectly with shiny satins and silks, in pastels or ice-cream colours.

✳ Keep foundation light and dewy and don't use heavy powder.

✳ Don't ever be tempted to put pink immediately around your eyes – it makes any woman look like a white mouse. Instead, smooth on semi-matte neutral colours which blend with your skin tone: try beige, ivory, deep grey, sand, pale peach. Brush deeper or contrasting colour – e.g. deep rose, honey, brown, taupe – into the socket line and under the lower lid. Add a hint of pink above the socket, and brown mascara.

✳ Remember, shine draws light, so don't put it anywhere you have lines. Use silver eyeshadow to highlight the centre of the upper lid and browbone. Line with silver, right behind the lashes, top and bottom.

✳ Lips should be pale but interesting; try applying a rosy colour, then rubbing or blotting off so just a stain is left. Then outline lips, and top with pearlised or silvery gloss. (Experiment mixing eyeshadows in lip gloss.)

✳ Wear toning pale nail varnish – frosted, if you like.

THE MIDAS TOUCH

Intense golds, coppers and bronzes are wonderful in the evening. Wear this rich Renaissance look with black, velvets, metallics – or go angelic and wear it with white or cream. You can adapt this make-up at any age by varying the intensity. Use a foundation that matches your skin or, for fresh, flawless skin, try a tinted moisturiser mixed with a little foundation.

✳ Teens to late 20s can go for all-over shimmer and kohl-rimmed eyes, with soft light gold dusted over lids and up to the brow, with a deeper colour (e.g. gold bronzer) on the lids.

✳ Older skins look better with softer shades smudged into a smoky effect, plus subtle touches to add sparkle – e.g. gold shadow dotted over your usual eyeshadow to highlight the arc of the brow, or gold gloss mixed with your favourite lipstick.

(See DIRECTORY for evening make-up sources.)

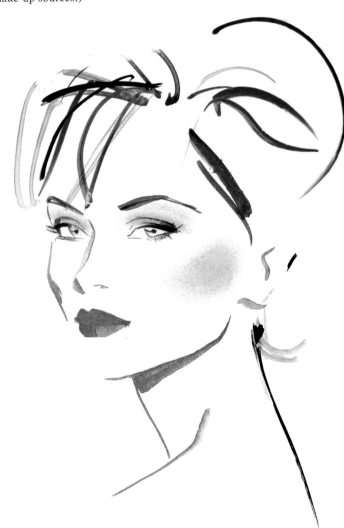

BRIDAL MAKE-UP

It's hard work being a bride. Not only does everyone expect you to look beautiful on the day itself, but the results must stand up to scrutiny for years afterwards, in photos and on video. So it's worth the extra effort to perfect your appearance.

 Most local hairdressing salons (as well as big city salons) can put a bride in touch with a professional make-up artist to make the bride look ravishing on the big day. It is vital to have a rehearsal well ahead of time, to ensure that both you and the make-up artist are happy with the results, advises Beryl Barnard, Principal of make-up school The London Esthetique, which offers two-hour face-to-face make-up lessons for brides as well as specialist courses for make-up artists.

'If you're using a make-up artist, establishing a good rapport is vital,' says Beryl. 'It means the bride has one less thing to worry about and enables her to enjoy having her make-up done.' Some brides, she points out, 'May not be used to wearing make-up at all, and if they feel like a painted doll they won't be relaxed on the day.'

Turn up wearing your usual make-up (or no make-up, if you don't normally wear any) so that the make-up artist can see how you like to look. Keeping make-up subtle – so that you still look like you – is the key to success. The effect, explains Beryl, should be similar to your usual style, with slightly more impact – and staying power, as your make-up will have to work hard and you probably won't have time to touch it up.

Foundation is the most important element of all, believes Beryl. 'It must be beautifully blended so that there are no tide marks. The pale colour of a wedding dress will emphasise poor blending or skin-matching, as there may be a lot of skin on show around the shoulders and neckline.' (For tips on finding your foundation match, see *Foundations*, page 16.) 'If someone has an oily skin,' she adds, 'we sometimes suggest using lacto-calamine on the T-zone under foundation, to help skin stay matte.'

Brides should, of course, blush – but not excessively. 'We tend only to use blusher if a girl is very pale. More often, we'll use a green under-base cover-up, to tone down natural flush.'

Lips should be outlined in a soft, nude lip pencil: Beryl likes to cover the whole lip area with the pencil, so that if the lipstick itself wears off, there's longer-lasting colour underneath. 'I like rosy lip shades, rather than bright reds, which contrast too strongly with the white or cream of the dress,' advises Beryl.

Eye make-up should be slightly more intense than usual, but stick to a natural palette of browns and taupes, not garish blues or greens: 'A touch of white highlighter on the browbone can look stunning.'

Nails, which should be immaculate, can be painted with clear varnish, as French manicure or in a delicate, pale shade of pink – whichever you prefer.

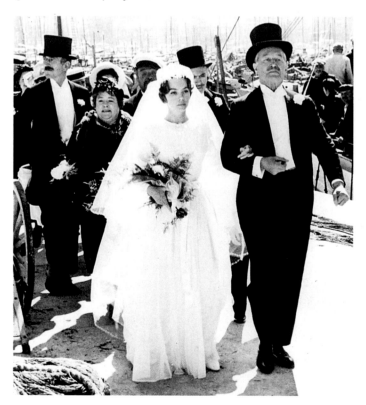

The most flattering element of all should, of course, be the dress itself. It's worth spending time trying several different shades of white/cream/ivory to find the one which best complements your skin tone. 'A cream or magnolia dress uplights the face beautifully. It's the kind of effect that Hollywood employs lighting cameramen to achieve, bouncing light onto the face so that it looks utterly radiant.' So much so, Beryl adds, 'That if I could afford the dry cleaning bills, I'd dress in cream and white year-round.' (Which is exactly what legendary natural health and beauty author **Leslie Kenton** does.)

GOOD IMPRESSIONS – INTERVIEWS AND FIRST DAYS AT WORK

Just three seconds is all the time it takes for a first impression to register on an interviewer – or a new work-mate. Your make-up, hair and hands are speaking for you before you even say a word, say psychologists and image professionals.

That certainly doesn't mean you have to be stunning to get the job. 'But it does mean that you have to look like you care,' stresses Judith Kark, Principal of London's Lucie Clayton Grooming & Modelling School, where women of all ages and nationalities are taught body language and posture, among other 'life skills'.

There is an art to projecting a winning interview image. Judith Kark's years of experience have led her to advise girls, 'To err on the side of polite caution.' (In other words: no nose rings, vampy nail polish or false lashes.) Neatness counts a lot. Hair should be off the face – 'Interviewers like to see your eyes' – but should look natural or bouncy. A new cut or a trim can do wonders to clean up your act – but do it a week in advance to give you and your hair a chance to settle in together.

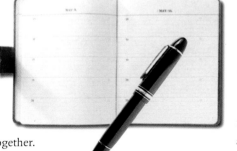

It may be too late to give up biting your nails, but that's no excuse not to reach for the anti-nail biting lotion. According to New York image guru Virginia Sullivan, of Image Communications International, 'Hands and shoes are the two most telling non-verbal clues which corporate recruiters look at.' Clean fingernails really do go without saying. Nails should be short, neat and, if you like varnish, polished in a clear or neutral colour.

For a smooth handshake, carry a tube of hand cream in your bag.

Just in case clamminess is a problem, Judith Kark counsels carrying a hankie to wipe hands on, or brushing your hands with the same powder you use on your face, which dries them off. (Be warned: only carry pressed, not loose, powder – it could spill and ruin your suit.)

Even though young skin tends to look wonderfully fresh, subtly-applied make-up is a must, for interviews and in the workplace. (At many companies where image matters – like The Disney Store and British Airways – make-up is actually mandatory.) 'No make-up at all is as sloppy as too much,' points out Judith Kark firmly.

Top make-up artist Ariane recommends a natural, neutral look, 'At least until you've found your ground.' Her essentials: start with an all-in-one foundation and powder, which can be touched up during the day. (N.B. in the washroom, not at your desk.) Judith Kark recommends matte-finish make-up. 'Because if you're nervous, you'll be quite shiny enough.' If you have blemishes or dark circles, put a skin tone-matched concealer on them, before your base. Next step is a camel-coloured blusher (she likes M.A.C.'s *Biscuit*), 'But don't put it just on the apples of cheeks or you'll look like a dairymaid; sweep it along the cheekbone, too.' (See *Blushing Beauty*, page 34.) Light eye make-up is another must (see *Getting Your*

47

Eyes Right, page 29), and good grooming definitely means plucking stray brows. Lips should be a near-natural pink, with maybe a dab of gloss or shine. (Ariane is a fan of Colourings Complete Colour all-in-one sticks, which work on cheeks and eyes, too – see *Double Duty Beauty*, page 50.)

If you're still insecure about the art of cosmetic face-perfection, the pros are agreed: a make-up lesson is a terrific confidence-booster. Choose one where you can get hands-on experience, rather than simply watch while you're transformed.

Finally, before any big interview or the first day at work, Judith Kark tells her girls to try on the clothes and the make-up they'll be wearing, in daylight, not last thing at night. 'Stand in front of the mirror and really try to see yourself as others will.'

TIP

■ The attitude to make-up and clothes is different in every workplace. Judith Kark suggests that when you're at the interview you take a good look at the make-up and hairstyles favoured by future colleagues. 'It's important to play by the rules when you're starting your career,' she believes. When you've gauged the attitude to appearance you can decide whether to be more daring.

Workplace Beauty – Where to Look
You don't need to spend a fortune to find wearable – and affordable – neutral make-up products. Ariane recommends checking out L'Oréal Perfection, Bourjois, Colourings (at The Body Shop) and Max Factor.

BODY LANGUAGE – WATCH WHAT YOU SAY

The way you walk, the way you look at the interviewer and the way you shake hands can have a positive or a negative impact. Body language expert Julius Fast (author of Penguin's *Body Language in the Workplace*) offers a few reminders: slouching suggests depression, while good posture points to a take-charge attitude. Looking the interviewer in the eye (without staring) signals honesty.

Leaning *forward* to talk and *back* to listen conveys involvement and enthusiasm. Keep your feet flat on the floor and knees together, rather than crossing legs. Folding your hands in your lap looks immature, but folding your arms is too defensive. Instead, rest one arm on the arm of your chair, the other in your lap. Use hands to gesture, but don't overdo it. The clincher is your handshake: not limp, not overly firm, just brisk and friendly.

INTERVIEWS AND THE WORKPLACE

DON'T...
...show any cleavage (sew bra-level buttonholes with an extra couple of stitches at each side to stop them popping open embarrassingly)
...repair your make-up in the office (that's what the Ladies is for, even if the lighting is dreadful)
...wear coloured nail varnish – it looks terrible when it chips
...go completely bare-faced – unless you are perfect-looking
...play the vamp – or the siren
...drench yourself in scent

DO...
...wear light, subtle make-up
...secure your hair off your face
...take a spare pair of shoes and tights – it's no fun sitting around with wet feet after a dash from the station in the rain
...buy a good hanger for your jacket/coat, and keep it at work
...keep a small make-up and hair kit, with an emery board for emergencies, in your desk drawer
...wash your hands often (and keep a tube of hand cream at work – handling paper really dries out hands)
...wear an effective deodorant/anti-perspirant. A new job can be nerve-racking and leave you feeling hot and sweaty. Mitchum is a good brand if you have problem perspiration

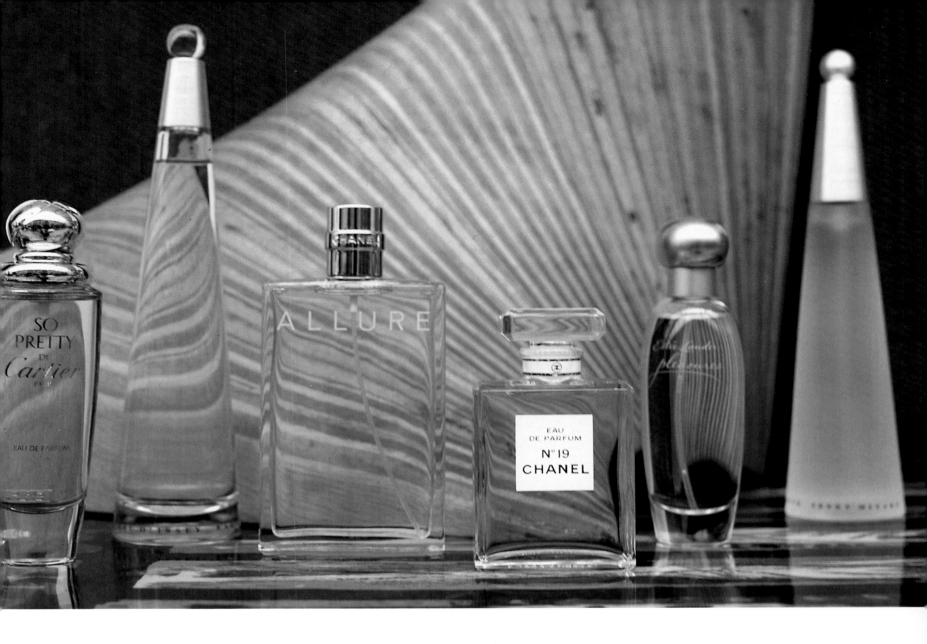

SAFE (BUT LOVELY) SCENTS

Chanel No. 19 or Chanel Allure

Joseph *Parfum de Jour*

Estée Lauder *Pleasures*

Cartier *So Pretty*

L'Eau d'Issey

4711

O de Lancôme

(Always wear the eau de toilette – save full-strength perfume
for Saturday night.)

DOUBLE DUTY BEAUTY

Most beauty products are designed with one use in mind, but some canny make-up artists and customers have discovered that a cosmetic – or sometimes a store-cupboard basic – can perform two, or even three tasks. Here are some of the cleverest we've found.

DOUBLE DUTY COSMETICS

works as...

Eyeshadow pencil	brow liner
Creamy-coloured eyeshadow	under-eye concealer (dot skin-matching foundation on top)
Eye make-up base	blemish concealer
Rosy lipstick or gloss	blusher (particularly good in summer when powder blusher often looks too heavy)
Bronzing powder	eyeshadow
Facial sprays	pre-styling hair dampener
Eye cream	lip moisturiser
Clay face masks	hand/foot masks
Elizabeth Arden 8-hour cream	lipgloss
Sloughing/exfoliating cream	shaving cream
Bottles of nearly finished scent	fragranced bath oil, when filled with baby oil
Intensive moisturisers	cuticle softeners for hands/feet

TRIPLE DUTY BEAUTY PRODUCTS

works as...

Vaseline	make-up remover, lipgloss, hair glosser (just use a *touch* – smooth a tiny spot on one palm, then stroke lightly over finished hairstyle)
Baby lotion	make-up remover, face and body moisturiser
Baby oil	eye make-up remover, bath oil
Eyeliner	brow liner, lip liner (choose soft, auburny-brown pencils)
Apple cider vinegar	bath softener, hair shiner in final rinse
Lemons	skin beautifier (put a slice in hot water and drink), elbow restorer (rub halves around elbows to brighten skin), hair rinse for blondes (put juice in final rinse)
Olive oil	with sea salt as an exfoliant (use 1 tablespoon olive oil to 1 teaspoon salt), without salt on hair as a D-I-Y mask (massage generously into dry hair, wrap with cling-film and leave as long as possible), as a skin and health enhancer (take 1 tablespoon daily, in salads or neat, to ease constipation and for general health)

NAMING NAMES

✪ The Body Shop Complete Colour = eyeshadow, lipstick, blusher ✪ Bobbi Brown Essentials Stick Foundation = foundation and concealer

✪ Kiehl's Ultra-Moisturising Eye Stick SPF18 = protection for eyes and lips

✪ Estée Lauder Just Blush! Eye & Cheek Mosaics – says it all ✪ Guerlain Issima Ivoire eyeshadow = concealer

✪ Bourjois Pastel Eyeshadow Brun Essential (a matte brown) = eyeshadow, liquid liner (used wet), brow colour

✪ Clarins Revitalising Moisture Mask = hand mask (pat into skin afterwards)

✪ Guerlain Issima Midnight Secret = cuticle softener, hand mask ✪ Kiehl's Pink Shine (lip froster) = lip, cheek and eye colour

✪ Stephen Glass Light Fantastic = eyelid foundation, under-eye concealer, all-over primer to lift dull skin

✪ Guerlain Lip Balm with Port = ointment for nipples (nursing mums use it!)

AND THERE'S MORE...

■ If you're out of wool wash, you can use any shower gel to handwash woollens, lingerie and sports clothes.

■ Aveda's Curessence (an intensive hair conditioner) can be used to wash knitwear, leaving it smelling fresh and baby-soft. Their Anti-Humectant Pomade (for hair) also works as a lip balm.

■ In an emergency, good old Nivea Cream will give ordinary leather shoes a gleam as bright as any upmarket leather polish. In fact, anything designed to make your skin more supple – a moisturiser containing shea butter or plant waxes, for instance – is likely to do the same for your leather loafers, provided you buff with plenty of elbow grease.

■ When locked away at a health farm writing part of this book, we tried Christian Dior's Svelte anti-cellulite treatment as a hairstyling gel. It worked.

■ Use hand lotion on your legs for shaving; it leaves skin ultra silky. (Hair conditioner works, too.)

■ Next time you blow out a candle, rub some of the still-warm wax on your cuticles; it works like an instant paraffin treatment.

■ The Body Shop's Honey Beeswax Almond & Jojoba Oil Cleanser works as a great furniture polish. (It's the beeswax that does it.)

■ Dog owners swear by Neutrogena's T/Gel Shampoo for washing their hounds!

■ For a light orange flavour in cookies and cakes, sprinkle a teaspoonful of Crabtree & Evelyn's Orange Water into the dough.

■ You have to wonder precisely how the marketing minds at Aveda stumbled upon the fact that their potent Active Formula Balancing Composition – effective as a massage oil, a bath additive and an invigorating inhalant – also acts as 'an ace toilet cleaner', in the words of an Aveda insider.

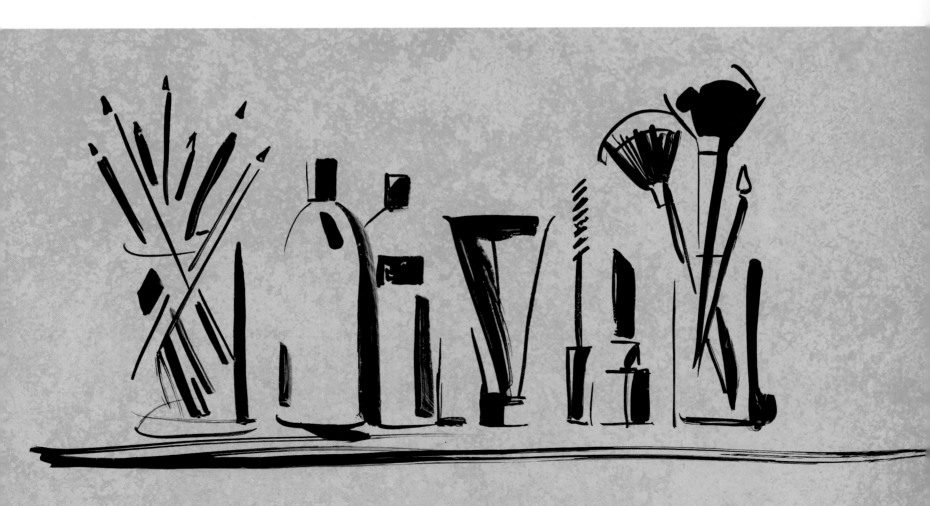

FIRST AID FOR MAKE-UP MISTAKES

Here are five remedies for make-up goofs which ensure you won't have to cleanse and start over:

Lipstick overdose... You hoped that red lipstick would make you look like a movie star. It does: Jack Nicholson as The Joker. Blot gently with tissues until they come away clean. If there's still a stain, apply moisturiser to your lips, leave it for a couple of minutes and blot again. Then apply a more neutral shade.

Foundation tide marks... You put your foundation on in the gloaming and in the cold light of day it looks unalluringly two-tone along the hairline or jaw. Blend with a clean, dry make-up sponge until the line disappears. If it won't shift, try blending with translucent powder, dusted onto a soft puff.

Too much blush... Instead of a fetching flush, you look like you've just run up Everest. Clown cheeks also call for a clean, dry make-up sponge – just rub gently over your brush strokes to take the colour out. You can soften colour even further with translucent powder, and redo with a new, subtler blush shade.

Smudged mascara... Happens all too easily, especially if you sneeze mid-application. If you're wearing waterproof mascara, dip a cotton bud in eye make-up remover and dab gently at it. If it's non-waterproof, just dampen the Q-tip with water, instead. You can use the other, clean end to reapply foundation and/or concealer.

The Groucho Marx brow... Strengthening the browline is a vital part of face-shaping – but you can overdo it. To remove excess pencil or powder, all it may take is a few strokes with a clean eyebrow brush. Failing that, wipe with a cotton bud.

FIRST AID (FOR FACES) KIT

What every woman should have on hand for emergencies:

- Tissues
- Round and wedge-shaped make-up sponges
- A powder puff
- Translucent or pale powder
- Eye make-up remover
- Eyebrow brush
- Cotton buds like Q-tips (rounded and with pointed tips, available from specialist make-up supply stores such as Screenface, see DIRECTORY)

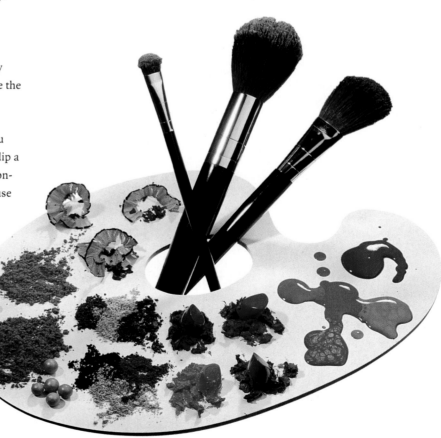

MAKE-UP THAT LASTS AND LASTS

There is an alternative to the daily grind of putting on and wiping off at least some of your make-up. Recent developments in semi-permanent make-up can give you back tweezed-out eyebrows, can ink in eyeliner, or can contour and/or stain lips a long-lasting rosy hue.

Semi-permanent make-up is a form of tattooing, so it's probably not for the squeamish. Minute, specially developed, coloured pigments of iron oxide are injected into the skin so that the tiny dots join up and form a band or patch of the desired colour.

Semi-permanent make-up may suit you if:
- your eyebrows are thin or non-existent
- you suffer from alopecia or have lost your hair through chemotherapy
- you have poor eyesight and find it difficult to apply make-up
- you play a lot of sport or swim a great deal, and do not want to reapply make-up endlessly
- you have a scar or other mark in your eyebrows
- you have had plastic surgery which has altered your eyebrows
- you are allergic to eye make-up
- you just want to save time

First of all, you should have an expert consultation at which you discuss your face shape and your individual requirements. Word of mouth is usually the best way of finding a reputable and reliable practitioner. We recommend you go to a medically trained practitioner such as a nurse; some already offer these services in beauty salons, others work with cosmetic surgeons. Always ask for before and after pictures of other clients and also contact numbers if you wish to talk to them.

If you agree to go ahead, the next step is an allergy test to make sure your skin won't react against the pigment. Before the first session, you should be asked to sign an informed consent paper, to acknowledge that you understand any risks.

Most practitioners ask you to draw in the shape of brow-/eye-line/lip line you want yourself. There is a wide colour range, so an experienced practitioner should be able to choose one which will look natural. An anaesthetic cream is used to numb the area and the process is not painful, although it may be uncomfortable. The first session may last one to two hours, depending on how much you need done.

You will need to apply an antibiotic cream (provided by the practitioner) for a week to prevent any infection and keep the area clean with cotton wool soaked in warm water. The tenderness may last for several days, or more, and the area may look quite red.

A top-up session is usually necessary after six or nine weeks, when the skin has renewed itself and the practitioner can judge how the pigment has faded. The effects normally last between six months and two years.

N.B. Bear in mind that any invasive treatment near the eyes carries some risk, however small.

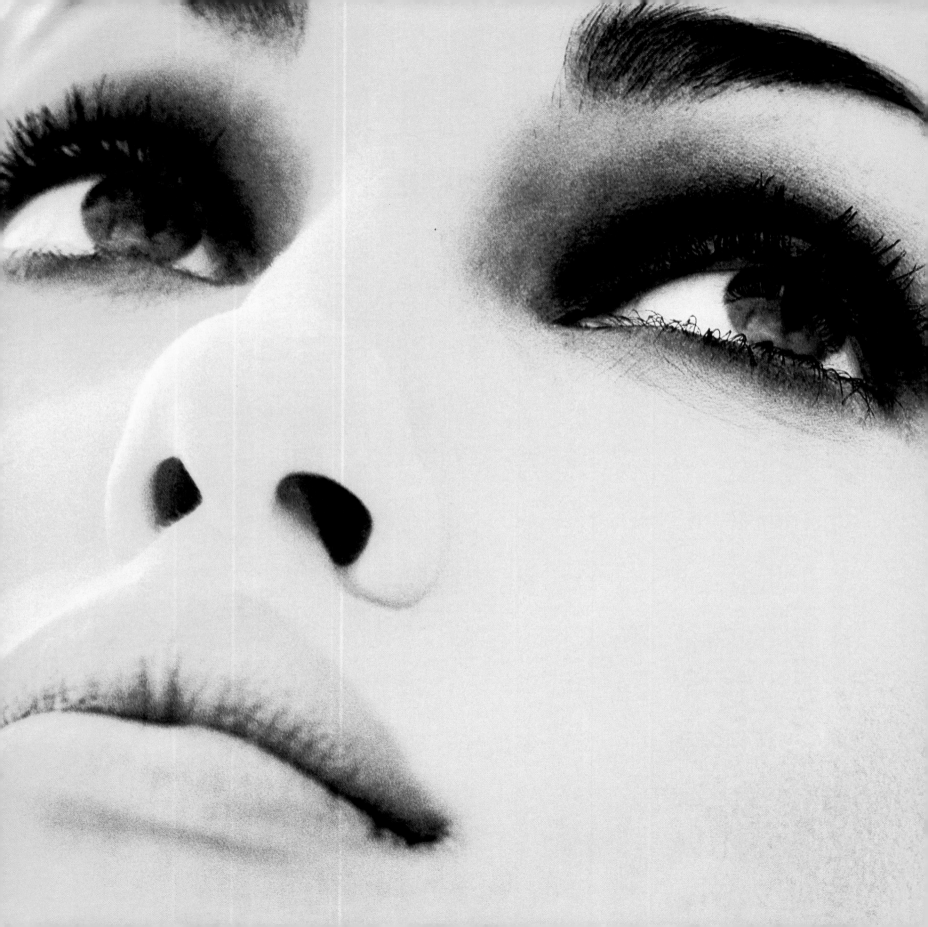

2
Eyes

Eyes cannot lie. About our feelings, about our health – and about our age. **And since up to 80 per cent of the information we receive from the world comes to us through our eyes, it is vital not to neglect them.** The conventional wisdom is simple: wear specs (or contacts) if you have poor eyesight, don't sit close to the TV, read under a good light, take off your eye make-up at night – and eat lots of carrots. But there is much more you can do to protect your vision, banish bags and keep the eye area beautiful.

HOW TO BE A BRIGHT EYES

Puffiness, bloodhound-type bags and dark circles can all provoke morning-after eye dramas. Fortunately, even small lifestyle changes can make a big difference to the state of the 'mirrors of your soul'.

Problems can be due to lifestyle or nature, or a mixture of both. Lack of sleep, or, conversely, too much, over-indulgence in alcohol, allergies such as asthma or hayfever, food sensitivity, water retention or even the common cold can all wreak havoc on your eyes. Heredity plays a significant part, too. In some women, dark circles are simply the result of a high amount of pigment under their eyes, and there is undoubtedly a familial tendency to under-eye bags and folds.

EYE BAGS

Bags are unlikely to disappear permanently unless you have surgery (see page 141), but these simple remedies can reduce excess baggage:

◆ Our grandmothers swore by cold teabags and slices of cucumber to reduce puffiness, but it is now clear that it's the chill factor – not the ingredients – which diminish bags by constricting the blood vessels; try holding an ice cube wrapped in cling-film to the puffiness, or wrap some crushed ice in a tea towel and lie under an ice eye-mask for a few minutes (but be careful if you suffer from broken veins). Or experiment with ice-cold teaspoons, kept in the freezer. (Stainless steel is better than silver, which warms up too fast.) We have also heard good reports on the effects of raw potato.

◆ Practise a 'tapping' massage to disperse bags: with your middle finger, tap the under-eye area lightly but swiftly, moving from the inner corner to the outer corner of your eye and back again in a semi-circular movement; just a minute of this can lead to visible results.

◆ Vigorous exercise reduces general puffiness; so does cutting down on salt and alcohol.

◆ Dr Goldwyn advises using an extra pillow; the angle keeps under-eye fluids from accumulating overnight and so prevents puffiness.

◆ You may be sensitive to certain eye products: drops, make-up, contact lens solution. Switch to different brands (one at a time

to identify the culprit). Look for 'fragrance-free' or 'hypoallergenic' on the label – although this is no guarantee that these will be trouble-free, just an indication that known irritants have been screened out.

◆ Your regular skin creams may be triggering puffiness; on the eye area substitute special eye gels which are light and cooling, instead.

◆ If you prefer the richer feel of an eye cream, proper application will prevent it seeping into the eyes at night: rub a dab between thumb tip and forefinger to soften it, so that you smooth on only a thin layer. Then pat along the bony ridge beneath your eyes, not directly under the lashes. Next, very lightly dot cream along the browbone, under the eyebrow. It will still deliver benefits, without irritating eyes.

◆ Food allergies and sensitivities can also be a cause of puffiness and dark circles.

DARK CIRCLES

Some people are born with dark circles under their eyes but these only really become noticeable as skin ages and loses elasticity. Irritants such as cigarette smoke, dust and other pollutants may cause dark circles – as well as red-eye – by triggering the release of chemicals in the body which enlarge the blood vessels in and around the lids, in an attempt to dilute the aggravating substance. As blood enters these vessels, it darkens the area under the surface skin and puffs it up. Some eye products may provoke a similar sensitivity reaction in susceptible women. Lack of sleep is famous for having the same effect, although when you catch up on lost zzzs, the circles usually disappear like magic.

Meanwhile, your best bet may be camouflage. Your usual concealer isn't ideal for under the eye because it's heavy, and may well be the wrong colour. Look for words such as 'lightweight' and 'light-reflective' on the packaging. Make-up artist Jenny Jordan advises dabbing a tiny dot onto darker areas and blending carefully.

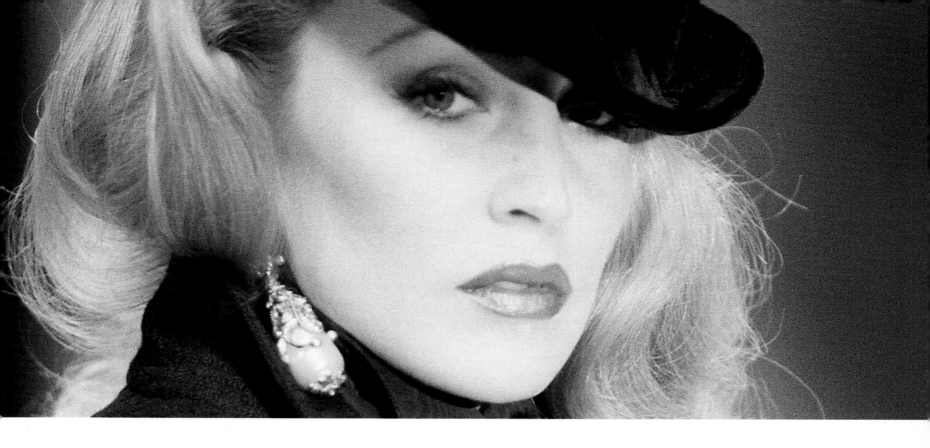

TRIED & TESTED

TREATS FOR TIRED AND PUFFY EYES

This is the *short-term* approach to combating eye problems after, say, too little sleep, a smoky party or working day-after-day at a VDU. We asked our testers to score products for puffiness reduction, eye-brightening power and instant refreshment.

Top Treats

E'SPA Soothing Eye Lotion

This light, blue lotion with soothing chamomile can even be applied over make-up without disturbing it, some testers reported.

COMMENTS: 'this feels deliciously cooling as it goes on and calms the whole area', 'easy to use and not sticky', 'great for waking you up!'

Px Prescriptives Eye Specialist

This is a lightweight eye cream designed to combat ageing which scored well for its soothing and anti-puffiness qualities.

COMMENTS: 'my eyes felt really clean when I used it', 'very smooth and easily absorbed', 'my eyes felt fresh for hours afterwards and the skin was very soft'.

Ultima II Brighten Up, Tighten Up

Several of our testers, although not all, felt that this product lived up to its catchy name.

COMMENTS: 'made eyes much brighter', 'the slight hint of colour is very good', 'also good at reducing dark circles'.

RoC Melibiose Anti-Ageing Eye Contour Cream

Again, designed for anti-ageing, but testers scored its soothing properties very highly.

COMMENTS: 'refreshing and hydrating', 'my eyes looked clearer and brighter', 'make-up went on as usual afterwards'.

Best Budget Buys

Of the less expensive products tried, those based on plant ingredients did best.

Boots Botanics Revitalising Eye Masks

These fast-acting eye pads, made to place over eyes after a tiring day or before a big event, scored especially well for their power to refresh.

COMMENTS: 'very relaxing and soothing on tired eyes', 'particularly refreshing', 'I felt revived after using these'.

Blackmore's Cornflower Eye Balm

This natural product features cornflowers, a well-known botanical eye-waker.

COMMENTS: 'very refreshing – particularly in a hot climate', 'liked the feeling – seemed to tighten up the eyes a bit', 'felt good and helped smooth out some wrinkles'.

PUT THE SPARKLE BACK

Most of us have woken up at some time with rabbity-red eyes. They usually go away once you get some sleep and fresh air. But if your eyes are often red (unless it's due to a hangover), try these steps:

◆ First, embark on a little detective work. Experiment with different brands of make-up and skincare, or go without, then add products one at a time. Even hair products, and nail varnish, can be culprits.

◆ If you regularly use eye drops to get rid of bloodshot eyes, you may want to think about trying a different make. Some contain decongestants or vasoconstrictors, which temporarily shrink blood vessels; these should be used sparingly because it's possible that, in time, the blood vessels will come back bigger and redder than ever. You may get on better with 'artificial tears' instead, which simply lubricate the eyes, giving them the chance to recover.

◆ There are common-sense ways to prevent red-eye: wash your hands before applying make-up, use disposable eyeshadow applicators, cotton wool swabs or washable sponge applicators. (And if they're washable, *do* wash them regularly).

◆ If you work at a VDU, remember it can bring on red-eye, because the static it gives out attracts dust to the area in front of the monitor. You could invest in a screen for it, and an ioniser for your desk.

EYE CARE

Should we use special eye creams? Some ingredients regularly used in facial moisturisers – fragrance, emulsifiers and emollients – may cause smarting in the ultra-sensitive eye area. So if you slather your usual moisturiser around the delicate eye area, you could end up with weepy, irritated eyes. Rich moisturisers can block the oil glands around the eyes, where glands are fewer in number, and smaller. The result can be unsightly little white or yellow cysts. So, the answer is yes; the eye area does need special attention, and an everyday moisturiser may not be the best choice.

TRIED & TESTED

TRIED AND TESTED EYE MAKE-UP REMOVERS

The bottom line for these products is: do they really remove every last trace of mascara, which is the hardest eye make-up to budge? Because stinging is often a problem with eye make-up removers, we asked testers to be alert for any soreness or irritation. On the whole, our testers found that the inexpensive products they tried were more likely to cause irritation. So – especially if you have sensitive eyes – it may be worth investing in one of the more expensive products, as none of our testers experienced any irritation with the top-scoring 'treats'.

Top Treats

Clarins Eye Make-up Remover Cream-Gel
This innovative formulation worked well on waterproof mascara as well as other eye make-up. All the testers agreed it removed eye make-up quickly and easily with no rubbing.
COMMENTS: 'very soothing for tired eyes', 'an excellent product – I wear contact lenses and have sensitive eyes.'

Bobbi Brown Eye Make-up Remover
This product was developed by make-up artist Bobbi Brown, who needed a really effective product for her work. Also works well on waterproof mascara. No irritation reported.
COMMENTS: 'lovely to use and the most effective I've tested', 'it took my eye make-up off really easily'.

Chanel Dual Phase Eye Make-up Remover
This needs to be shaken before use to mix the ingredients, which are formulated to remove all kinds of mascara.

COMMENTS: 'it left my eye area feeling very soft and silky', 'the best I've ever used'.

Best Budget Buys

Body Shop Camomile Eye Make-up Remover
Our testers reported this was a really effective option, which required very little effort to swipe away make-up. The gentlest of the inexpensive products tested.
COMMENTS: 'very gentle but definitely does the trick for me', 'removed make-up effortlessly'.

Blackmore's Gentle Eye Make-up Remover
The fact that this product contained only natural ingredients made it popular with many of our testers.
COMMENTS: 'it took my eye make-up off swiftly and easily', 'compact, lightweight bottle good for travelling'.

BROW BEAT

Think of your brows as face architecture. Well drawn eyebrows really do frame the face, attracting attention to the eyes and making them appear larger and more defined.

Brows should always be well groomed. Even 'Brow Queen' Brooke Shields plucks her strays. Make-up artist Carol Shaw (creator of the LORAC range) suggests having your brows shaped by a professional first, to get the right arch, and then maintaining them at home, plucking stragglers that fall below the curve.

THE SECRETS OF A GREAT TWEEZE...

▲ Natural daylight is best, so sit near a window and use a hand-held magnifying mirror.

▲ Cleanse the area thoroughly, removing any last trace of cleansing product with toner or rosewater, so that the surface isn't greasy.

▲ Using a brow pencil, draw in the brow's natural line, to act as a guide and prevent over-plucking.

▲ Gently pull the skin of the outer edge of your eyebrow up and out so that you can see the browbone, and use it as a guide. Brows should extend a bit beyond each corner of your eyes, so don't pluck too much from either end – and don't pluck more than one hair at a time,

or you'll end up with bald patches.

▲ Pluck stray hairs first, using a sharp tweezer with fine points. Make-up artists all swear by Tweezerman's.

▲ Always tweeze from underneath the brow, never the top, following the natural shape and plucking hair out in the direction it grows.

▲ Start at the middle of the brow and work towards your ear, then work from the middle in towards your nose. Make sure the arch is highest at the centre of your eye.

▲ Swipe tweezed brows with a cotton bud dipped in pure tea tree oil – nature's perfect antiseptic.

▲ Be warned: continual plucking will eventually make the hairs grow more and more slowly, until they stop growing altogether. Avoid over-zealous plucking, because you're bound to want to change the shape of your brows at some stage in the future – and you may not be able to grow them back. (See *Make-up that Lasts and Lasts*, page 53, for details of semi-permanent make-up to 'tattoo' lost eyebrows back in place.)

If you can't get to a salon for a first-time tweeze, make sure that your chosen brow shape suits your face:

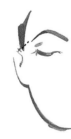 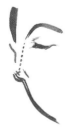 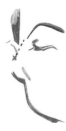 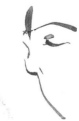

If it's **round**, aim the end of the brow towards the tip of the ear.

For an **oval** face, the brow should curve down towards the lower ear.

For a **square** face, slope it towards the middle of the ear.

For a **long** face, shape the brow in a straightish line towards the tip of the ear.

GROWING THEM OUT

If you change your mind about the shape of your brows, that in-between stubble can be unsightly. Kevyn Aucoin advises: 'With a brush, paint facial hair bleach onto the little hairs and it'll disguise them till they grow back. Then you can give them a new shape.' (We recommend Jolen's facial bleach.)

PERFECT BROWS

● Should the colour of your eyebrows match your hair? 'I prefer brows the same as hair or a little lighter,' declares Carol Shaw. 'If brows are much darker, you look like you're scowling.'

● Kevyn Aucoin likes brows a couple of shades lighter than hair: 'I take a cream bleach and apply it to the eyebrows, leaving it on anywhere from one to 15 minutes, depending how light I want them to be. I check by wiping the bleach from a tiny part of the eyebrows. Leaving it on too long can irritate the skin, so I err on the side of caution. If the skin is sensitive, I remove the bleach early. If I go too far in the other direction, the eyebrows can always be dyed back easily to their normal shade.'

● To define brows, 'Use light, feathery strokes whether you're using a pencil – which shouldn't be too soft – or powder, which you should apply with an eyeliner brush following the direction of the hairs,' advises Mary Greenwell.

● Make-up artist Vincent Longo uses pencil first on brows, then matching powder shadow. 'That fixes the brow for the whole day.'

● To highlight the browbone and define the brow, some make-up artists draw a line underneath the brow with a fat concealer stick, then blend it with a Q-tip.

● Many make-up artists prefer brow colour in powdered form, rather than a pencil, to get a softer and prettier finish. There are now special brow powders – try Colourings, Estée Lauder and Chanel – which all have a higher wax content, for staying power.

● If you do want to use a pencil, look for one with a built-in brush, so you can groom any wandering hairs.

● Once you've made up your brows, you may want to use a special brow gel – although a touch of hairspray, sprayed onto a toothbrush and very lightly brushed through the brows, also does the trick.

TIPS FROM THE TOP

Actress **Patsy Kensit** actually snips off the straggly hairs which stick up above the top of her eyebrows: 'I was terrified when this was first done to me, but suddenly I had the sort of super-neat eyebrows I'd seen on Yasmin Le Bon and wanted myself. Now I do it to all my girlfriends. You have to go very carefully, one hair at a time, and just trim off the tip of the brow hair right where it reaches the outer line of your brow.'

Actress **Jaclyn Smith** shares her brow-plucking secret: 'I've discovered that it's best done first thing in the morning, before my shower. That way, any puffiness or redness has a chance to subside before I get ready to put on make-up.'

Black supermodel **Veronica Webb**: 'If I'm going out at night, I'll intensify my brows by making the shape more dramatic. I elongate the tail just slightly with a pencil and lift the arch a little by drawing it on top of the brow, instead of underneath. A super-sharp pencil is the only way to get a clean line.'

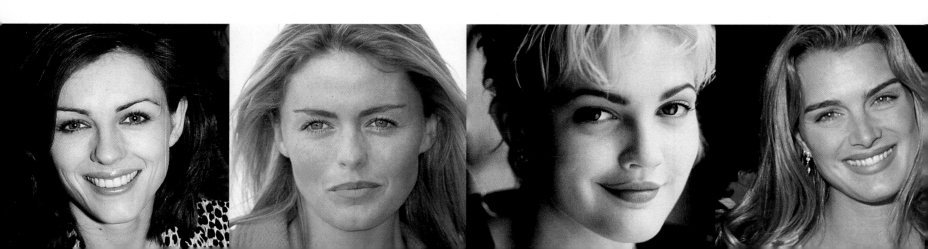

SPECS APPEAL

Faces, like bodies, come in a variety of different shapes and the quest for the ultimate in flattering frames can be an uphill struggle. So, how to find your perfect match?

Which Glasses Suit You?
The main rule is simple: avoid the same shape of frame as your face, e.g. if you have a round face, don't choose round frames, while square or angular faces should steer clear of square or angular frames.

Do you have an oval face? (i.e. vaguely egg-shaped)
You'll look good in just about any frames because there's no pronounced forehead or jaw to work around. Try angular or rounded aviator shapes, or John Lennon-style wire frames. The only ones to sidestep are those that don't feel comfortable or simply look odd.

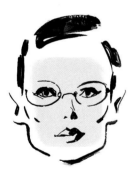

Do you have a square face?
(i.e. strong, angular – or short and wide)
This face looks best with thin frames in oval or round shapes, which give a slightly softer, more rounded appearance to the jawline. Frames to avoid are those that emphasise squareness.

Do you have a round face?
(i.e. short and fairly wide with full cheeks and a rounded chin)
The right shape will slim down the appearance of your features: choose angular frames – cat's eye, rectangular, square shapes. Frames to avoid are small and circular, or else very large, both of which will make the face look rounder.

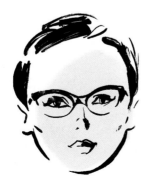

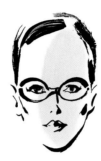

Do you have a long face? (i.e. high-cheekboned, often with a deep forehead and a strong, sharp or chiselled jawline)
Look for wide, large frames that counteract the face's narrowness. Frames with a strong top bar or rounded 'owl' shapes can work well. But steer clear of small, square styles.

✳ If your eyes are close-set, avoid big frames as they'll emphasise the fact.
✳ If you have a long nose, be careful of glasses with high 'bridges', as these will emphasise the length of your nose. A high bridge can give length to a short nose.

FIT TIPS
✳ Eyes should appear in the middle of the lens, to avoid looking cross-eyed.

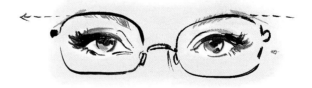

✳ Eyebrows should line up perfectly with the top bar of the glasses; if they're higher or lower you'll look double-browed.
✳ Glasses shouldn't touch your cheeks.
✳ Choose frames which fit comfortably and are the right width for your face; opticians can do a lot to make glasses fit better.
✳ If your glasses leave pinch-marks on the nose, they're too tight. You can probably get them 'eased' at the optician's.

Glamour and Glasses

Glasses call for an eye make-up rethink.

✳ If your prescription is for nearsightedness, your eyes will seem to recede a bit behind spectacle lenses. So accentuate them by using a pale, neutral shadow on eyelid and browbone; contour with a slightly darker shade in the crease and follow with liner (on top lid only) and mascara.

✳ Specs for farsighted women exaggerate everything – even make-up mistakes! – and eyes can seem to protrude. So play eyes down with a genuinely shadow-coloured eyeshadow – soft brown or perhaps a greenish-grey – with a darker shade in the crease. Avoid light, bright or shiny shadows.

✳ Since frames cast shadows on the face, use concealer – a shade lighter than foundation or skin tone – to camouflage any circles.

✳ Wear quite a strong-coloured lipstick, so your glasses don't overpower your other features.

✳ Eye make-up is hard enough to apply at the best of times, but when you can't see a thing without your specs it becomes a nightmare. Try using a shaving mirror that will magnify your face. Cut the end off your make-up brushes and slice eye pencils in half, so you can get closer to the mirror.

✳ Avoid liquid liner unless you feel naked without it; a pencil is easier to control. But if you like liquid, use the brush to feel your way along your upper lashes and then switch to a pointed sponge-tipped applicator to trace over the liner with a shadow in the same colour, smudging the line to make it look more natural.

TIP large and/or wraparound frames help protect the sensitive skin around your eyes from sun-induced wrinkling and lines.

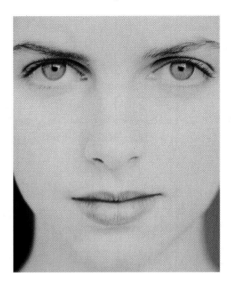

QUICK-CHANGE EYES

Just as you can metamorphose your hair colour from mouse to mink or ash blonde, so now you can enhance the natural colour of your eyes. And it's simple.

Whether you want plain or prescription coloured contact lenses, many good high street stores, including Dollond & Aitchison and David Clulow in the UK, offer a consultation and fitting service which can morph dishwatery puddles into flashing violet orbs.

The most time-consuming factor, according to one black-eyed beauty who swopped to azure blue, is learning how to put the lenses in – and, crucially, take them out. It took her a good half hour at the shop with some uncomfortable moments ending in watery red eyes, and then a fair amount of practising at home. She loved the result, though.

Expect to pay about £30 for the initial consultation, which is mandatory. Brand leaders in non-disposable coloured contacts are Durasoft and Elegant, both of which do a wide range of shades costing around £150 per pair; these lenses will last about nine months to one year. You can wear Freshlook disposable lenses (which come in green, brown, blue or violet) up to 30 times; a pair costs about £25 and the thinner lenses give much less risk of infection. (Generally, the shorter the wear time the better the lenses are for the eyes, whether coloured or not.)

These lenses are all available internationally.

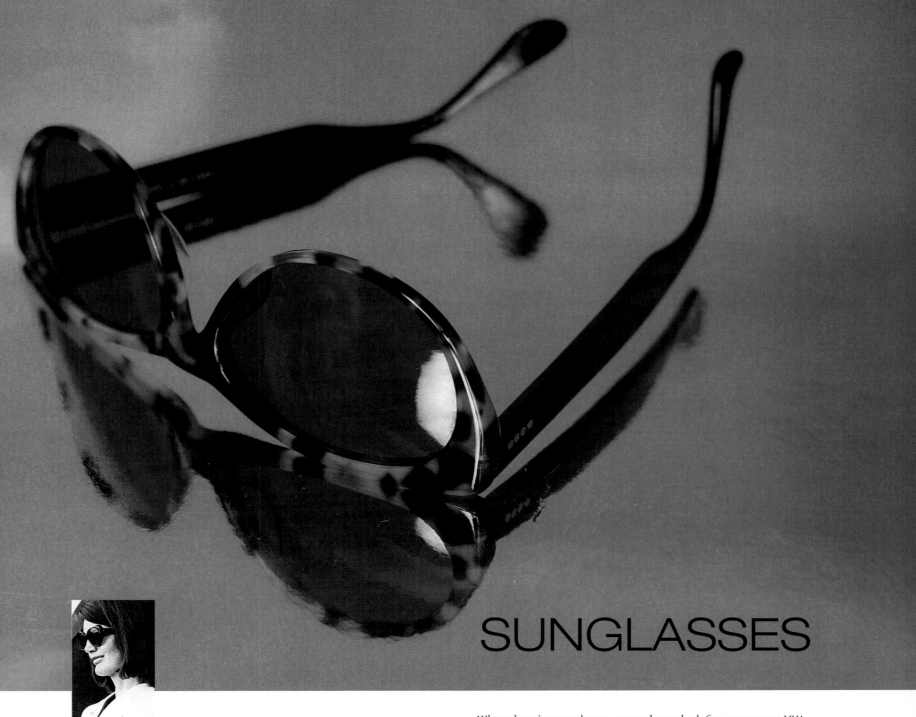

SUNGLASSES

Sunglasses won't just save you squinting – they should also protect your eyes from damage.

When choosing sunglasses, remember to look for 100 per cent UVA and UVB protection to prevent harmful radiation affecting the eye lens. Radiation can cause 'opacity', where vision becomes hazy and unclear. If you are going to be in a very hot climate, look for infra-red protection, too: it will help keep your eyes cool and comfortable. (See page 63 for guidelines on choosing flattering frame shapes.)

65

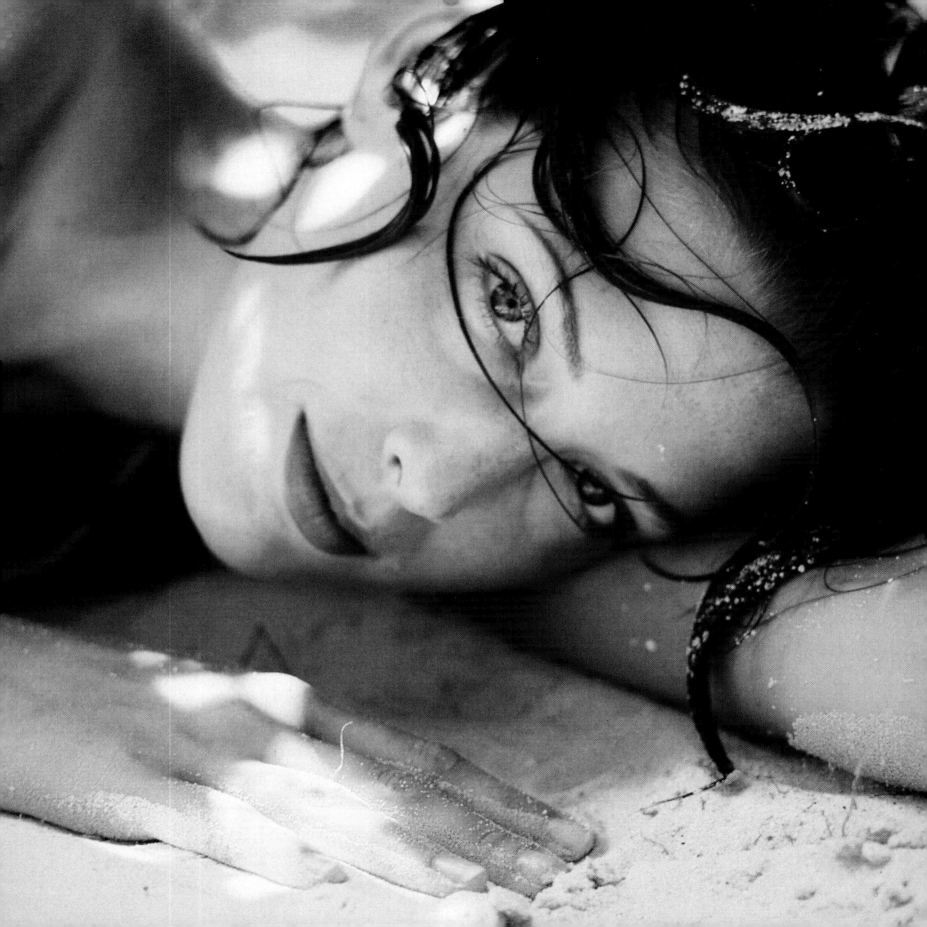

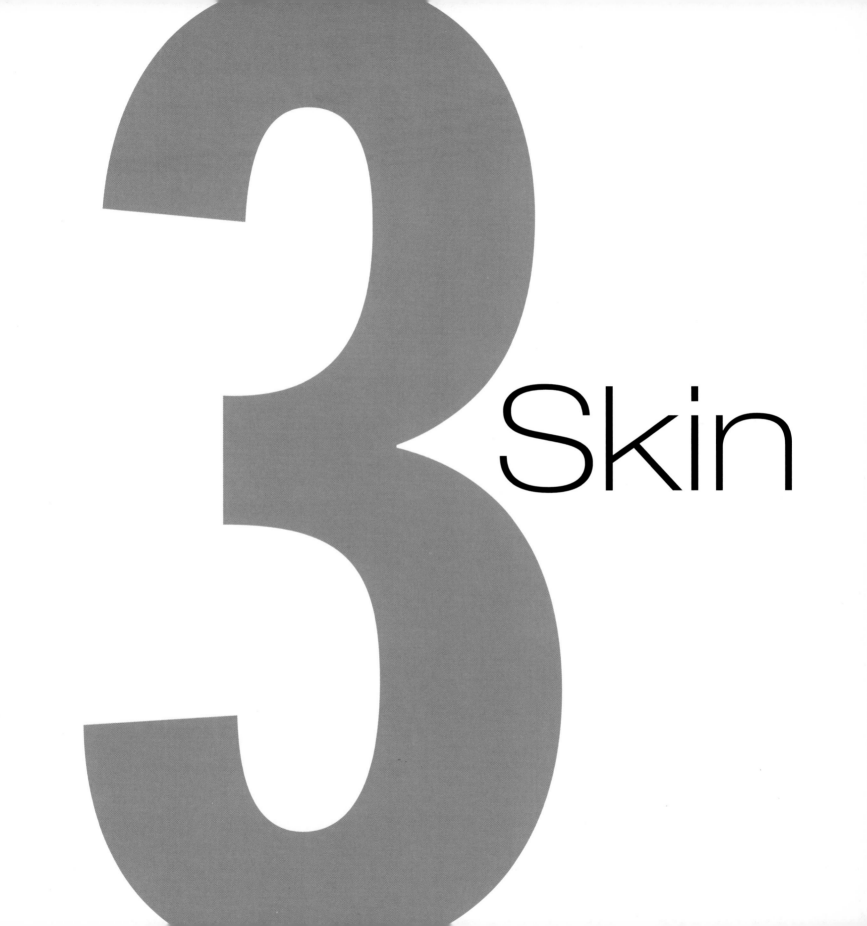

3 Skin

Beauty at any age isn't just about looking young: it's about wearing your age happily and healthily. If you don't work at beauty from the inside-out, even the most expensive skincare isn't going to make a difference. **Taking care to look after your skin is a mark of self-respect, not a sign of vanity**. Here's what you can do to ensure beautiful skin at any age. We tell you everything that's important: the no-cost beautifiers, lotions, potions, what works and what doesn't. Here are the right skincare – and lifestyle – choices to get you glowing.

FROM BABY TO BAG LADY

Virtually everyone, whatever their age, genes, environment or bank account, can have clearer, brighter, more healthy-looking skin. Here's how.

Spots, blackheads (comedones), whiteheads (milia) and skin bumps erupt; pores open; moles and freckles and blotches of all kinds gather; dark rings appear under puffy eyes. Then, from the age of about 25, it can seem like a downward descent into the sags, bags and wrinkles of middle age. Think of a baby's skin. After the odd bumps and blotches of birth have died down, it's picture-perfect – pink, translucently clear, even and smooth all over. Then something happens, particularly to the most visible part – our faces.

Composition of Skin

First, to make sense of it all and understand, for instance, why water is so vital, you need to know how your skin works. Your skin is a living, breathing organ. The billions of cells in your skin float in watery liquid which has the same amount of salt as seawater. Seventy per cent of your body is water and, of that, 35 per cent is found in your skin.

A cross section of skin looks a bit like a jam sandwich, with the upper layer, the epidermis, and the lower layer, the dermis, sandwiched around the thin basal layer. It sounds as simple as nursery tea, but in fact what's happening in your skin is a complex, never-ending saga of activity.

Skin renews itself every two to three weeks in young women (up to twice as long in older women), giving repeated opportunities for improvement. The visible outermost layer of skin, which protects the inner layers from the world, is made up of hardened rigid skin cells. As these die, they loosen and are shed, then instantly replaced by their fellows queueing up behind. Every day we shed about four per cent of our total number of skin cells; during our lives we lose about 13.6kg (30lb) of skin. (Dead skin cells, incidentally, are a huge component of household dust.)

The headquarters of skin renewal lies deep in the thick squidgy cushion of the dermis. Although we can't see what's going on, this governs the outer layers and thus the appearance of our skin. Here, beavering away, are the blood vessels, sweat glands and hair follicles, the connective tissue (containing the all-important collagen and elastin which keep our skin plump and youthful), as well as our sebaceous glands.

Sebaceous glands are one of the key factors controlling facial skin because they are targeted by androgens, the male hormones which women also have in lower levels; these trigger acne, whiteheads, blackheads, skin bumps and the waxy yellow lumps of seborrheic hyperplasia. (See *Problem Skins*, page 104.)

Ageing

Why does skin age? In a nutshell, it occurs as collagen and elastin, the two major components in the underlying support structure of the skin, degenerate. The major factors in this degeneration are ultra violet (UV) light from sun and sunbeds, and damage by nasty little single molecules called free radicals, which cause cellular havoc as they race round looking for a mate. (See *Cracking the Cosmetic Code*, page 80 for more details.) Both UV light and free radicals cause the collagen fibres, which should lie straight and orderly, to twist and mat so that the skin begins to line, sag and wrinkle. Sun exposure at least can be avoided where possible: since much of the harm is done before you are 18, start using a sun preparation early and make sure your children do too.

From the age of 50, the number of elastin fibres declines tremendously, accelerating the drooping, bagging and sagging. At the same time, the skin becomes drier because oil production diminishes, as does the skin's ability to hold water. As if that weren't enough, the rate of cell renewal also reduces.

So, as the years go by, skin becomes increasing fragile and vulnerable to the skin villains listed opposite. But not all damage done to your skin is irreversible – give it some extra tender loving care and your skin will respond quickly and positively.

Skin Facts

✳ The average adult has some 300 million skin cells, covering up to 2sq m (21sq ft) of skin, weighing 3.2kg (7lb).

✳ Facial skin is about 0.12mm (0.005in) thick; body skin about 0.6mm (0.02in); and the thickest areas on palms and soles about 1.2mm (0.05in) or more, up to 4.7mm (0.19in).

✳ The thinnest skin is on the lips and eyes.

✳ Each square half inch of skin contains, on average, at least ten hairs, 100 sweat glands, 1m (3.2ft) long of tiny blood vessels and 15 sebaceous glands.

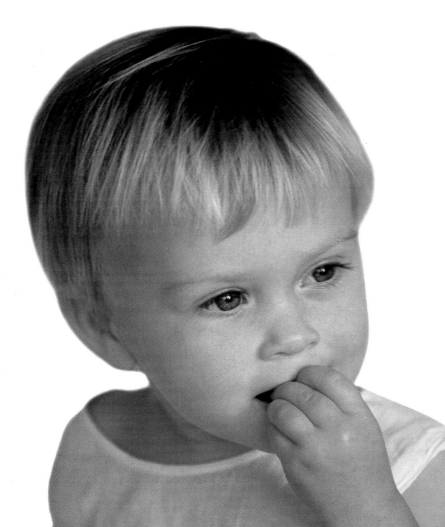

SKIN HEROES AND VILLAINS

HEROES	VILLAINS
Fresh air	Tobacco smoke (yours and others)
	Air conditioned offices and modern office technology, e.g. VDUs
	Air travel
Sun preparations	Ultra violet light (sun and sunbeds)
	Climate changes
Fresh food, particularly fruit and vegetables	Processed or refined foods, e.g. white sugar/flour
Water	Coffee, alcohol
Good digestion	Poor elimination (constipation, etc.)
Relaxation and sleep	Stress

Your skin's daily tasks include:

◆ Keeping your insides in!

◆ Repelling foreign invaders, e.g. chemical and bacterial agents

◆ Regulating body temperature

◆ Getting rid of waste matter through the pores

◆ Manufacturing essential vitamin D from sunlight

◆ Housing our senses of touch and pain

FOUNDATIONS OF GOOD SKIN

Family Matters

Dermatologists tend to joke that if you want great skin you should choose your parents carefully. Not a very helpful thing to say, but genes do play an important part in how your skin behaves and ages, so it is useful to look at your parents and forewarn yourself about any problems that may come your way. Although you can't change your parents, you can take steps which could significantly improve the outlook for your skin.

Family habits matter almost as much as genes. So when you're scanning your parents' faces, look at frown furrows, nose to mouth lines and tramlines around the mouth. It may well be that you have a tendency (which you can now try to avoid) to move your face in the same way. Facial exercises (see page 92) can help put this right. If you already have lines and furrows caused by bad face habits, see HELPING NATURE, page 141.

Let It Breathe

You need to breathe, and so does your skin. Seven per cent of the oxygen you take into your lungs is used directly by your skin. Breathing in supplies your cells with essential oxygen, breathing out removes carbon dioxide (which would poison cells if left long enough) and waste from your body. Babies and animals breathe perfectly: long, slow, deep breaths which oxygenate the whole body and take away all the nasties. As we get older, most of us breathe incorrectly, only taking air into the top of our chests and not expelling it fully. Failing to breathe properly makes us feel less than well and our skin and every part of our bodies ages more quickly.

Start with a simple breathing technique. Wherever you are, uncross arms and legs. Let your shoulders sag downwards. Now take a deep, slow breath in through your nose, right down into your stomach, to a count of four or more (N.B. don't let your shoulders rise to the heavens), hold it for one, and push it right out again to a count of four or more. Do this at least four times and see how much better you feel. Then practise this as often as you can during the day and in bed at night. It's a wonderful de-stresser too. (See *Instant Stressbusters*, page 185.) Consider also taking lessons in techniques such as yoga, autogenics, t'ai chi or qigong (see DIRECTORY for contacts), all of which focus on correct breathing.

Most of our oxygen intake comes through the bloodstream but the skin also absorbs a small amount directly through the pores. It's important, therefore, to let your skin breathe by spending a part of each day or night without anything on your skin – particularly on your face. Some women – even 50-somethings – are now discovering that they do not need to use a night cream regularly. Another option is to apply your night cream half an hour earlier than usual, allow it to sink in for 20 to 30 minutes, then blot off any excess with a tissue. It will have done its work and your skin is then left free to breathe. Incidentally, it's always a good idea to clean your face before exercising to stop sweat blocking pores.

Skincare companies such as Lancaster and Jil Sander are now making products which claim to transport oxygen directly to the skin. But nothing is as effective as a good brisk walk...

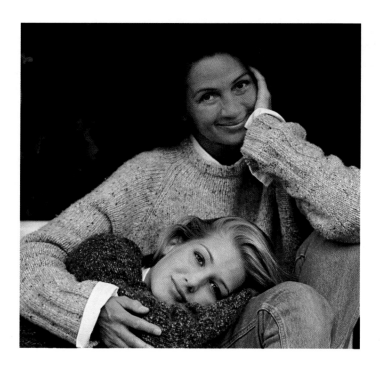

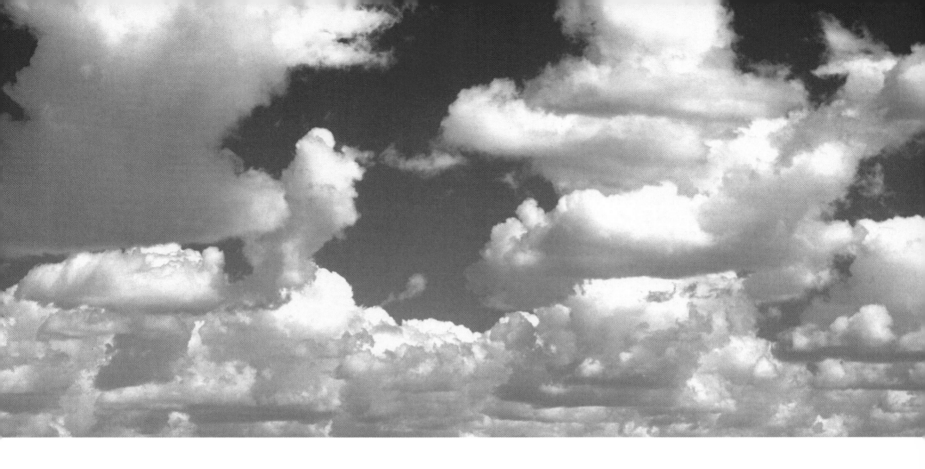

Fresh Air

No one doubts that fresh air keeps your skin looking blooming. There's fresh air and 'fresh' air though. The benefits of walking by the sea, in a park full of trees or in the mountains is strikingly different from a walk along a crowded city street. So aim to exercise in the least polluted place you can get to easily.

If you work in a hermetically-sealed office, particularly if it's filled with technology (VDUs, photocopiers, etc.), you might like to invest in a plug-in ioniser. The negative ions put out by these small gizmos are said to help counteract pollution, including cigarette smoke. You can certainly feel the difference when you are near one – and it's shocking how much dirt and dust they attract. Many users swear by them. Bowls of water can also make a very simple but potent difference if the air is dry.

Carry On Moving

Regular exercise is essential to the overall good health and functioning of our minds and bodies. When you exercise, oxygen surges to every cell in your body, allowing nutrients to be absorbed more efficiently and cells to grow faster. This means more collagen production, which leads to improved texture and moisture retention, and a thicker, more resilient dermis.

Researchers at the University of Wisconsin have discovered that the more oxygen you take in, the less likely you are to suffer free radical damage, which is linked to premature ageing. Aerobic exercise – brisk walking, jogging, running, bicycling, swimming or dancing – will stimulate the circulation, prompt a sluggish digestion to eliminate waste and toxins, and bring an instant glow to your skin.

In addition, says legendary beauty guru Lesley Kenton, exercise helps to stimulate sex and steroid hormones, and is one of the most effective ways of dispelling stress – one of the greatest skin villains.

Feed Your Skin

Some dermatologists dismiss the food you eat as if it couldn't possibly affect the general state of your skin, although few could deny the connection between specific foods and skin reactions, from rashes and itching to eczema. (Dr Jonathan Brostoff's *Food Allergies and Intolerance*, see BEAUTY BOOKSHELF, gives detailed information if you're interested in following this up.) Most would also have to agree that a diet rich in fresh foods – particularly fruit, vegetables and

73

grains – and low in processed and refined foods will benefit your whole system, skin included.

Clear, bright, healthy-looking skin is dependent on the efficient functioning of kidneys, intestines and liver. The liver not only manufactures the substances which help remove waste products from the body but also filters out any harmful chemicals from, say, non-organic food and drink, alcohol and tap water, prescription drugs, and the toxins produced in the body by bacteria and viruses. A sluggish system which allows all these toxins to create havoc in the body leads to pasty, blotchy, blemish-ridden skin.

If you have great genes and the beauty of your skin never wavers, you can probably afford to eat and drink what you like. If, however, heredity has been less gracious, listed below are suggested foods and supplements to benefit your skin. (See also *Problem Skins*, page 104.)

Eat Plenty Of...
Fresh fruit and vegetables, especially green and orange ones (including avocados and apples), also bananas, garlic, onions – with skin/peel where possible/palatable

Dried fruit

Cereals, pulses and grains

A few eggs weekly, if you like them

Oils, e.g. olive, sesame, walnut, hazelnut, safflower and sunflower (look for unrefined, cold-pressed oils – try health food shops – and store in a cool, dark place)

Dairy products

Wheatgerm and wholewheat bread

Brown rice, wholewheat or rice pasta

Soya

Nuts (store in a cool, dark place and grind in a coffee grinder)

If you aren't vegetarian:
Organic meat

Fish (oily, e.g. mackerel, salmon, sardines, tuna)

Seafood, i.e. shellfish

TIP Organic food is a great beauty – not to mention taste – investment. (See DIRECTORY for sources.)

More Could Be Better
Nutritionist Kathryn Marsden, author of *Superskin* (see BEAUTY BOOKSHELF), also suggests supplementing with:

vitamin B6	magnesium
vitamin C	essential fatty acids, e.g.
vitamin E	evening primrose oils
zinc	fish oils
silica	micro-algae
sulphur	lecithin
calcium	

(For preferred brands see below and *Can Supplements Help?*, page 165.)

Kathryn says: 'My absolutely top skin supplement is Co-enzyme Q10 (by Pharma Nord or BioCare). It's expensive but really worth it. Studies show that Q10, a powerful antioxidant and free radical scavenger, has a positive effect upon the ageing process. I take 30mg every day with my midday meal. Oil-based capsules are best; dry tablet forms, although cheaper, don't seem to reach the bloodstream. I certainly found that powdered Q10 didn't work.

'I'm also a great believer in an occasional course of probiotics (acidophilus or bifidus, by either Blackmore's or BioCare). Probiotics are the "good bugs", or bacteria, also found in some kinds of yoghurt. I use a 90-day course every 12 months and recommend it to anyone with eczema, psoriasis, herpes, acne and always following a course of antibiotics (which wipe out all bugs, good and bad). For eczema sufferers, probiotics work especially well when combined with Evening Primrose Oil (3g daily) or a similar oil (e.g. borage or starflower) containing gammalinolenic acid.

'I also take Femforte, a general multivitamin/mineral by BioCare, designed for women and containing all the other skin vitamins including vitamins A, C, E, all the B group and essential minerals.'

Sleep
Scientists now believe that skin cells regenerate as we sleep, and it's undoubtedly one of the greatest free beautifiers. We also have a theory that a sound sleep relaxes your facial skin, so that lines and furrows are softened by the morning. (See *Beauty Sleep*, page 88.)

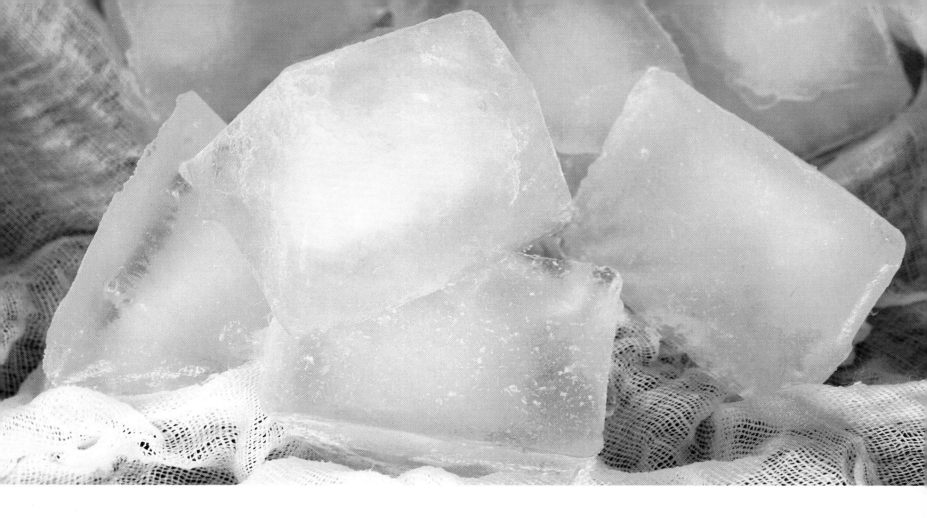

Water, Water Everywhere

Dermatologists are usually sceptical about what they regard as extravagant claims for the beautifying powers of water, but every woman with stunning skin that we know puts it down to drinking at least 1.5 litres of water daily. Filtered or bottled is best, we think (unless you live in an area of outstanding natural water), but tap is definitely better than nothing. Experts advise that still, room-temperature water is most compatible with your body.

Spraying your face with spring water (Evian is the best known) can make it dewy fresh on a hot day. Also try spraying after cleansing but before moisturising; the creams then seem to lock in the moisture.

Ice cubes wrapped in cling-film, a cotton hanky or a napkin make a wonderful de-bagger for puffy eyes: just smooth them over the offending area and watch the bags shrink. Ice-cold water splashed on your face (or, if you're the Spartan type, a cold shower) can also get the circulation zinging round on a bad morning. (N.B. Don't try these if you have broken veins on your cheeks.)

Hormones

Oestrogen is an important skin regulator. The ups and downs of your skin may simply be due to waxing and waning hormone levels, as with the onset of acne at puberty. A good supply of oestrogen means that skin tends to be supple, soft, healthy and resilient. Any major changes in hormone levels can create havoc to the beauty and health of women's skin.

Hormone levels (both oestrogen and progesterone) rise and fall throughout the menstrual cycle, peaking during the last ten days, the usual time for flare-ups. When women first go on the Pill, it can suddenly lead to spots and even stretch marks, which are in fact hormone, not weight related. Conversely, as oestrogen levels decline drastically at menopause, HRT (Hormone Replacement Therapy) is noted for putting the glow back.

Since hormone function is also dependent on nutrition, Kathryn Marsden emphasises the importance of eating the healthiest diet possible.

SKINCARE

In addition to working on beauty from the inside-out, good skincare and sun screening are vital.

THE DIRT ON CLEANSING

How to Pick the Perfect Cleanser

Cleaning your skin properly is the single most important favour you can do for your complexion. Everything your mother ever told you about not falling into bed with your make-up on is true. Legendary London skincare professional Eve Lom actually believes that so long as you cleanse skin properly, you can use any old moisturiser. 'Poor cleansing,' she explains, 'allows bacteria to grow, and sebum – the skin's natural oils – to accumulate, leading to blackheads, whiteheads and even the dreaded zit.'

The cleansing cosmetic you use should be more than what takes your fancy: you should first determine your skin type, then decide on your cleanser accordingly. Most women assume that if their skin feels taut, it's an indication of dry skin. Not necessarily. In fact, pore size is a more reliable indicator of your skin category. Look in a magnifying mirror: if your pores are open (i.e. look like miniature craters), then you probably have oily skin. Small, almost invisible pores usually signify skin that's on the dry side. If you have combination skin – usually with an oily, large-pored T-shaped panel across forehead, nose and chin, with normal or dry skin everywhere else on your face – you should ideally use two appropriate cleansers. (This might sound expensive but they will last twice as long!)

GOOD FOR DRY/DELICATE/MATURE SKINS: cream cleansers have a rich consistency and leave a light, moisturising film. Susan Ciminelli, whose Manhattan Day Spa is a Mecca for frazzled models such as Christy Turlington, stresses that any surplus should be removed gently with water and a warm, wet, clean washcloth.

GOOD FOR NORMAL AND NORMAL-TO-DRY SKINS: lotions consist of a combination of mild detergents (a.k.a. surfactants) and moisturisers, so they won't strip skin of its natural oils. The drier your skin is, the thicker the cleanser you will need. If your skin is normal, you may want to try a gel cleanser, instead. Gels are particularly popular with skincare specialists because they rinse off easily and leave practically no residue.

GOOD FOR NORMAL-TO-OILY/OILY SKINS: foaming cleansers help dissolve any oil-based material on the skin. Gels are another good bet for oilier skins, and an excellent alternative to soap or soap-style bars.

GOOD FOR ACNE-PRONE SKINS: use a gentle cleanser – a gel or foaming version – and go easy on the scrubbing, however satisfying it feels; abrasive exfoliators can irritate lesions.

How often should you cleanse? Look before you lather: the morning wash should be dictated by the amount of sebum that's built up on your face overnight. If there's no shininess and your face feels dry, simply swipe your face gently with a warm, wet washcloth and then moisturise. But if your face is shiny, use a cleansing product to remove the dirt and dust which adhere to surface oils and can get trapped under make-up.

You still love soap?

If you can't wean yourself off that lathery texture, do at least switch to a special soap-free cleansing bar (otherwise called 'beauty bar'/'facial bar'). Dr Daniel Maes, PhD, Vice-President of Research and Development at Estée Lauder Worldwide, maintains that the alkaline residue left by many soaps is hard to rinse off, which can interfere with the efficiency of your moisturiser. And beware of any cleanser that leaves your skin feeling tight; that's not cleanliness, that's dryness.

Remember: at 25, oil production starts to slow. In pregnant or menopausal women, hormonal shifts can make a difference. So be alert to changes, ready to make a clean sweep of your beauty regime as soon as they occur...

The Secret of Coming (Perfectly) Clean

❧ Wash your hands first, so that you aren't transferring bacteria to your face.

❧ Start with your hairline (hairstyling products attract dirt), then sweep cleanser over face and lips and down the neck to beyond where you apply foundation.

❧ After you've applied your cleanser, gently massage it in with the balls of your fingers and leave it on for a minute or so to allow make-up to melt away. This will sweep away dirt, pollution and cosmetic build-up without tugging at the skin.

❧ The same cleanser may not be right for you year-round; harsh weather and cold temperatures can zap the body's moisture level, so each skin type needs a corresponding shift to the milder side (women with oily skins may want to switch to a cleanser for normal skin, and so on). (See *Weather-Beating Beauty*, page 98.)

Exfoliation: Here's the Scrub

Exfoliation with a facial scrub is claimed to perk up the complexion by sloughing off dull surface cells and revealing shiny pink ones underneath. (This is how AHA creams work, too, see page 85.) But do you really need to exfoliate? Internationally-renowned facialists like Eve Lom and Jo Malone say not. And Eve Lom even argues that exfoliants can do more harm than good: 'If used wrongly, scrubs can abrade the living layer of skin. Most people scrub too vigorously, especially around the cheeks, so they remove more skin there than around areas that are more difficult to access – like the folds around the nose – where cell build-up can be worse.'

If you still like to use a scrub, look for those with granules that dissolve in water as these cause the least amount of irritation, and do not exfoliate more frequently than once a week. Some dermatologists advise that grainy scrubs – made from crushed fruit kernels, for instance – may be too harsh; rough face puffs likewise. California skincare salon owner Sylvie Archenault declares: 'If you look at your skin under a microscope after you use these types of exfoliants, you'll see the skin has the texture of a cat scratch right before it bleeds.'

TIPS FROM THE TOP

Eve Lom recommends cleansing with wet muslin washcloths (she suggests a baby's Harrington nappy cut into squares), which can be washed with your laundry every couple of days. 'Use one for removing cleanser, one for eye make-up remover,' she advises. 'You need never buy cotton wool again. What's more, it's all the exfoliation your skin needs, without ever scratching.' (See *Here's the Scrub*, right.)

We all know what **Marilyn Monroe** wore to bed – just a veil of Chanel No. 5. But to remove every last trace of greasepaint beforehand, she loved ShuUemura's Utowa Cleansing Oil (see Directory).

Martina Navratilova and **Brooke Shields** are both reputedly fans of Neutrogena's no-nonsense, no-alkali transparent Facial Cleansing Bar, which is widely available.

SKIN TONERS – THE MYTHS AND THE FACTS

Your first astringent is like a rite of passage. It feels so incredibly satisfying to wipe that cotton wool ball over your face and see it come away grimy. But as skins mature, should women still reach for toners as the final stage of their clean-up regime?

The biggest reason for their popularity is the sensation of freshness which toners give. 'Toner' and 'astringent' are often taken to mean the same thing, but do make sure you're using the type that's right for your skin.

Toners traditionally contain little or no alcohol and, these days, are sophisticated products formulated to do everything from soothing irritated skin to exfoliation. Exfoliating lotions, often called clarifying lotions, are designed to make your face look fresher by dissolving dry, dead skin cells.

Astringents are usually alcohol-based and should really only be used by women with truly oily skin – and, even then, some women may only need to use them premenstrually, when skin tends to get greasier. If you have dry, sensitive, mature – or that rare commodity, normal – skin, then look for an alcohol-free toner; alcohol is much too drying and makes your skin more prone to irritation.

> How can you tell if a toner is alcohol-free? Ingredients are not always listed, so quiz the consultant if you're at a beauty counter. Many labels will specify 'alcohol-free' or 'gentle', or that they are targeted specifically at dry or sensitive skin, in which case they're almost certainly alcohol-free. And if your skin's really sensitive, remember that good old rosewater – or orange flower water – will give you that 'clean sweep' sensation (inexpensively) without stripping any of your skin's precious oils.

Don't believe any of that baloney about pores opening and closing. Pores are the openings for sebaceous (oil) glands, not lift doors which can be closed from the outside, and any beautician who says she's about to use something on your face 'to close the pores' isn't worth the paper her diploma is printed on. Toners can only ever make the pores look smaller *temporarily* by causing the capillaries (tiny

blood vessels) to dilate, and the tiny erectile muscles of the pores in your skin to tighten.

Eve Lom is convinced that nobody needs a toner or astringent if they've cleansed properly, especially if they have open pores as it will ultimately make the pores more noticeable. 'Just avoid putting moisturiser on that area and the pores will start to appear less obvious. They do get better with patience and care.'

THE MOISTURISER MAZE

Buying a moisturiser used to be easy. But now that more research money goes into developing moisturisers than almost any other skincare product, deciding which of the avalanche of possibles is right for you can be a baffling, time-consuming and expensive business. So here's how to find your perfect match.

The natural oils in skin stop dehydration but, if there is too little oil, the skin becomes dry and flaky. Moisturisers are designed to correct this imbalance and also to act as a barrier against outside elements. Your first step is simple: choose a moisturiser specifically targeted at your skin type.

DRY SKIN calls for a fairly rich moisturiser with a high oil and/or fat content, which should be used at least once a day on the cheeks and forehead. Use a special eye cream on the eye zone to prevent irritation.

OILY SKIN also benefits from a moisturiser lightly applied around the eyes, the edges but not the apples of the cheeks, and the neck. Daily moisturising enhances the barrier function of the skin and makes it easier to apply make-up. Look for products labelled 'oil-free' and/or 'non-comedogenic', which means they won't block the skin's pores and cause blackheads.

If you have COMBINATION SKIN, you will need a moisturiser for the dry bits.

According to Eve Lom, 'Nobody needs a moisturiser around their nose, or their chin.' In those areas, she explains, even parched skins produce enough lubricating moisture and adding any more will, in time, lead to larger-looking pores.

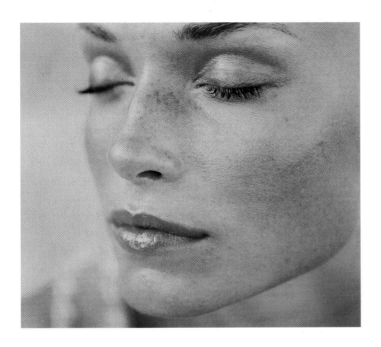

Dermatologists believe that we should all be wearing a daily dose of sun protection on our faces. Increasingly, skincare companies are responding by adding sunscreens to their daytime moisturisers. Look for SPF15, the recommended protection level even for city-living in mid-winter in temperate climates. Some moisturisers now contain anti-oxidants for protection not only against sun damage but also against pollution. Dermatologists at Estée Lauder are among those who are now convinced that pollution and smoke cause just as much premature ageing as the sun. So consider switching to one of these 'new generation' ultra-protective moisturisers. That way you won't have to double up by wearing moisturiser, then sunscreen on top.

TRIED & TESTED

NECK CREAMS

As the neck has only a small number of fat cells and meagre supplies of sebum, it is the area most prone to dryness and crêpiness. There is a case for using a specially enriched neck cream.

Top Treat

Clarins Firming Neck Cream
Another area where Clarins emerged ahead of the pack for a skin-softening, anti-ageing product.
COMMENTS: 'the lines looked less visible and my neck felt firmer', 'it seemed to take the tension out of my neck', 'general softening and less crêpiness – I love the smell and am hooked for life'.

Gatineau Throat Gel
This was considered by some of our testers to have an especially firming and softening action.

COMMENTS: 'refined my skin's texture', 'felt like a tonic to the skin', 'slight decrease in fine lines and definitely less dry'.

Estée Lauder Re-Nutriv Firming Throat Cream
This comes from Estée Lauder's luxurious anti-ageing range and moisturised even very dry, older skins.
COMMENTS: 'my neck was very much softer, with fewer fine lines', 'certainly smoother and softer', 'I will use this religiously because at my age (76) my neck really needs it'.

Mary Cohr Neck Firming Cream
From a top French name in salon care that is becoming more widely known.
COMMENTS: 'neck certainly felt smoother and less dry', 'I noticed a huge improvement and less crêpiness', 'whole area felt smoother, softer and looked younger'.

Best Budget Buy

The Body Shop Neck Gel
A fraction of the price of the upmarket ranges, this product was considered to perform well in its price bracket.
COMMENTS: 'my skin was smoother, slightly tighter and softer', 'I liked the texture, packaging and the smell'.

Natural Choice

Elemis Tissue Toning Neck Cream
This mid-price, pump-action product, based on plants, scored well for softness and smoothness.
COMMENTS: 'less crêpiness', 'smells great', 'the place I noticed a definite reduction in crêpiness was on my chest area, which the instructions suggested I include'.

Italian supermodel **Carla Bruni** believes: 'Prevention is the only thing you can do to help skin. I wear sunscreen every day, even in the city, even in the spring, even on cloudy days; I use Clinique City Block as a make-up base. It's more like an "environment cream", good not only for sun protection but to keep dust and pollution away from the skin.'

Make-up maestro Kevyn Aucoin has developed his own technique of applying moisturiser (he loves Kiehl's Imperiale Reparateur Moisturising Masque, or Chanel's Hydra-Système) to maximise its efficiency and to plump up the areas where the skin is dry: he applies a thick coat to the face while it's still damp, lets it sit for 10–15 minutes, blots it off with a tissue, and then applies an oil-free foundation on top.

DO YOU REALLY NEED A NIGHT CREAM?

Daytime skincare is all about protection – against dehydration and pollution – but at night, skin needs to regenerate and rest. Sleep does more for your skin than any cream can ever do. Some experts such as Eva Fraser (see her *Instant Face Saver Tips*, page 92) maintain that you shouldn't put anything at all on your skin at night, in order to let your skin breathe. But many women would feel their skin is then uncomfortably dry. Whether you apply a special night cream (usually thicker and richer than daytime creams) or simply use the same moisturiser as you do for the day is really a matter of personal preference. And remember, it really doesn't matter if your p.m. cream doesn't match your a.m. cream in terms of manufacturer (although skincare sales people would hate to admit it).

CRACKING THE COSMETIC CODE

What's in skincare – and what do the ingredients do? For all those of us without a degree in rocket science, these are the most common (and often most confusing) beauty terms and ingredients:

ALPHA-HYDROXY ACIDS, often called fruit acids. AHAs are now appearing in an ever wider range of products, and are derived from natural ingredients, including grapes, apples, olives and milk. They act to speed up exfoliation by dissolving the 'intercellular glue' (which bonds dead, flaking cells to the skin's surface), uncovering the smooth skin beneath. When first launched they were touted as the wonder anti-ageing ingredient for the nineties. But it has since emerged that they should be treated with caution as they can prove too harsh for fragile, sensitive and delicate skins; at any sign of irritation or lingering redness, discontinue use.

ANTIOXIDANTS, found mostly in moisturisers, make-up and sun preparations. These are vitamins – betacarotene (the precursor of vitamin A), C and E – that help combat damage from free radical attack, which is triggered by exposure to sun, pollution and cigarette smoke. (According to research from Estée Lauder's laboratories, smoking is at least as damaging to skin as the sun.) Free radicals act like 'cellular terrorists', attacking collagen, cell membranes and the skin's lipid layer, while antioxidants 'mop up' free radicals in the skin. Experts are still divided over the effectiveness of antioxidants when mixed into moisturisers, although beauties have long sworn by the benefits of breaking open a vitamin E capsule and smearing it on the skin. But for anyone who's exposed to sun/smoke/pollution (and that means all of us), they would seem to be worthwhile insurance.

BETA-HYDROXY ACIDS: These natural acids are close relations to AHAs and work in much the same way, speeding up cell turnover. The best known is salicylic acid (from willow bark). The same cautions apply: BHAs are acknowledged irritants, and anyone who experiences irritation should stop using them straight away.

CERAMIDES, mostly used in skin creams. These lipids, found in the skin's intercellular cement, help stabilise skin structure by retaining moisture. They are therefore primarily of benefit to older, dry or damaged skins and are not necessary for healthy, young skins.

COLLAGEN/ELASTIN are vital elements in the skin's supporting structure, required for skin elasticity and smoothness; over time, production slows, leading to sags and bags. Collagen-containing creams and masks may be useful as surface moisturisers.

ENZYMES, mostly found in moisturisers and masks. Enzyme exfoliants are a relatively new type of naturally derived 'anti-ageing' ingredient (often from papaya); they gently and thoroughly rid the surface layer of dead cells without harming living cells or irritating the skin.

HUMECTANTS are ingredients which attract moisture from the air to the surface of the skin, and are valuable ingredients in moisturisers or facial sprays for dry skins. Humectants include glycerine, sorbitol, squalene and urea.

LIPOSOMES are high-tech skincare 'rockets' which can be launched into the epidermis and deliver their moisturising cargo deeper than would otherwise be possible, so helping to fill in the gaps between the intercellular cement. Afterwards the skin should feel – and look – intensively moisturised.

NANOSPHERES, a fancy term for small, rounded particles, which are 'second generation' liposomes.

NATURAL MOISTURISING FACTORS: Hyaluronic acid, sodium PCA and linolenic acid are all naturally present in the skin and come under the umbrella of NMFs. When applied in a cosmetic cream, they act as a natural, light moisturiser.

OXYGEN is now in some skincare formulations. Oxygen delivered to the skin's surface is supposed to improve cellular activity and turnover. But the best way to provide your skin with oxygen remains a brisk walk, or other physical activity (including sex).

PANTHENOL/PRO-VITAMIN B5 is derived from vitamin B. Gentle and non-irritating, it can have a cosmetic and temporary 'skin-plumping' effect, is highly conditioning and is also an ingredient in hair products.

pH is a term often seen on packaging denoting acid balance. Your skin is naturally slightly acid, with a pH between 4.5 and 5.5. The correct balance can be disturbed by the use of soaps (most of which are strongly alkaline) and some cosmetics which are not acid-balanced. This is particularly the case if your skin is sensitive, excessively dry or oily, or is prone to acne.

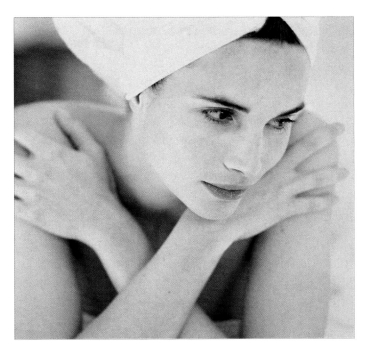

HOW QUICKLY SHOULD YOU SEE RESULTS?

We buy beauty products hoping for instant results. Some do deliver in a flash, but other treats take longer because their effects are cumulative.

According to Gary Grove, a Philadelphia-based skin physiologist, 'So many manufacturers shoot themselves in the foot because they say something will work instantly and it doesn't. Consumers who stick with the products a little longer have a better chance of getting the results they're expecting.' But – while you're twiddling your thumbs – here's how long you may have to wait before different products start to make a difference.

FACIAL MASKS: deep cleansing masks should give brighter skin after just one treatment, and moisturising masks should show (temporary) improvements immediately.

AHA CREAMS: softness, texture and brightness should improve within a few days – or even as quickly as 24 hours; any smoothing of fine lines may take up to a month.

HAND CREAMS: temporary softening should be immediate, with optimum benefits after about two weeks of regular use.

IS THERE SUCH A THING AS A MIRACLE CREAM?

The traditional line on such creams from sceptical dermatologists has been that nothing you apply to the skin can get past the *stratum corneum* (underlying the epidermis). As research delves deeper, this attitude may change – particularly now that skin permeability is being exploited by drug companies and manufacturers of skin patches which deliver, for instance, HRT or nicotine into the bloodstream.

Medical experts tend to be unimpressed by the claims of cosmetics companies, principally because their findings are rarely published in scientific journals. The cosmetics companies counter that they are reluctant to give away secrets to their rivals. But they may also fear that if their more extravagant claims *were* substantiated by the medical establishment, their products might have to be licensed as pharmaceutical drugs, not cosmetics – which would be much more expensive and time-consuming. (It takes about ten years and well over US$15 million to research and develop a drug.) Some prefer instead to understate what their products achieve. So, there could well be creams out there that deliver more than the hype promises.

Things are scheduled to change in Europe, however. European Community law is due to make it mandatory for companies not only to list ingredients fully, but to back up any claims with hard data. So if your moisturiser says it 'removes wrinkles and fine lines', that will have to be proven, as already happens in America.

Alongside a good diet, exercise, stress reduction, sleep and a good cleansing routine, however, creams can play a valuable part. Cosmeto-dermatologist Dr Andrew Markey suggests that the only way to find *your* miracle cream is to try out a number of creams and not be afraid of switching. And bear in mind that there will probably always be a gulf between marketing hype and the reality.

An expensive price tag certainly doesn't guarantee wonders, and sometimes women find bargains are still best. Fashion designer **Ronit Zilkha**, who confesses to buying every skincare product that comes on the market, says the most effective skin cream she has ever used is Nivea. TV presenter **Liz Earle** swears that piercing a capsule of natural vitamin E and anointing her skin is her favourite face treatment. Other products we have heard impressive reports of include a serum called Cellex-C which contains five per cent vitamin C with tyrosine and did make a noticeable difference to the skin over a six-week test period, Guerlain's Issima Super Aquaserum and OxyPeel's Revital Cream Special. But again, what seems miraculous to one woman may leave even her best friend less than impressed...

TRIED & TESTED

'MIRACLE' CREAMS

These products are designed to reverse skin-ageing. Ambitious, maybe, but many testers were impressed. We have not included a Best Budget Buy because none of the inexpensive products made the grade with our panel.

Top Treats

Revlon Eterna 27+ Instant Wonder Cream
This re-worked old favourite scored the highest of all. All our testers said they'd buy it.
COMMENTS: 'the improvement is amazing', 'my skin feels velvety and the lines are nowhere near so apparent', 'after two weeks my face felt softer and a dry spot had definitely improved'.

Chanel Serum Extrème Anti-Rides Raffermissant
This is a pump-action serum formulation, to be used with a moisturiser on top.
COMMENTS: 'the texture was just right', 'pump action made it very easy to apply', 'smoother, firmer skin apparent after just one application'.

Decleor Timecare Cream
This fast-growing French skincare company had particularly good reports from women with sensitive and problem skins. This is Decleor's star anti-ageing product.
COMMENTS: 'fine lines miraculously vanished', 'I felt my skin looked slightly more youthful and softer', 'made my skin appear less dingy'.

Natural Option

Jurlique Herbal Extract Recovery Gel
This light, gel-textured product – from one of the purest skincare companies in the world – scored the highest marks of any product tried.
COMMENTS: 'this has to be one of the nicest products I've ever used', 'skin seemed firmer, plumper and even rosier', 'definitely something I'll always have in my beauty regime'.

Neal's Yard Frankincense Nourishing Cream
This all-natural product earned especially good reviews for its scent.
COMMENTS: 'I like the jar, texture and smell very much', 'my skin looked smoother, felt softer'.

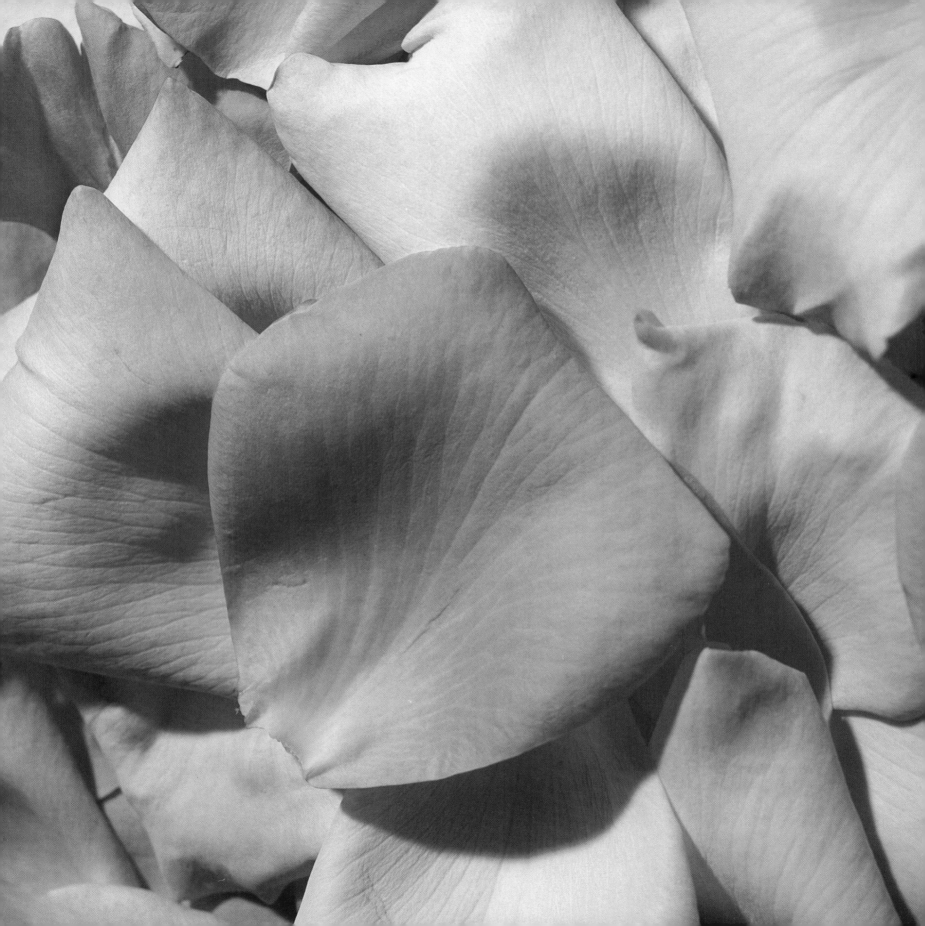

IS YOUR SKIN HAVING A NERVOUS BREAKDOWN?

Do certain products ever sting, burn or bring you out in a rash? Welcome to the club. Skin sensitivity has become a beauty buzzword and cosmetic companies are now racing each other to launch products that soothe skin.

Although some 60–70 per cent of women believe their skin is sensitive, skin sensitivity remains stubbornly hard to pin down, and even experts have trouble agreeing on a precise definition. You might find, for instance, that you react to products most women have no problems with. Or your system may be allergic to an ingredient in a skincare product, and irritation is the sign that your body is fighting back. Many of us also suffer temporary bouts of sensitivity, set off by anything from pollution to mental stress.

Skin pros are agreed that the best way to handle sensitive skin is by acting as if it's very dry skin. So don't scrub or exfoliate, go for facials or use masks unless you are certain the products suit you, and steer clear of aggressive treatment products, especially anything containing AHAs, see page 80 and opposite.

Although sensitive skin undoubtedly needs protection from UV rays, certain types of sunscreen are common rash-catalysts because of the interaction between chemicals and the sun's rays. Suncare ingredients to be avoided are PABA, benzophenone and methoxycinnamate; instead, look for sunscreens containing titanium dioxide, which create a physical barrier to keep the sun's rays out. These used to be like slathering yourself in white gunk, but the new generation of titanium dioxide products are virtually invisible.

Sensitive skin can have a thousand causes. The more likely culprits in cosmetics are alcohol (used in toners and astringents), surfactants (detergents used in soaps and cleansers), and high levels of propylene glycol; if your skincare carries full ingredient listing, look out for these. Perfumes and preservatives can also set off reactions – but be wary of anything labelled 'unscented' or 'fragrance-free'. That really means that more chemicals have been used to mask the scent. Any kind of stress is likely to exacerbate reactions. 'Whatever your tendency is – oiliness, dryness, hives,' explains Diana Bihova, M.D., Clinical Instructor of Dermatology at New York University's School of Medicine, 'stress unmasks and exacerbates it.'

Action Plan For Sensitive Skin

■ Look for hypoallergenic and allergy-tested products – although they are no absolute guarantee against problems...

■ Avoid the sun or protect your face from it with a physical sunblock containing titanium dioxide, rather than chemical sunscreens, which can prompt photosensitive reactions.

■ Don't use soap, which can alter the skin's natural pH balance, so leaving it vulnerable to irritation.

■ Steer clear of exfoliants and high-concentration AHA creams (ideally, avoid AHAs altogether).

■ Always do a 'patch test' first, before using new products. Apply some to your inner elbow and repeat for several days. If there's no problem, try it out on a corner of your face – say, near the ear, which you can cover with your hair if it reacts.

■ Consider investing in a humidifier. Parched skin is more prone to sensitivity.

■ Always, always stop using any product at once if it creates an irritation – regardless of how much you want it to work...

■ If your skin reacts, try some simple first aid: rinse the area with cold water for about 30 seconds, then apply aloe vera gel (available from health food stores).

■ An extra caution: if your skin is inflamed enough to prompt a visit to your doctor, our experience is that while the hydrocortisone creams often prescribed can help temporarily, but with long-term use skin may flare up ever more frequently – as if it almost gets 'addicted', and forgets how to heal itself.

If your skin is behaving badly, look on it as a warning signal that your whole body and mind may be on overload. As life becomes more complicated, so does the interaction between what we put into and onto our bodies and what happens as a result. During a typical day, we ingest hundreds of chemicals (preservatives, additives, pesticides) which our systems haven't learnt to cope with properly. According to L'Oréal, contributing factors can be internal (food, alcohol, spices or

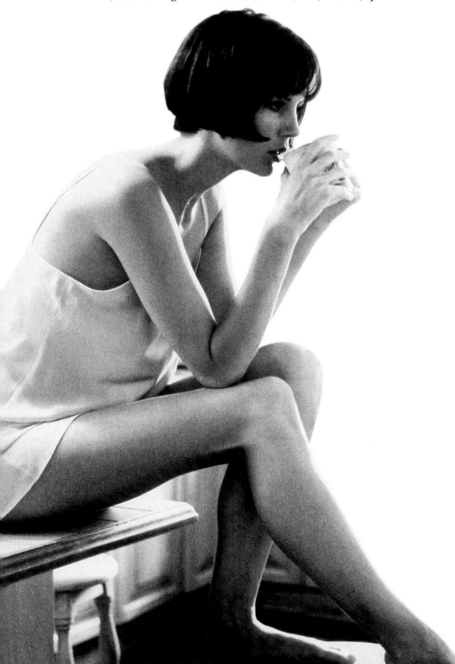

hormone levels), as well as external (wind, sun, pollution, dust, air conditioning or detergents). And then, of course, there's stress itself. 'In times of stress, skin gets the short end of the stick,' observes Dr Peter Pugliese, a skin physiologist from Bernville, Pennsylvania. Blood is directed to the major organs, so the result is a pale, ashen look that emphasises under-eye circles. Chronic strain slows skin cell turnover, encouraging a build-up of metabolic by-products (toxins) which make skin look sallow. Meanwhile, the proliferation of adrenal 'stress' hormones can cause pimples. 'High-level stress is enough to bring on blemishes in an adult, even if she never had acne as a teen,' warns Dr Bernard A. Kirshbaum, Clinical Professor of Medicine in the department of dermatology at the Medical College of Pennsylvania in Philadelphia.

The sensible answer: reduce your emotional stress, get more sleep and eat well, focusing especially on fresh fruit and vegetables. Your skin is less likely to suffer a nervous breakdown. And so is the rest of you...

AHA CREAMS

Alpha-hydoxy acids (AHAs or fruit acids) have been heralded as the latest 'wonder ingredient' in anti-ageing creams. They are a group of natural chemicals – found in fruits, wine, sour milk and sugar cane – which exfoliate the skin's top layer, accelerating the production of new cells and leaving the complexion noticeably smoother, cleaner and brighter. On Asian and black skins, they also reduce ashiness. But many of the creams which incorporate AHAs treat the skin without adding moisture, so you may need to apply a moisturiser on top.

It has been suggested that there may be a link between some AHA products and skin sensitivity. When we've tried AHA creams on our sensitive skin (and 60–70 per cent of women say they have sensitive skin), we have experienced short-term improvements – a definite brightening of the skin – but soon noticed some irritation and redness. From the experience of other women we know, this is not uncommon (see *Cracking the Cosmetic Code*, page 80).

Basically, as with any so-called 'miracle cream', apply common sense when using AHA creams. If your skin is unhappy, and it tells you so with a rash or irritation, ditch the cream. End of story. Even if it cost you a small fortune.

MASKMANSHIP

These facials-in-a-flash can act like first aid for faces – if you choose carefully and don't use them too often. (Once a week is maximum – and only if you feel your skin needs it.)

Always apply facial masks to cleansed skin, and only leave on for as long as the instructions recommend. 'Mask ingredients are more concentrated than those in lotions or cleansers, so they produce more noticeable benefits,' observes Aida Thibiant, whose European Day Spa in Beverly Hills attracts famous faces like Rachel Hunter and Bette Midler.

THE PERFECT FAST FIX FOR:

Oily skin, or skin that's broken out
KEY WORDS IN THE NAME: *Deep Cleansing, Clarifying, Mud, Clay.*
INGREDIENTS TO LOOK FOR: kaolin (oil-absorbing clay), aluminium magnesium silicate (talc), bentonite (white clay), witch hazel or zinc oxide (antiseptics), eucalyptus (draws out impurities).
HOW TO USE THEM: most oily skin masks start off as a thick paste and then dry on the skin to a hard crust. Apply, avoiding eye area. A clean, hot washcloth is best for removing all traces – the skin feels temporarily tightened.
HOW THEY WORK: these clean the skin and absorb excess oil, so cutting down shine. Antiseptic ingredients inhibit the growth of bacteria, while clays cause the skin to perspire, bringing out impurities with the sweat.

Dry skin that's rough, flaky and feels tight
KEY WORDS IN THE NAME: *Moisturising, Hydrating.*
INGREDIENTS TO LOOK FOR: buttermilk, milk protein, vegetable proteins, collagen, vitamin B Panthenol, amino acids, water, oil, lanolin, hyaluronic acid, urea, algae.
HOW TO USE THEM: apply, and tissue off after the recommended time. Masks for dry skin shouldn't set hard.
HOW THEY WORK: by delivering a concentrated mix of moisturising ingredients to parched surface cells, the mask temporarily reduces the appearance of fine, dry lines.

Dull skin that looks tired, greyish, lacks translucency
KEY WORDS IN THE NAME: *Perfecting, Botanical, Replenishing.*
INGREDIENTS TO LOOK FOR: menthol, peppermint, eucalyptus. N.B. avoid masks containing AHAs unless you know for sure your skin can cope with them without triggering sensitivity.
HOW TO USE THEM: smooth on; if the mask is a cream, tissue or wipe off. Some of them are peel-off formulations: once the mask has set, pull downwards (gently), starting from the forehead.
HOW THEY WORK: plant ingredients slough off dead surface cells and dirt partly responsible for the dull look, and stimulate the skin, giving a (pleasantly) tingly feeling.

Blotchy skin (i.e. sensitive)
These masks are appropriate for any skin type suffering tightness or red patches.
KEY WORDS IN THE NAME: *Gentle, Soothing, Relaxing.*
INGREDIENTS TO LOOK FOR: kaolin, caffeine, azulene, chamomile, aloe, grapefruit seed extract, honey (all soothing).
HOW TO USE THEM: smooth onto skin; wipe away with tissues or a hot washcloth.
HOW THEY WORK: caffeine and grapefruit seed extract reduce redness. Chamomile extract and aloe tackle inflammation (which is why they're often found in after-sun treatments), and have a cooling effect on the skin.

Actress **Bernadette Peters** and supermodel **Stephanie Seymour** both love Donna Karan's Natural Exfoliating Mask (see DIRECTORY), which they slather on once a week.

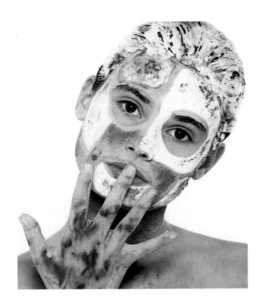

MAKING THE MOST OF YOUR MASK

* Cleanse first: using a mask on a dirty face is like putting polish on a dirty floor.
* Read instructions carefully: for best results, pay close attention to suggested masking time and proper removal technique.
* Be generous: most masks work best when laid on thick.
* Avoid the eye area: nearly every mask advises you to apply it well away from sensitive under-eye skin.
* Put your feet up so that oxygen is redirected from lower body to your head, oxygenating facial skin to facilitate the mask's actions.
* Moisturise immediately: now that you've removed dead skin cells and unclogged pores, your moisturiser will penetrate more deeply, for maximum results. Women with dry skin may want to seek out one of the newer cream masks, which can be left on the skin to sink in. Lingering traces of the mask can simply be smoothed in like a moisturiser.

TRIED & TESTED

FACE-SAVERS

These products are designed for those times when your face needs a fast pick-me-up – before an important meeting or party, when you have a cold or haven't had enough sleep. Products were marked on uplift, improved tone and whether make-up could go on as normal afterwards. Testers found that some were even more effective if left on overnight.

Top Treats

Guerlain Issima Midnight Secret

We're not surprised this product came out best, since it has consistently been described by beauty insiders as 'eight hours sleep in a jar'. It achieved top marks for instant uplift and improved skin tone, but worked best when left on overnight.
COMMENTS: 'skin felt hydrated and smooth', 'my complexion was smoother and softer', 'the improvement was continual'.

Guerlain Issima Aquamasque

This should be left on skin for ten minutes. Some testers reported that it had a warming action as it got to work.
COMMENTS: 'my skin looked fresher and stayed looking good all day', 'a very good moisturising treatment'.

Clarins Beauty Flash Balm

This is another well-known and bestselling face-waker; it works within minutes, so it's good when you're in a hurry. All our testers agreed that make-up went on normally.
COMMENTS: 'my skin felt soft and fresh', 'the results lasted most of the day'.

Best Budget Buy

Vichy Lift Effet Lumière Instant Beauty Fluid

Although Vichy products are a little more expensive than most Budget Buys, they're still considerably cheaper than Top Treats.

COMMENTS: 'gave me a healthy glow – my skin looked as if it was sparkling', 'my skin appeared visibly enhanced instantly'.

Natural Choice

Elemis Tonic Fruit Cream Mask

This company is well-respected for its aromatherapy and plant-based products, and this fruit-based mask proved very popular with our testers.
COMMENTS: 'my skin felt soft, smooth and nourished', 'the results lasted most of the day'.

Anne-Marie Börlind Bi-Activ Vital Cream Mask

This Scandinavian range is another good choice if you like entirely natural products.
COMMENTS: 'my skin felt soft and hydrated all day', 'intensely moisturising', 'no messy washing off, because this mask is left to be absorbed by the skin'.

N.B. Always pay attention to instructions.

BEAUTY SLEEP

Twelve hours' sleep a night is what Claudia Schiffer insists she needs to look good. Fortunately, most of us can get by on rather less, or we wouldn't get much done. But it isn't called 'beauty sleep' for nothing; cut down your sleep rations for just a few nights and you will soon see that your skin looks drab and grey circles develop under the eyes.

This much we understand. Yet sleep remains one of the great medical mysteries, and its effect on our complexions is just beginning to be understood. According to dermatologist Robert A. Weiss of the Johns Hopkins University School of Medicine, 'The release of growth hormone [while we sleep] is likely to influence specific skin-growth factors: collagen and keratin production may be stepped up, and skin cells may replicate faster.' Studies have shown that hormone levels fluctuate when sleep patterns are interfered with,

and may be linked to acne flare-ups and excessively dry skin. That hollow-eyed look, which identifies the sleep-deprived, is due to circulation changes; when the body struggles to fight fatigue, blood is diverted to the major organs – draining the face of colour and highlighting under-eye circles. In the quest for health and beauty, it really is best to sleep on it...

The so-called 'average' amount of sleep we need is just a statistic. Sixty-six per cent of us regularly sleep for between six and a half and eight and a half hours a night. Some 16 per cent sleep for longer, and 18 per cent skimp on under six and a half. Professor Jim Horne, who runs the sleep laboratory at Loughborough University, says: 'The acid test for insufficient sleep is whether you have trouble staying awake during the day.' But it's *quality* of sleep, not merely quantity, that is emerging as a chief factor in the sleep/health/beauty equation.

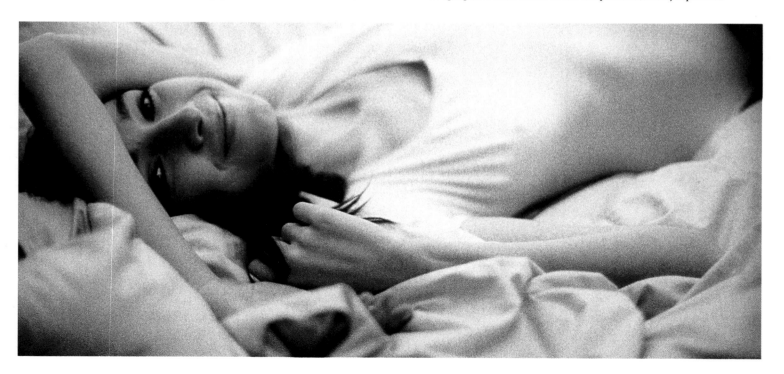

Just what does constitute perfect sleep? Dr Deepak Chopra, bestselling health author (whose works include *Restful Sleep*, see BEAUTY BOOKSHELF) observes: 'It seems to happen by itself. You don't have to fight for it against restlessness or anxiety, or take drugs of any kind to experience it. You rarely wake up in the middle of the night from good sleep, but if you do, you get back to sleep quickly without worrying about it. You wake up naturally in the morning. You're neither sluggish and groggy nor anxious and hyperalert. Finally, good sleep provides you with a sense of vitality that lasts through the day. You don't feel you've been deprived of rest during the preceding night, and you don't feel anxious about what's going to happen the next time you try to fall asleep.'

ACHIEVING PERFECT SLEEP

◗ Aim for a regular wake-up time and bedtime. If establishing a bedtime pattern is a problem, make a point of always getting up at the same time.

◗ Avoid napping; instead, a relaxation technique – meditation, Alexander Technique or yoga (see DIRECTORY) will give you the benefits of a nap without disturbing your sleep/wake cycle.

◗ Try not to harbour tension, anger or resentment. If sleep is elusive, try to relax (using deep breathing techniques, for instance), and don't worry about not sleeping. Unless there's a medical problem, everyone gets the amount of sleep they need, in the end.

◗ Try to fit in at least half an hour of exercise a day; walking is fine. It's often stress hormones that keep us tossing and turning, but exercise helps to stop their build-up in the system. Avoid vigorous exercise in the evening, although an after-dinner stroll can help digestion.

◗ Keep the bedroom warm but not stuffy; allow fresh air to circulate.

◗ Caffeine interferes with sleep. It isn't just an after-dinner espresso that will disturb sleep patterns; caffeine consumed at two in the afternoon can still have an effect. N.B. there is some caffeine in cola, tea, chocolate, and even in decaffeinated drinks.

◗ The herbs valerian and passiflora have long been popular insomnia cures. They are now available as Valerina, Natrasleep and Natural Sleep tablets, which are non-addictive alternatives to sleeping pills. Kava, another herb, is also a sleep remedy. Look for all of these in health stores.

◗ Heavy alcohol drinkers may fall asleep quickly but suffer a disturbed pattern of sleep later and wake up – unable to doze off again – in the small hours.

◗ *Where* you sleep, and the furniture arrangements, may also be a factor in optimising sleep quality. Alternative therapists sometimes suggest that sleeping with the head facing magnetic north will enhance sleep. (It works for Terence Stamp.)

TIPS FROM THE TOP

◗ Legendary French beauty **Catherine Deneuve** says: 'I try to respect my basic needs; eight hours of sleep at a minimum. Rest is the unassailable beauty treatment.'

◗ **Katie Boyle** keeps a bottle of Dr Bach's Rescue Remedy by her bedside. 'It stops the mind whirling. If I wake up at 5.30 and take a few drops on the tongue, I go straight back to sleep and don't feel groggy when the alarm goes off.'

◗ Supermodel **Paulina Porizkova** says: 'I try always to get eight hours' sleep a night, even though I consider sleep a total waste of time: I'd rather be playing the piano, listening to classical music or painting. But my mother always told me that I'd age more quickly if I don't sleep a lot – and since she's absolutely stunning, I take her advice!'

FINDING THE PERFECT FACIAL

Few other sybaritic pleasures compare with a good facial; beauticians and even some medical experts believe that your complexion will improve as much as your mood. US cosmetic surgeon Stephen Bosniak is not the only expert to acknowledge that 'people who get facials definitely have softer and more pliable skin.'

'The main purpose of a facial is to have the type of deep cleansing you can't do at home,' explains Beverly Hills-based facialist Aida Thibiant, who has a long list of celebrity clients including **Candice Bergen**. A facial consists of at least six steps, starting with skin analysis and make-up removal. Steaming and/or deep cleansing of blackheads and whiteheads is central to the proceedings, once skin has been carefully warmed and prepared for 'extraction' of built-up skin debris and white- and blackheads. A mask follows, then finally rehydration of the skin with a moisturiser or protective cream. Many facialists massage the skin with their fingers, while some salons instead include an electrical treatment with a wand rather like a cattle-prod. This stimulates the face in much the same way as massage, but it may give sensitive skins just too much of a jolt.

Facials aren't cheap, but devotees look upon them not just as pampering but as preventive treatment, like going to the doctor or the dentist for check-ups. Most beauticians recommend a monthly facial; according to Isabelle Reiser, Director of Training at Guinot Paris (a leading international salon treatment company), 'the skin's cells regenerate about every 21 days, so it makes sense to get rid of the accumulation of dead skin cells.'

There is a wealth of wonderful facial treatments available. You may want to try a couple before you settle on one that strikes the perfect balance of de-stressing and deep cleansing. You will know when you've found your perfect facialist – just by looking in a mirror immediately afterwards. You shouldn't be blotchy or red. You should be relaxed. And your skin should look instantly great.

FACIALS WE LOVE

Yasmin Le Bon swears by skincare from London skin queen Jo Malone: 'I've never found anything better. She has a blissfully simple but effective approach; her Cleansing Milk, Juniper Skin Tonic and Orange & Geranium Night Nourishing Cream are unbeatable.' **Natasha Richardson** and model **Gail Elliot** are also fans of Jo; like many top facialists, her regime focuses on massage – but never to the point of over-stimulation and redness. You can buy her skincare by mail order, even though she is so much in demand that her appointment list is now closed.

Eve Lom uses lymphatic drainage massage to help eliminate toxins that cause a dull complexion. Eve dishes out good lifestyle advice to clients, advising them to eat as much garlic as possible to boost their immune system: 'I'd put garlic in my creams, if I could!' Her wonderful creams, including a unique cleanser, are also available by mail order.

Decleor aromatherapy facials always start off with a de-stressing half-hour back massage, a real bonus. Elemis facials are also aromatherapy-based, and blissfully relaxing. Dr Hauschka's homeopathic facials, using extracts of flowers and plants organically grown and processed without synthetics or additives, have reached cult beauty status in America; they're now available in many countries including the UK. (**Cher** is a Dr Hauschka regular.)

Thalgo treatments use products rich in seaweed and sea minerals – and so do Repêchage facials; their 'Four Layer Facial' has a celebrity following that includes **Robert de Niro**, who likes to give the hardened seaweed 'cast' of his face to friends! Clarins is one of the top international names in facials, offering a wide range of botanically-based treatments. Their Paris Method treatment, featuring a unique circulation-boosting facial massage, is world-famous.

(For contacts, see DIRECTORY.)

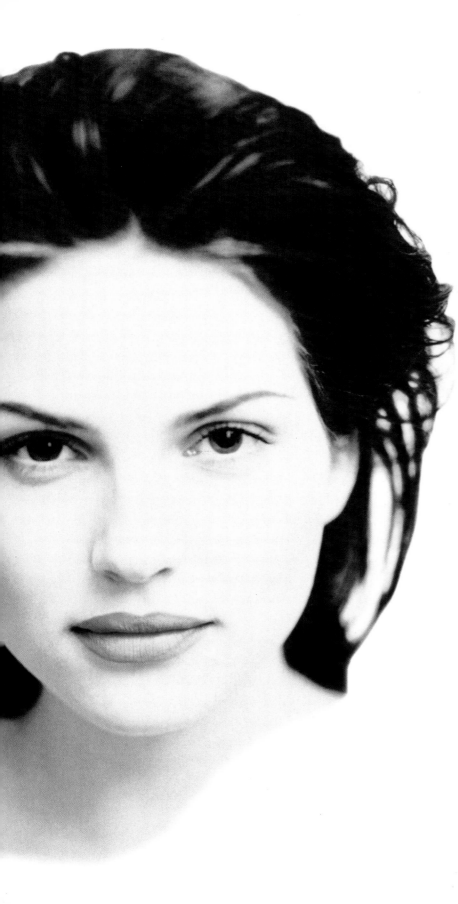

Finding the Perfect Facial – a 10-Point Plan

❶ Ask around for friends' facial recommendations – word of mouth is always best.

❷ Avoid booking a facial around the time of your period; skin can be more sensitive then.

❸ Before you make an appointment, ask two key questions: what's the training and experience of the facialist?

❹ Enquire whether any instruments or machines are used during the facial; if so, what – and why? (Most of the leading facialists we know advise against the use of vacuum extractors or metal tools for removing blackheads/whiteheads, as they potentially damage the skin.)

❺ Find out not only how much the facial costs, but how long the treatment will take. Also ask whether you need to leave your face clean to 'breathe', or if you'll be able to apply make-up straight afterwards, so you can either plan an evening in or go out and party.

❻ Once there, the beautician should take a full skincare history. Mention any skin troubles and whether you're on any medication.

❼ Ask to be talked through the facial step-by-step; you can feel rather trapped just sitting there, not knowing what comes next.

❽ Remove contact lenses before any facial treatments.

❾ You may well be left alone during the face mask part of the proceedings. Again, this can feel quite claustrophobic if you're not used to it, so ask the beautician to pop back half-way through and check you're OK.

❿ Once you've found the perfect facialist, stick with her; don't chop and change. Ideally, you should only have one pair of hands that touches your face – apart from your own...

AHA Peels

A variation on the salon mask is the exfoliating peel with alpha-hydroxy acids,or AHAs; of these, glycolic acid is often used, in concentrations which can range from just four to 40 per cent. We believe that these are best carried out by dermatologists, because they have the potential to damage the skin's natural protective barriers. Before any kind of AHA peel, a patch test should always be carried out to check for sensitivity.

EVA FRASER'S INSTANT FACE SAVER TIPS

Eva Fraser is 67 and looks 20 years younger. Her face-saving, skin-saving secret is facial exercises which she has developed over many years. We asked her to share her favourites with us here. Practise one, some or all of these as a daily routine to wake up a tired face and prevent lines and sagging. For a more detailed workout, follow Eva's book or video, or consult her at her facial workout studio in London for your individual programme. (See DIRECTORY.) While doing the exercises, feel relaxed and breathe slowly and rhythmically.

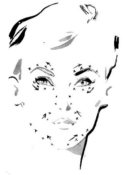

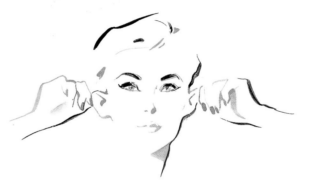

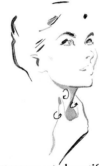

1 **Face tapping – to get the circulation going**
Tap 20 times on each dot with the pads of your middle fingers. From the bridge of your nose work out along your eyebrows, then in round the top of your cheekbone. Tap up from the sides of your mouth to each inner eye. Then out from the chin along the jawline to each ear. Make sharp, light, very quick taps as if you are testing a very hot iron.

> **TIP** Eva's preferred body exercise video is the Medau technique by Lucy Jackson (see DIRECTORY).

2 **Ear massage – to get your face glowing**
With index fingers and thumbs, hold the top rim of your ears and pull upwards. Massage, making small circles between fingers and thumbs. Move down all round the rim of the ears, pulling ears out gently and massaging, as above. When you reach the lobes, pull them down slightly and massage for about one minute. Repeat this sequence if you have time. Then, with small, quick circular movements, massage all the crevices and spirals of the ear. Use the surface of the nails of your index fingers, or the pads of your middle fingers.

3 **Throat massage – to beautify your neck**
Put the fingers of one hand on one side of your throat and the thumb on the other. Make rapid circular motions up and down the throat. Repeat with the other hand.

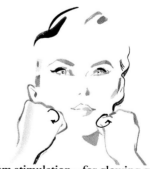

4 **Gum stimulation – for glowing gums**
With fingertips or knuckles, make circles just above the jawline along the gums.

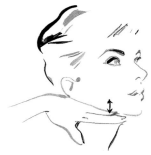

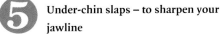

5 Under-chin slaps – to sharpen your jawline

Slap quickly and lightly under your chin 30 times with the back of one hand.

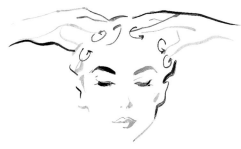

6 Hair massage – to stimulate hair growth and soothe headaches

With the pads of your fingertips, massage in small circles all along the front of your scalp for at least 30 seconds. Then take large fistfuls of hair and gently pull upwards. Now clench your hands into fists and lightly pound your scalp about 20 times.

7 Face stroking – to soothe, relax and generally uplift face and mind

N.B. This is not massage but very superficial stroking.

Start with the flat of your right hand against your chest and stroke up to your jawline, then immediately follow with your left. Continue alternating like this for at least ten strokes.

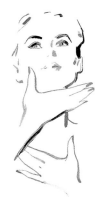

Next, immediately smooth the palms and fingers of your hands over your face – very, very lightly. Start at the jawline, move up and over your cheeks and each side of your nostrils, gently over the eyes and over the forehead to the hairline, then back down the sides of your face to your jaw. Repeat five to ten times in a continuous motion.

Now glide your middle fingers towards the bridge of your nose, out along your eyebrows, down your cheekbones and back to the bridge of your nose. Make ten of these light circular movements.

Then, with your middle fingers on the bridge of your nose, stroke up towards your forehead. Place all fingers (not thumbs) on your forehead and smooth outwards towards your temples; hold for a moment, pressing down slightly. Continue lightly down the side of your face, back along the cheekbones and up from the bridge of your nose. Do this ten times.

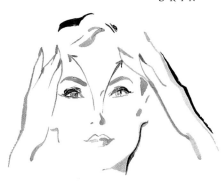

8 Temple pressure – to lift eye area and whole face

Leaning back in a chair, place the base of your palm or the pads of your fingertips against your temples and push upwards. At the same time, suck your tongue against the top of your mouth keeping your back teeth together. Hold this for a count of ten, increasing to 20. Slowly release and relax.

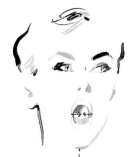

9 Exercise your mouth – to lift lip lines

Sit or stand, looking into a mirror. Open your mouth quite wide, as if about to yawn. Pull in the sides to form an oval. Now curve your lips over your teeth. Then, very slowly to the count of ten, close your lips until they are about 1.5cm (1/2in) apart. You will feel an upward pull. Release very slowly.

10 Finish by closing your eyes for a few moments, breathing deeply and gently and allowing yourself to drift off into a peaceful place – a summer garden, a warm deserted beach or, Eva's favourite, the clouds.

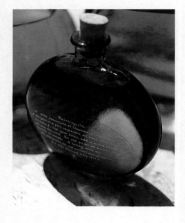

FACE MAGIC

We asked aromatherapist Kay Cooper to prescribe some facial oils specially for *The Beauty Bible*.

Kay, who describes herself as an alchemist, says that the joy of using oils rather than creams is that oils penetrate more deeply into the dermis. Meanwhile, the brain is awakened and soothed by the aromas. So aromatherapy is doubly potent.

Essential oils are the concentrated essences of fragrant plants and flowers, distilled into oils. For massage, the oils are mixed in minute quantities with carrier/base oils. Pure vegetable carrier/base oils are best for your face, ideally cold-pressed.

Mix a ratio of 30ml of carrier/base oil with no more than 15 drops of a single essential oil, or a combination of no more than four oils (again, not exceeding 15 drops total).

CARRIER/BASE OILS

Choose the one which seems most applicable to your skin:

PEACH KERNEL OIL — *rich in vitamin A; nourishing*

APRICOT KERNEL OIL — *rich in vitamin A; good for wrinkles as well as stretch marks on the body*

WHEATGERM OIL — *rich in vitamin E and phosphorus; soothes, heals and helps to smooth out wrinkles and lines*

ALMOND OIL — *lubricates and smoothes skin and reduces red veins; good for sensitive and dry skin*

COCONUT OIL — *acts as a cleanser, can have a drying effect on skin; good for oily skin*

ESSENTIAL OILS

Kay suggests choosing the oil or oils most appropriate to your skin. Or, she says, simply opt for the smells which please you most:

BENZOIN — *has a toning effect, acts as an antiseptic; very good for dry skin*

LAVENDER — *has a stimulating and antiseptic effect; good for oily skin and spots or any blemishes which need healing*

PATCHOULI — *soothes dry, flaky skin*

FRANKINCENSE — *rejuvenating and regenerating*

NEROLI — *rejuvenating and regenerating, this is the only one to use around the eye area; very good for broken capillaries*

MYRRH — *nourishes mature skin (aged 50+); especially good for any areas of inflammation*

GERANIUM — *balances combination skins, as well as your emotions*

TO APPLY, put a little of the mixture into the cupped palm of your hand or a small bowl, dip your fingertips in the blend and gently massage your face, working from the neck up to the hairline in small circles. Or stroke on the oils and practise the facial taps described by Eva Fraser (see page 92).

JUST HOW NATURAL IS NATURAL?

'About 60 per cent of any substance applied to the skin is absorbed into the body,' explains Rob McCaleb, President of the Herb Research Foundation in Boulder, Colorado. 'You should choose your bodycare products with as much care as you do the foods that you eat.'

About the only way that you can ensure that your cosmetics are 100 per cent natural, without chemical preservatives, is to whizz them up yourself in a blender at home. In fact at Kiehl's, the famous New York apothecary that's on every supermodel's beat (see DIRECTORY), they actively encourage customers to make their own cosmetics. 'There's almost nothing better for your hair or your face than egg yolk,' observes Kiehl's boss Jami Morse. 'But I don't use it in any products that are for sale, because if you want to keep it intact, the amount of preservative you would need would outweigh the potential benefits.'

When **Liz Earle** – the UK's best-selling health writer – was formulating her own signature skincare range (see DIRECTORY), discussions with potential manufacturers horrified her. 'What do you mean, you don't want to use formaldehyde to preserve your product?' asked one would-be manufacturer. 'Everyone else has it...' Liz shopped around until she found someone who was able to match her high demands. Which were: no petrochemicals, the minimum of preservatives necessary for a potential shelf-life of two years, and the highest possible levels of active natural ingredients. And absolutely no formaldehyde, thanks.

In the USA, where full ingredient listing has been compulsory for years, you can tell just what is and isn't natural. Similar legislation is due to be introduced in Europe shortly, although it may be several more years until it is enforced and fully operative. Another advantage of full listing is that if you know you're sensitive to an ingredient, you need never waste your money buying products that include it. In the meantime, there are plenty of ranges on the market which – while trumpeting their 'naturalness' – contain little more than traces of natural elements, mixed in with laboratory-made ingredients.

MORE NATURAL KNOW-HOW

If you'd like to know more about which ingredients – natural or synthetic – are most likely to trigger skin reactions, two good sources to consult are *A Consumer's Dictionary of Cosmetic Ingredients* and the Cosmetics Ingredients Decoder, an ingredient 'wheel' which tells you whether commonly used ingredients are 'unlikely', 'quite likely' or 'very likely' to set off problems(see BEAUTY BOOKSHELF for sources). If you have sensitive skin, you may want to seek out products, e.g. Kiehl's and Aveda, which already have full ingredient listings, to help you pin-point potential trouble-triggers.

Ultimately, we agree with Jami Morse, who says: 'even at their best, these are just cosmetics. If you really want to talk about taking care of yourself naturally, breathe clean air, eat right and exercise. That isn't something you can buy in a bottle.' Or even a greengrocer's, come to that.

FRIDGE-FRESH AND FABULOUS

Since the dawn of time, womankind has relied on ancient herbal wisdom for skincare and cosmetics. It is only in the last few decades that western women have been able to go to beauty counters – rather than the herb garden – and bought cosmetics. But there are still good reasons why we should consider concocting our own cosmetics – at least occasionally.

– It's great fun (and can be shared with children).
– It's a way of using up what's in the fridge before you head for the supermarket.
– It's the only way to be absolutely certain about what you're putting on your face or body.

The easiest and quickest face-treats to make yourself are masks. These are perfect for enjoying as part of our *At Home Spa*, page 190.

✳ Oily skins respond to whipped white of egg (dries, tightens), yoghurt (cleanses, nourishes), mashed strawberry (counteracts oiliness) and clay (absorbs oil).

✳ Yoghurt is used as a natural face mask in many eastern countries. It contains a form of lactic acid, which is a natural exfoliant, similar to the AHAs used in some commercial products.
✳ If your skin is blemished, experiment with a plum mask: boil six plums (enough for one application), strain and leave to cool. Mash with a teaspoonful of sweet almond oil.
✳ Dry and sensitive skins love egg yolk, crushed grapes, honey or glycerine (attract moisture), sunflower or sesame oil (soothe). In South Africa, mashed avocado pulp is rubbed onto the face to counteract the drying effect of the sun. Any good home-made mayonnaise, straight from the jar, also works.
✳ On combination skins, slather an oily skin mask on your T-zone, and a dry skin mask elsewhere. Mix and match ingredients to find out what is best for you.
✳ A winter salad face mask perks up skin: take fresh vegetables in any combination (e.g. cabbage, carrots, cucumbers, tomatoes, celery, lettuce, spinach, beansprouts). Whizz in a food blender or mash with a pestle and mortar, and add a few drops of jojoba oil if your skin is very dry. Apply to a cleansed face, then lay two tissues over the top (to absorb excess liquid). Leave for 15–20 minutes, then rinse.

TIPS FROM THE TOP

Barbara Carrera's stay-young secret? Forget expensive lotions and potions: 'I think you can find whatever you need in your own kitchen. Instead of throwing away watermelon rinds, banana peels, papaya skins, lie down and put them on your face for half an hour. It's incredibly reviving and feels yummy.'

Liz Earle whisks up her own face mask with one beaten egg white sprinkled with a teaspoon of vitamin C powder.

MORE BOTANICAL BEAUTY SECRETS

■ The old remedy for scaly elbows does actually work: cut a lemon in half, squeeze out the juice and rest your elbows in the lemon 'cup' for 5–10 minutes. This has a gentle bleaching action, and the fruit acids exfoliate.

■ Jo Malone, top international beautician whose clients include **Yasmin Le Bon** and **Viscountess Linley**, has a recipe for a wonderful body-buffer: blend one cup of coarse-grain sea salt with a teaspoon of almond oil and half a teaspoon of grated orange or lemon zest. Massage into damp skin, rinse off with warm water, then pat skin dry and apply body lotion.

■ Vegetable oil is a cure for dry body skin, which tends to plague women who wear opaque tights: rub a teaspoonful into each shin and other dry patches before bedtime.

■ Oatmeal baths are excellent for sore, cracked skins – and great for eczema sufferers. To avoid feeling like you're bathing in porridge, wrap the oatmeal in a square of muslin, secured with string, and hang from the hot tap so the water flows through it. (No muslin handy? A pop sock or the foot of laddered tights will do just as well.)

■ Oatmeal can also be used as an exfoliant for the face. Mix it with your normal moisturiser and then massage into the face in ultra-gentle, circular movements. Rinse after five minutes.

■ Cucumber juice – whizzed in the blender – makes an excellent skin freshener.

■ A slice of raw potato rubbed over the face is soothing, especially to areas of irritation. Laid on puffy eyes, slices are great de-baggers.

■ Unless you're prone to broken veins, stroking ice cubes wrapped in cling-film over your face acts as an instant 'lift', reducing puffiness and stimulating circulation.

■ Combine glycerine and rosewater (both available from pharmacies) in a ratio of 3:1 for a lotion to soothe delicate skin.

■ Deep clean dirty hands after gardening with a mixture of fine grain rock salt and a little olive oil.

■ A cup of apple cider vinegar added to the bathwater soothes itchy, flaky skin, and calms sunburn.

Recommended Natural-as-Possible Brands

Aesop	Blackmore's	Kiehl's
Aveda	Creighton's	Martha Hill
Beauty Through	Naturally	Neal's Yard
Herbs	Dr Hauschka	Rachel Perry
Beauty Without	Elemis	Urtekram
Cruelty	E'SPA	Weleda

WEATHER-BEATING BEAUTY

With each season your skin behaves differently. If you travel abroad, the change in climate may also call for skincare adjustments.

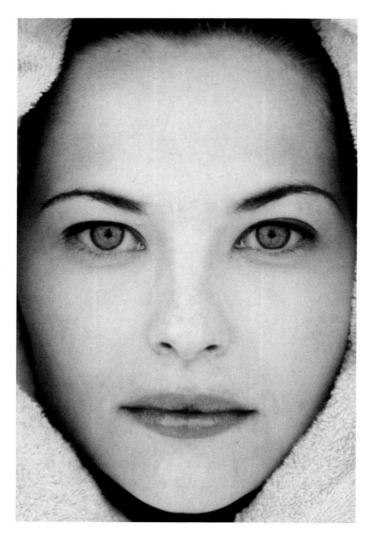

COLD WEATHER SKINCARE

Sticking to your usual regime when the thermometer plummets, cold winds whip up and central heating is turned up can mean lizard lips, alligator elbows and chapped cheeks. In summer, with the right sun protection, you can get away with minimum attention – and still look great. But in cold weather, skin, hair, body and make-up all need winter-proofing.

TLC for Faces

First step: skincare. The cold weather watchword, regardless of skin type, is more: *more* moisturising, *more* gently, *more* often.

More Gentle

In winter, those who cannot otherwise be dissuaded from using soap and water really should put their soap into hibernation. 'Soap strips the skin of its natural oily protection – and no cream can ever replace that moisture,' warns skincare pro Jo Malone. Cold weather can incite skin sensitivity, too – to detergents, fragrances, lanolin. So choose a gentle, water-soluble cleanser that's non-irritating to skin. After cleansing, if you feel you have to use a toner, make sure it's alcohol-free.

More Moisture

'Women often find that their make-up looks patchy in winter – it just doesn't stay put,' observes Creative Director of Givenchy Cosmetics, Olivier Echaudemaison. 'The right moisturiser fixes that.' All skin types need help. Lydia Sarfati, New York salon owner and creator of the Repêchage range, insists: 'It doesn't matter what your skin type – oily, dry, sensitive – everyone needs to moisturise in winter.'

According to dermatologist Dr Stephen Curtin, of Mt Sinai School of Medicine, the conditions in your bedroom may be more harmful than the great outdoors. 'Few people realise that due to better insulation, the heating in modern apartments and homes forces humidity down. The newer the building, the lower the moisture in the air.' Central heating dries out air and lifts moisture from skin into the atmosphere, so keep thermostats as low as possible (and cut fuel bills at the same time). Place small bowls of water near radiators to work as humidifiers, and if the air is really parched, drape them with damp towels. Turn your space into a jungle, with plants that thrive on regular misting. Best skincare investment of all? A cold water humidifier (from electrical stores).

Lip Lubrication

Lips boast only three to five layers of skin cells, compared with 15 elsewhere on the body, which is why a barrier between your lips and the environment is essential. Most lip balms are petroleum-based, but lips can actually become addicted to these, meaning that they wil have to be used more and more often to have any effect. (Non-petroleum lip balms we love include The Body Shop's and Kiehl's). One definite don't: habitual lip-licking. Once the moisture has evaporated, lips will feel drier than ever.

Beauty Barometer

❂ A tip from Bobbi Brown: 'During winter months, when skin tone may pale, try a lightly-tinted powder – translucent tends to make your skin pale and pasty. Pink offers a rosy cast; yellow or beige gives a healthy glow.'

❂ Paint concealer onto red, raw areas around the nose, lips and cheeks with a soft lip brush, then set with powder.

❂ Choose a lipstick with a moisturising formulation. (Look for the word 'moisture' in the name.)

❂ Avoid 'long-lasting' lipstick formulations, which can be extremely drying.

❂ Pick a rosy blusher shade which matches your cheeks after a breezy walk and won't compete with your natural colour.

WARM WEATHER SKINCARE

Just as you pack away your woollies and bring out the silk and cotton, your cosmetic kit-bag needs 'summerising'. If your skin is good enough, skip foundation and replace it with tinted moisturisers that include sun filters, mixed with a dab of concealer if necessary. Otherwise make sure to choose an oil-free foundation.

❂ Cheeks are naturally rosier, so skip blusher.

❂ Get your lashes dyed and leave the mascara on your dressing table: the sultry effects last for about six weeks.

❂ Look for cosmetics, particularly lipsticks and foundations, that do double duty as sun protection.

Safe Sunning

If you like contemporary horror stories, there is no need to reach for Stephen King. The reports from any dermatologists' conference make shocking enough reading.

FACT: skin cancer statistics are soaring. (In the UK, as many as 40,000 people a year are diagnosed with different types of skin cancer.)

FACT: skin cancer (notably malignant melanoma) can be fatal.

FACT: a tan does not protect against skin cancer.

There are several kinds of skin cancer related to sun exposure, including solar keratoses (wart-like growths) and malignant melanoma, now the most frequent type of cancer for young adult women. This is thought to be related to short, sharp overdoses of sun – just one bout of sunburn may be all it takes. But that still doesn't stop millions of us throwing caution to the off-shore breeze and racing to expose our vulnerable bodies to the sun at the drop of a wide-brimmed hat...

A tan is actually the body's defence mechanism against the threat posed by the sun. Sunlight stimulates the skin to step up production of melanin. Darker-skinned people have more natural melanin in the skin; someone with (naturally) blonde hair and light eyes will never be able to tan like someone with dark hair and dark eyes. As the melanin supply is activated, it moves up towards the surface of the skin, where it helps prevent burning and reduces penetration by damaging rays. The side effect of this protective mechanism is to make the skin turn brown. As Brigitte Bardot knows all too well, over-exposure to the sun accelerates the natural pace of ageing.

The Sunscreen Scene

To most dermatologists, no tan is a good tan. However, there's no denying that seeing the sun and being brown makes people feel good. *Everyone* who goes in the sun needs sunscreen. End of story. Since the ozone layer has thinned, and more of the sun's harmful rays reach our skins, many dermatologists insist that we wear a protective sunscreen all the time, even on cloudy days in the city.

Sunscreen factor numbers can seem baffling. The simple rule is the higher the number, the more protection a cream offers. Sun protection factor (SPF) numbers relate to the length of time you can stay in the sun without burning. Most fair-skins can tolerate ten to 15 minutes in full sun, according to consultant dermatologist Dr Tim Cutler. Multiply that baseline period of ten minutes by an SPF of 15, and you get two and a half hours' protection (150 minutes). After that you really should come in out of the sun; that's your daily ration. If you have naturally darker skin, you will safely be able to stay out longer, but the golden rule is to reapply sunscreen regularly. Once your body has acquired a protective tan, you could opt for a lower SPF, but Professor Rona Mackie, the UK's leading expert on malignant melanoma cancer, cautions nothing less than SPF10.

Always opt for a cream that screens out UVA *and* UVB (ultra-violet) rays. Initially, research scientists believed that UVA rays weren't as harmful to the skin as UVB. But, in fact, it has since emerged that UVA rays speed up ageing, damage elasticity and increase the long-term risk of skin cancer. UVB rays cause erythema (sunburn and redness). A simple memory device works: UVA equals *ageing*, and UVB equals *burn*.

Even with a broad-spectrum SPF and under a broad-brimmed hat, it is pure madness to put your face in the sun; because facial skin is thinner, it is the fastest track to wrinkles. (Conversely legs, where skin is thick, take the longest to tan.) Nowadays, with bronzing powders, tinted moisturisers and a new generation of excellent fake tanners, there is absolutely no reason to expose your face if you want a sun-kissed look.

SUMMER SKIN

Don't wear nylon or polyester sweatbands or visors; these fabrics can allow sweat to build up around the hairline, blocking sweat glands and encouraging little white bumps to come up, or spots to develop. Instead, wear cotton visors, baseball caps and sweatbands, and wash them regularly.

Do switch to an alcohol-free version of your scent, if available; the effect of sun on the alcohol can cause redness, even burning.

Don't expose just-waxed or shaved skin to the sun – or to sunscreens. Rashes can break out.

Do dry your skin thoroughly with a towel after swimming in the sea. It may feel cooling to lie on your beach towel and let the sun evaporate the water, but it'll leave a thin layer of salt behind – which can be extremely drying if you have sunburn or skin prone to feeling parched.

Don't apply foundation on top of sun cream on top of moisturiser; it not only wastes time and money but you run the risk of clogging pores with so many cosmetic layers, thereby triggering tiny pimples or rashes. Look for one product that moisturises, protects and gives skin a healthy glow. (See our *Tried & Tested Tinted Moisturisers*, page 22.)

Don't jump into the pool without waterproof sunblock; this protects against chlorine which can aggravate acne.

Do wash your beach towel every day; sweat, sunscreen and bacteria can build up on a towel, making it very unhealthy to dry your face on.

Don't wear certain acne preparations in the sun: benzoyl peroxide products can be altered by UV rays, triggering irritation. (Save them for after sun-down.)

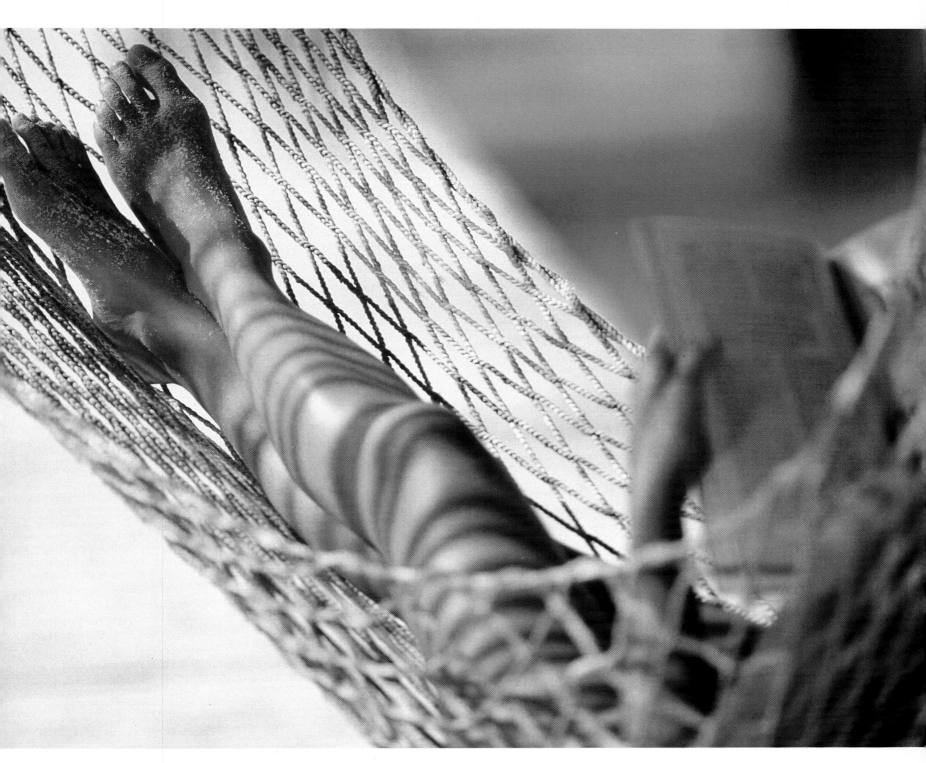

WHY A LITTLE DOESN'T GO A LONG, LONG WAY

☀ Be generous with sunscreen: one shot-glassful is the average amount a woman needs to coat her body. If you apply it too thinly, you can lose about half its SPF value. And don't rub too hard: being over-enthusiastic can reduce a sunscreen's potency by around 25 per cent.

☀ Always apply each day's first dose of suncare to cool, dry skin, paying extra attention to delicate areas like face, ears, neck, upper chest, arms and backs of hands and feet. (N.B. solar radiation penetrates lightweight material, too.) Then reapply, preferably every hour (i.e. even more frequently than the maximum time the SPF allows you).

☀ Follow instructions and slavishly apply sunscreen 30 minutes *before* going out in the sun. It's all too easy to spend the first half-hour on the beach locating your perfect spot and settling in – while the sun beats down on your unprotected skin.

☀ If you can't reach some parts of your body, ask someone to help you. (Be particularly careful to cover areas bordering your bikini/costume.)

☀ One of the quickest ways to burn is snorkelling; always wear a T-shirt to protect your back, and cover up with a water-resistant block.

☀ If you do go into the water and towel-dry afterwards, always reapply your sunscreen all over; even a waterproof lotion isn't *towel*-proof.

☀ Drink plenty of water and fresh fruit juices to keep your body and skin from becoming dehydrated.

☀ A word on hats – the bigger and more closely woven the better, to keep your face and the back of your neck covered.

☀ The combination of sun, snow and altitude when you're skiing or mountain-climbing is especially potent. Piz Buin and Ambre Solaire make special sunscreens for these conditions.

D-I-Y SENSITIVITY TEST

The chemical ingredients in sunscreens, combined with UV light, heat and sand, can easily irritate sensitive skins. As a safeguard, head for the ranges designed for sensitive skin. (These include Almay, Clinique, Estée Lauder, Lancôme, Piz Buin, Boots Soltan and Ambre Solaire's range for sensitive skin.) PABA (para-aminobenzoic acid) is one of the commonest sensitivity-triggers in sunscreens; products containing titanium dioxide (e.g. Estée Lauder's range) are less likely to irritate. Always carry out a D-I-Y patch test first: diligently apply a small blob of sunscreen to the inside of your elbow each day for five days. If you experience any redness/stinging/itchiness, abandon that product. Unfortunately, suncare companies seldom offer sample sizes, so always buy the smallest size first, just in case. If you continue to have problems, consult a qualified pharmacist.

Faye Dunaway – 50-something and fabulous – protects her skin daily with an SPF30 sunscreen.

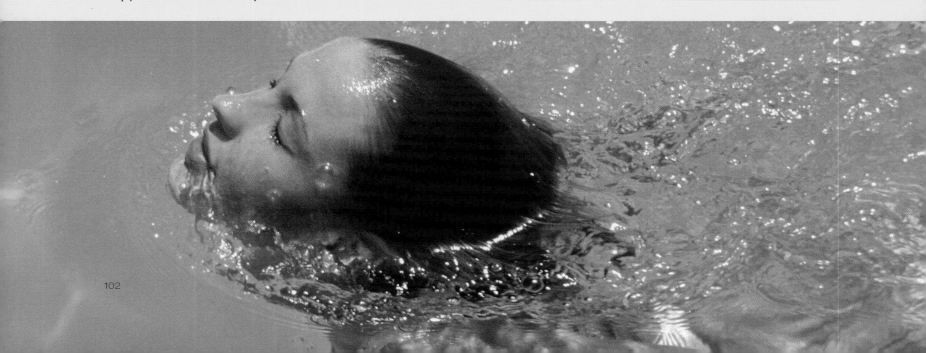

THE TAN COMMANDMENTS

The only safe tan is a fake tan, and sales of D-I-Y alternatives are booming. Clever fakers know that the new generation of self-tanners leaves yesterday's orange, streaky and smelly lotions in the shade. But there are still tricks for ensuring such a perfect tan that nobody will be able to tell you haven't just stepped off a plane from the Riviera...

1. Do a patch test the night before, to check you like the colour.

2. De-hair your legs 24 hours before to ensure smooth, even results.

3. Remove dry skin with a body scrub or loofah, concentrating particularly on dry patches like elbows, knees and heels.

4. If you're fake-tanning your face, exfoliate thoroughly first with a wet muslin square or washcloth.

5. Because dry areas are much more absorbent, use lotion sparingly on the thick skin around elbows and knees. After you've finished applying your fake tanner, remove any excess by swabbing lightly around these areas with a damp tissue.

6. Wash your hands immediately afterwards to avoid bronzed palms.

7. Allow at least four hours for colour to develop before reapplying.

8. Clothing can take on a fake tan, too, so remain scantily clad until it has sunk in properly, and avoid sitting on good furniture or sheets. Some products take up to an hour before they stop being tacky.

N.B. Fake tans offer no protection from the sun, so always apply a sunscreen before going out into the sun.

TRIED & TESTED

SELF-TANNERS

These products really do give a natural-looking, flattering glow. Those designed for the face can also be used on the body, but not always the other way round.

Top Treat

Clinique Self-Tanning Body Balm
The body version of the facial self-tanner which also scored very well with our testers.
COMMENTS: 'the best-tanning product I've ever used', 'smelt refreshing and pleasant, not synthetic', 'everyone said it looked totally real'.

Lancaster Quick Action Self-Tan Golden Glow
The colour of this spray-action self-tanning product develops extremely fast, even in an hour.
COMMENTS: 'I liked the subtlety of colour – more of a glow', 'very natural colour – my favourite', 'nicer than any I've used before, but you do need to use plenty'.

Helena Rubinstein Golden Beauty For The Face
Our testers reported that this product could be used on the complexion without any qualms, as it really did give natural results.
COMMENTS: 'lasted for ages', 'was absorbed quickly', 'great comments from other people'.

Lancôme Sôleil Tanning Spritz
The spray action makes this really easy to apply, and it's free of any trace of the 'morning-after' smell common to many self-tanners.
COMMENTS: 'left skin soft but not greasy', 'this product gave the best colour for me'.

Best Budget Buy

Vichy Moisturising Self-Tan For Body
This is a new and even better version of Vichy's successful self-tanner for the body.
COMMENTS: 'blended well, with no smearing', 'realistic shade', 'no patches and easy to apply'.

Yardley Easy Bronze Self-Tanning
This product tints the skin as it goes on, making it easier to see straight away exactly where you're applying it.
COMMENTS: 'best I've ever used – brilliant', 'very good colour', 'developed instantly'.

Vichy Autobronzant Visage
This is one of the products specifically targeted at the face zone. It scored very highly.
COMMENTS: 'good instructions', 'very faint, pleasant smell', 'suitable for very pale skins, as you can build colour up gradually'.

Natural Choice

Elemis Sunwise Bronzing Cream
Our testers agreed that this was the best bet for a plant and aromatherapy based product.
COMMENTS: 'I have a fair skin and the colour looks natural – not too yellow', 'easy to apply'.

103

PROBLEM SKINS

At some time in our lives, most of us have less than perfect complexions. Here's the lowdown on skin trouble-shooting.

Conventional dermatologists and their counterparts in unconventional medicine tend to disagree about the causes and treatment of problem skin conditions. For instance, most dermatologists argue that diet makes no difference to acne, whereas nutritionists and other alternative practitioners say their experience shows otherwise.

We suggest you talk to your doctor but also try using pure, natural skincare products (see *Just How Natural is Natural*, page 95), overhaul your diet, make sure you get plenty of sleep, fresh air and exercise, take stress management seriously, and consider consulting a qualified nutritionist, naturopath or Chinese herbal medicine practitioner.(For contact details, see DIRECTORY.)

ACNE is an inflammation of the sebaceous glands and occurs where the glands are most active; on the face, neck, back and chest. Excess sebum (see *Composition of Skin*, page 70) blocks the hair follicles and pores, bacteria builds up and spots and pimples erupt. The sebaceous glands are controlled by androgens, the male hormones also found in women. Hence the eruption of acne at puberty and other times of hormonal upset – although at least one woman in 20 has acne after the age of 25.

TREATMENT: most dermatologists suggest over-the-counter preparations for four to six weeks, then, if the condition doesn't clear up, antibiotic creams and/or long courses of oral antibiotics or drugs which influence the way the skin responds to hormones (see page 75). If you get an unexpected breakout after years of clear skin, change your skincare products and be gentle with your skin, i.e. no scrubbing or exfoliating. Also rethink your diet. In a small study conducted recently, three out of four acne sufferers found a clear improvement using the pure, organically-grown Dr Hauschka skincare products combined with a low fat, vegetarian diet, rich in salads, vegetables, whole grains, Quark (a curd cheese), yoghurt and sour milk. At the same time, they cut down

on alcohol, nicotine and caffeine, and avoided meat, processed meat pulses, processed sugar and margarine, and juice concentrates. They also took regular exercise.

BLACKHEADS, WHITEHEADS and those funny little WHITE SKIN BUMPS which can appear on your face are not caused by dirt but are due to sebum blocking the hair follicles. Blackheads are their colour because the sebum oxidises when exposed to the air, just as a cut apple turns brown.

TREATMENT: steam your face under a towel over very hot water (add chamomile, sage, echinacaea herb or tincture). Use gentle masks, particularly kaolin (see page 86). Regular facials from a good beauty therapist may also help. Never squeeze blackheads, whiteheads or skin bumps: it may cause cross infection and can leave scars.

RED PATCHES, as opposed to a flattering rosiness in your cheeks, are often due to enlarged blood vessels, which may be an inherited condition or caused by rosacea. This usually occurs on the cheeks and nose in women of 30 plus. Rosacea, which is sometimes activated by the menopause, is a particularly unkind skin disorder since sufferers are often thought, quite wrongly, to be drinkers. The cause is a mystery, although heat or sunlight probably stimulate the release of chemicals which encourage the blood vessels to enlarge. Rosacea seems to run in families, particularly Northern Europeans and Southern Celts whose pale faces tend to flush and blush easily. However, this apparent trend may simply be because the enlarged blood vessels are more noticeable in pale skin as it has no pigment to act as camouflage.

TREATMENT: avoid extreme heat or cold, chocolate, spicy foods, coffee, oranges, orange juice and red wine which may irritate it. Take supplements of Vitamin B1 and B2. Soothe irritation with Bach Flower Rescue Remedy Cream. If you have found

conventional medicine unhelpful, try consulting a qualified
naturopath or Chinese herbal medicine practitioner.

FACIAL ECZEMA is another possible cause of red patches and rosacea
keratitis, pustules and acne-like rashes can affect the eyes and
eyelids. Consult a dermatologist, qualified naturopath or Chinese
herbal medicine practitioner.

YELLOW PATCHES, medically called xanthelasma, which are usually
found around the eyes (particularly on the lids), may be a result of
fatty deposits. In about 50 per cent of cases, they are a sign of
abnormal fat levels in the blood; others are caused by recurrent sun
damage, which distorts the elastin fibres in skin. The fibres mat
together, resulting in waxy yellowish lumps, often on the upper lid.

TREATMENT: although this condition is not unique to smokers, it is
greatly increased in habitual puffers, so first of all stop smoking.
Consult your doctor and ask for a referral to a dermatologist.

SHINE OFF

**If you have greasy skin – which tends to get worse during the
summer months – how should you absorb the oil surplus?**

■ Use a kinder cleanser. Skin doesn't need industrial-strength
scrubbing to combat shine. Oily complexions are often sensitive, and
aggressive cleansers or exfoliants can irritate them.

■ Don't always reach for the powder puff to banish shine. Layers of
powder can form a 'cement' with oil and sweat, triggering breakouts.

■ Look for the magic word 'matifying'. An amazing armoury of
ingredients – from microscopic sponges to nylon, via seaweed and
clay powder – are deployed in 'matifying lotions' designed to repress
oil production and blot shine. Apply after your cleanser – and only
where necessary: with combination skin, put it on the T-zone only.

■ Give it time to dry before applying foundation and other make-up,
which should go on ultra-smoothly – and stay shine-free for hours.
(Some foundations and powders contain matifying ingredients, too.)

> **TIP** For extensive spotty problems – i.e. backs and/or
> chests – we've heard good reports on naturopaths and
> practitioners of traditional Chinese medicine.

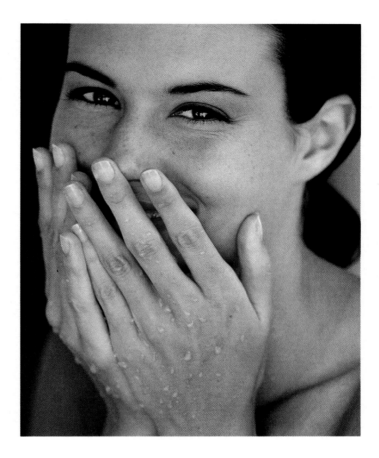

DOS AND DON'TS FOR ACNE SUFFERERS

Do make absolutely sure your hands are clean every time you
touch your face.

Don't touch or squeeze spots. Ever.

Do use a cover-up or camouflage. You might want to try one
that's camphor-based, such as that produced by the Sher skincare
regime. According to Helen Sher, creator of the Sher system,
'with a camouflage, any redness goes away instantly. And if it's
camouflaged, it doesn't bother you.' Acne can have a
tremendously inhibiting effect, psychologically. But if it's less
visible, then it will worry you less.

Don't ever go to bed without removing your make-up; left on, it
will cause blocked pores.

4 Hair

Nobody ever died from a bad haircut – but plenty of women have walked out of the salon wishing they had a paper bag to cover the damage. **How good (or terrible) you feel about your hair can have a dramatic effect on your morale**. When it's wonderfully cut and shimmering with light, women feel able to conquer anything. When it's droopy and you can't do a thing with it, it can throw your whole day. But, with insider information from the hair world's leading professionals, bad hair days can be history. Here's how to find the best cut, colour and haircare for you – and your lifestyle.

HAIR HEALTH

More than a great cut or glamorous style, healthy hair is what makes heads turn. In a perfect world, hair would be clean, glossy and bouncy all the time.

Hair is a perfect barometer of your general health. When you're fit and happy, your hair will swoosh, bounce and shine just like in the ads; if you're ill, tired, stressed out or eating poorly, it will show up in your hair.

Each hair is made up of overlapping layers of the same substance, keratin, that makes up dead protein cells. When the layers lie flat and smooth, each strand reflects the light, making it shine. When the layers are damaged, no light is reflected and your hair is left looking dull and lifeless. The apparently strange but common combination of greasy scalp with dry hair may also be the result of damage – hair's natural oil (sebum) is prevented from travelling down the hair shaft.

So the first step to shiny hair is to get yourself healthy, physically and emotionally: eat well, take plenty of exercise and fresh air (your hair needs oxygen too), and make sure you get enough sleep. Reduce stress levels wherever possible and, in addition, learn and practise relaxation techniques (see page 196). Remember, healthy hair depends on a healthy scalp, which is of course another part of your skin, so all the suggestions we make for healthy skin in SKIN apply to your hair and scalp as well. Overprocessing of all sorts or overheating your hair (with a hairdryer, etc.) can also do considerable damage.

The good news is that, unless you have a medical condition, tender loving care from you, in tandem with today's technologically advanced formulae, can give you great hair in a relatively short time.

HAIR VILLAINS

Any and all of these are likely to damage the condition of your hair and scalp:

Over-exposure to sun, salt air, wind and chlorinated water
Pollution
Central heating
Chemotherapy/radiotherapy
Some pharmaceutical drugs including the Pill, thyroid
  drugs, cortisone, sedatives, tranquillisers and
  barbiturates, amphetamines, antibiotics
Poor diet/nutrient deficiency (particularly iron)
Crash dieting
Stress, anxiety, depression
Head and neck tension, which disrupt supply of blood and
  vital nutrients
Illness, shock or trauma
Thyroid problems
Not enough rest and sleep
Shallow breathing
Perming, bleaching, tinting
Curling tongs/heated rollers
Blowdrying at too high a temperature
Too much brushing with a sharp bristled brush

HAIR FACTS

◆ We are born with a specific number of hair follicles which cannot be changed.

◆ The size of the dermal papilla (at the bottom of the follicle), which may change through illness, for example, or hormonal fluctuations, determines the thickness of the hair.

◆ We each have about 120,000 hairs; blondes more, redheads less.

◆ We lose up to 100 hairs naturally every day.

◆ Although the hair we see is technically dead, with no blood, nerves or muscles, healthy hair can stretch up to 30 per cent in length, absorb its own weight in water, and swell up to 14 per cent in diameter.

◆ Hair grows an average of half an inch (13mm) each month, faster in summer than in winter.

FEED YOUR HAIR

No miracle shampoo and condition regime can compensate for the wrong diet. Not only do healthy hair cells need the right nutrients and plenty of fresh water, good digestion is also vital, according to nutritionist Kathryn Marsden. 'Dull, oily hair may be the result of poor elimination of wastes and toxins, poor circulation, inadequate fluid intake, a sluggish bowel – or of simply being below par.' In these circumstances, she suggests a regular cleansing diet (see page 162) with herbal and vitamin supplements.

Foods to help your hair are live yoghurt, plenty of fresh vegetables, salads and fruits, cold-pressed oils (e.g. olive, safflower, sesame – but don't cook with them as it alters the chemical composition), linseeds, pulses, sunflower/pumpkin/sesame seeds, sea vegetables (seaweed/samphire), wholegrains (brown rice/oats), buckwheat, millet, almonds, figs and dates. If you're not vegetarian, fresh oily fish (e.g. mackerel, herring, tuna, salmon, sardines). Plus plenty of pure water.

Try to cut down on cow's milk products, caffeine, cola, chocolate, sugar, salt, saturated and hydrogenated fats, processed foods.

Try to give up smoking. (This, of course, goes for every single facet of health and beauty.)

Supplements: All the B vitamins, gamma-linolenic acid (GLA), fish oil, linseed oil, antioxidants including vitamins beta-carotene, C and E, and minerals, selenium and zinc (see also page 165).

TIP After much research, hair colourist Jo Hansford recommends a supplement called Nourkrin. One bonus: as hair and nails are made of the same protein (keratin), eating for healthy hair also improves your nails.

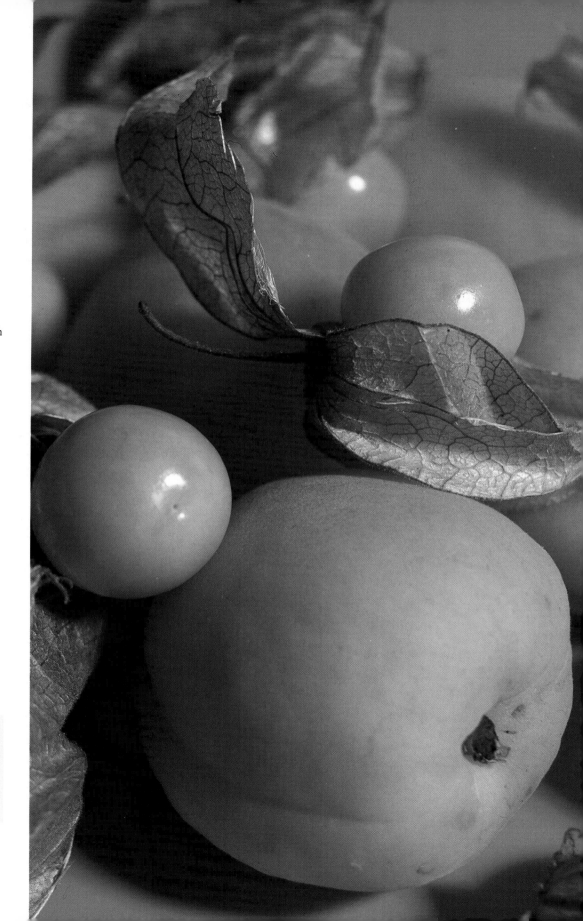

HAIR ANALYSIS

Once upon a time, the nearest we came to hair analysis was when the hairdresser took a strand of hair, pronounced it split beyond repair and prescribed a cut. Today your hairdresser will probably, if asked, go into far more detail about your type of hair and its individual needs.

Expert analysis can also determine products which will improve our crowning glory. Companies including Lazartigue, La Biosthetique, Shiseido and Redken (see DIRECTORY) offer hair, and sometimes scalp, analysis at their own salons and at counters in big department stores. The usual method is to remove a few hairs from your scalp and magnify them, showing up any damage. The products they prescribe are, of course, their own (and in some cases they're expensive) but they can help deal with a range of hair problems such as dry or unmanageable hair.

If you have long-term or acute hair problems, we suggest you ask your doctor to refer you to a dermatologist with a particular interest in hair (see *Thinning Hair*, below). You may also consider consulting a trichologist privately. Some trichologists, for instance Philip Kingsley (probably the best known and one of the most respected hair gurus), have created their own range of products.

Otherwise, a reputable nutritionist who combines hair and other tests (e.g. blood, sweat, urine) with a detailed medical and lifestyle examination should be able to guide you on improving your health from crown to toe, by suggesting eating plans and, if necessary, nutritional supplementation. (See DIRECTORY for how to find a qualified practitioner.)

THINNING HAIR

Thirty per cent of women will notice some thinning of their hair by the age of 50; in comparison, 50 per cent of men will notice some change before 30. In men, the hair loss is more severe and concentrated in specific areas (e.g. the crown, temples etc.), whereas in women it tends to be a general all-over thinning. Although it's a well-accepted fact that male pattern baldness is due to the activity of testosterone (the male hormone, also present in women), prescribed hormones are a greatly overlooked cause of thinning hair in women, according to biochemist and trichologist Dr Hugh Rushton. Many women are suffering hair loss, he says, through taking various types of HRT (hormone replacement therapy). Meanwhile, the contraceptive pill can affect hair in both ways: hair loss or its opposite, hirsutism. Philip Kingsley says he has also found that women with irregular menstrual cycles or with polycystic ovaries (which, research indicates, may affect more than ten per cent of women of reproductive age) often suffer hair loss.

The sudden bald patches of alopecia areata (AA) are thought to be stimulated by an auto-immune response (where the immune system acts against itself); some experts believe this is exacerbated by stress, combined with genetic susceptibility to AA. If there are just one or two patches, they will usually grow back within six to nine months, according to Dr Rushton.

So what can be done? Fortunately, for women, inherited female hair loss is much easier to treat medically than male pattern baldness. With specialist advice, supported by a good general health regime, virtually all women with genetic hair loss can normally expect a 30 to 40 per cent regrowth. Treatment is usually a combination of hormone therapy (oral or topical) and topical drug therapy, together with nutritional supplementation; blood tests are necessary to determine nutrient levels. Treatment must be given under medical supervision; Dr Rushton suggests you ask your doctor to refer you to a gynaecologist, endocrinologist (hormone expert) or dermatologist with a specific expertise in this field.

More extensive hair loss may respond to topical corticosteroid creams. Meanwhile, really good wigs and hairpieces are now available, and support organisations such as Hairline International can offer further information (see DIRECTORY).

TIP Women who experience thinning hair during menopause should have their thyroid levels checked, especially if they are also feeling tired, advises Dr Rushton. (See also *The No-Wash Regime*, page 117.)

WIGS AND HAIRPIECES

Whether you are looking to disguise hair loss, or simply see a wig or hairpiece as a fun way of changing your look for a party, there is a wide range available at reasonable prices. Wigs and hairpieces have improved enormously in the last decade and now even top international stylists such as Nicky Clarke offer a wig-cutting service. But do seek expert advice and do shop around. Support organisations such as Hairline International offer information. Leading suppliers are listed in the DIRECTORY.

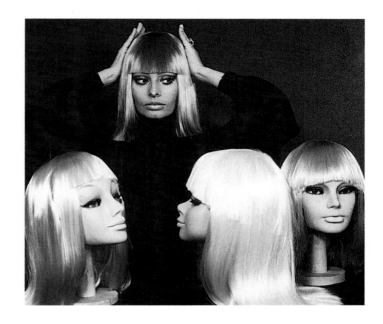

HOW TO HAVE MORE HAIR

Not so long ago, there was only one way to acquire longer hair – and it entailed months of angst, frustration and battling against the urge to snip it all off again with the nearest pair of secateurs or nail clippers, before the desired length had been achieved. But increasingly, women – from **Madonna** to **Tina Turner** to **Carly Simon** – are opting for hair extensions. Top hairdresser Orlando Pita believes extensions are a fabulous way of experimenting with a new hair look, not to mention the only way to go from short to long in an afternoon. 'I think of it as the ultimate in versatility,' explains Orlando. 'And if you don't like it, you can go back to how you were – fast.' Hair extensions are also useful for adding extra body to thin or fine hair.

There are two sorts of hair extensions. The first is made either of monofibres (acrylic) or real hair, which is then heat-bonded to your own hair, lasting for weeks or even months before it needs replacing.

The extensions are then 'snapped' out of the hair, leaving your own hair as before. The alternative is the temporary, clip-in, clip-out hair extensions, which stylists such as Orlando like to play with on the catwalk and for photo sessions.

Extensions can be colour-matched to your own hair, or used to provide lowlights or highlights. They are styled with your own hair, though obviously they don't grow as your own hair does, so you need regular salon upkeep. Although they are popular with young, fashion-conscious women, Orlando thinks they are a great way for older women to overcome the problem of thinning hair.

A big fan of hair extensions is **Naomi Campbell**. Actually, reveals Orlando, she has what we call a 'weave', 'But a very, very good one, which is actually sewn into her own hair.' This explains why, when she was growing it out, Naomi didn't have to endure the same agonies as most of us.

For details of where to get extended, see DIRECTORY.

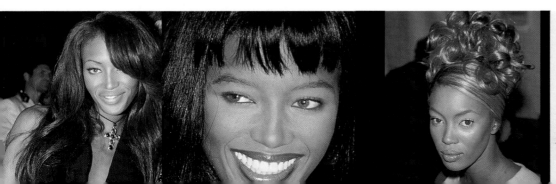

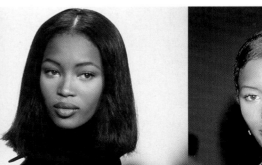

SHAMPOOING YOUR HAIR

It sounds like kindergarten stuff, but experts say that many hair problems occur because people don't know how to wash their hair properly (see *Dealing with Dandruff*, page 116). An estimated one in three people don't use a shower attachment to wet and rinse their hair, relying instead on dunking it under the bathwater or pouring over a few jugs of water. To work effectively, most modern haircare formulations need plenty of water to remove the dirt and release the conditioning agents.

How often should you wash your hair? Expert advice differs between daily and twice a week. The sensible solution is that if it's looking good, don't change your routine. If it isn't and you are washing it every three days or so, try washing it daily in a gentle shampoo and always follow with a suitable conditioner. If you wash it every day and are disappointed, first of all try different products, then less frequent washing, starting with alternate days.

Many people believe their hair gets used to one product and will benefit from frequent changes. This is, in fact, true, says trichologist and biochemist Dr Hugh Rushton – particularly with some of the newer polymer volumising products. So do switch every so often.

How to Wash Your Hair

◆ Wet hair in the warmest water your scalp can stand.

◆ Apply about a dessertspoonful of shampoo – less for short hair, more for really long. Using more shampoo than you need won't result in cleaner hair. Always apply from the palm of your hand, not the tube, so you can judge the amount. In soft water areas, or if you have a water softener, you won't need so much.

◆ Use the pads of your fingers, not your nails, to massage shampoo into the scalp, then work through to the ends of the hair – massaging, rather than rubbing, to avoid tangles.

◆ Rinse thoroughly.

◆ Repeat the whole process if you don't wash it daily.

◆ Squeeze out the extra moisture with your hands before you apply conditioner. Massage conditioner onto your hair

(especially the ends, not your scalp) and leave on for the recommended time.

◆ Blot hair dry with a fluffy towel – don't rub or wring hair as it is at its weakest when wet. Use a second towel to wrap around your hair; leave it on for a few minutes to absorb excess moisture.

◆ To prevent split ends, apply a dab of conditioner to the ends of the hair before using a hairdryer, curling iron or heated rollers. (Try to avoid using these last two too often.)

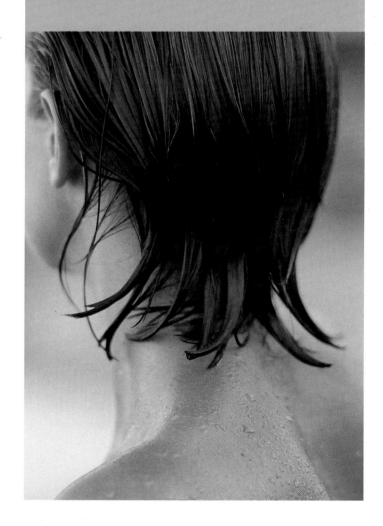

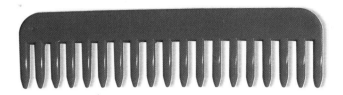

TIP Wash your brush/comb frequently – at least once a week – with warm water and a little shampoo. Or dissolve a tablespoon of washing soda in warm water, add a little antiseptic and agitate your brush/comb briskly in the mixture.

COMING CLEAN

What's in a shampoo? The main constituents are water, surfactant (soapless detergent) and perfume. Surfactant breaks down the natural sebum (oil) on your hair, so when you rinse it this goes down the plug-hole along with the dirt and grime that's collected on your hair. Lathering, incidentally, has nothing to do with a product's efficiency – it's purely cosmetic. (Some of the home-made shampoos we suggest in *Botanical Hair Beauty Secrets*, see page 135, hardly lather at all, but they work perfectly well.) Preservatives are added, to guard against contamination. Thickening agents bolster the texture. There may be other additives: keratin (*Hair protein*), amino acids and hydrolised protein, which is picked up by the hair and fills out gaps in the cuticle, boosting shine and making hair appear thicker. On the whole, manufacturers' claims for hair products are a pretty accurate guide to what suits your hair type – whether fair, fine or dry, etc.

Will a shampoo with vitamins help my hair? Hair can't absorb vitamins – with the exception of vitamin B5 (panthenol). Studies have shown that B5 penetrates the hair shaft, which is why it is increasingly used in shampoo formulations to improve condition.

Will a time-saving 2-in-1 product do the trick? These are fine when you're in a hurry, but if you use them on a regular basis your hair may not be getting all the conditioning it needs.

How quickly should you see results?

Intensive conditioners/hair masks: Immediate improvements, but long-term results are cumulative, if used once or twice weekly.
Dandruff shampoo: Two weeks for an improvement, six weeks to banish symptoms.

What's in a conditioner? When we say hair is 'out of condition', this refers to the state of the cuticles or surface scales on the hair shaft. If these are damaged through styling, drying, chemicals, etc., the result is lack of shine and bounce. Conditioners make hair shiny by depositing a lubricant on the hair, together with a 'cationic agent', techno-speak for an ingredient which delivers a positive electric charge to the lubricant, enabling it to cling to the hair. It also reduces static electricity, making styling easier and preventing flyaway hair.

Does greasy hair need a conditioner? First question is whether you really have greasy hair: try shampooing daily and see if it improves. If you still have a greasy scalp, use a very light conditioner, just scrunching it onto the ends, then rinse with head forward so the conditioner doesn't run down onto the scalp.

Should you buy your shampoo and conditioner from your hairdresser? This depends on how much you trust your hairdresser. On the plus side, no one else knows your hair as well, and so he/she should be able to suggest a tailor-made haircare prescription. But remember you may pay more for salon products. (And if you don't like them, you could be stuck with something expensive that seems to last forever because products tend to come in salon sizes.)

What about 'designer haircare'? Most top hairdressers – from Vidal Sassoon onwards – have now started formulating their own ranges: partly because they are anxious not to splash their name across inferior products and partly because they may reap rich rewards. Unless you get to see the great man (or, less likely, woman), it's pretty well pot luck if a product suits you, as with any other range whatever the source – supermarket, chemist or salon. The best advice is to ask your hairdresser what he/she suggests, have an expert hair analysis (see page 118) or, for real problems, consult a trichologist.

DEALING WITH DANDRUFF

Dandruff affects nearly everyone at some time in their lives. The word itself is used as an umbrella term to describe every kind of scalp condition which leads to visible flaking. Real dandruff, however, is caused by an increase in a natural yeast, *Pityrosporum ovale*, which results in a disturbance in the normal shedding of skin cells – and so leads to 'shoulder snow'.

Dandruff is not the only reason behind flaking: skin cells shed all the time, but the process can be speeded up for a number of reasons. Stress is one trigger for an almost immediate downpour. Another common culprit is using a shampoo with too high a surfactant (detergent) content.

As a first line of attack, biochemist and trichologist Dr Hugh Rushton suggests washing hair every day or every other day with a mild shampoo (not a specifically formulated anti-dandruff shampoo). Most medium-priced products do a good job; choose one which leaves your hair feeling fresh and shiny. Soak your hair thoroughly, then apply a good blob of shampoo, about a dessertspoonful. Rub into the scalp well, then rinse very thoroughly. Flaking can also be the result of inadequate rinsing because the shampoo residue disturbs the inter-cellular cement, or 'glue', which binds the skin cells together. If you shampoo your hair every day, use one application; if you prefer to shampoo less frequently, use two applications, with a slightly smaller one to start with. You may notice some flaking at first but this should soon settle down. If you wish to use a conditioner, apply it to the hair ends only.

Try this washing regime for four weeks; if after this time the condition doesn't improve, you may have real dandruff. Try using an anti-dandruff shampoo such as Head & Shoulders or Vosene twice a week, on alternate shampoos. (There are suggestions that high levels of coal tar in shampoos may be implicated in cancer; you may wish to check your anti-dandruff shampoo does not contain it.) Some sufferers have even found a 'no-wash regime' beneficial (see opposite). Dandruff can be triggered or made worse by stress, so take sufficient exercise, get enough sleep, eat a good diet and consider learning stress reduction techniques (see page 185 and DIRECTORY).

If, however, the flaking is associated with red patches on your scalp or eyebrows, or down the folds running from nose to mouth, possibly accompanied by itching, you don't have dandruff but a mild form of eczema. Try cutting out all dairy products for a month. If the condition doesn't improve, ask your doctor to refer you to a dermatologist or trichologist.

Trichologist Philip Kingsley suggests making your own anti-flaking tonic with equal quantities of any mouthwash and witch hazel. Shampoo, then apply conditioner to the ends of hair only. Rinse well, dry gently with a towel and, before styling, sprinkle the mixture all over your scalp.

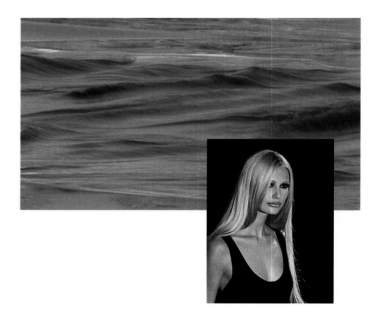

TIPS FROM THE TOP

To prevent hair product build-up, every few months actress **Jaclyn Smith** whips up a deep-cleanser: half a cup of white vinegar mixed into a quart of boiling water. Shampoo the cooled solution into just-washed hair, then rinse with ice-cold water.

THE NO-WASH REGIME

Some people, including dandruff sufferers, swear by not washing their hair at all. You will need, however, to groom it by combing and rinsing with water daily. It may look awful for the first four to six weeks but should then recover; hair has its own natural balance which is disturbed by washing and conditioning, but in time it settles down and becomes literally self-cleaning. This method is fine for people with thick hair but may not work so well for the more sparsely endowed who need the extra volume given by shampoo, or for women who like to style their hair. However, we have heard of some extraordinary results in men with thinning hair who have adopted a 'no-wash' regime; their hair has started to grow back.

TRIED & TESTED

HAIR MASKS

These used to be called intensive (or deep) conditioners, but are now increasingly marketed as the once- or twice-a-week hair equivalent of a face mask. We asked testers to mark on ease of application, instant gloss, manageability, bounce and body. There were a lot of good products, of which the following excelled.

Top Treats

Estée Lauder Herbal Hair Pack

Although it's expensive, this was considered to be the best all-round treat, with rave reviews for the deliciously herbal smell.
COMMENTS: 'non-messy and easy to use, with great condition, shine and bounce', 'it didn't drip down my neck even though I had it on for 20 minutes', 'my hairdresser – who makes his own range of products – said how impressed he was with the results'.

Lancôme Fluance Extra Rich Cream Conditioner

This intensive conditioner is from a small new range of hair products by the top French skincare name, and scored very well all round.
COMMENTS: 'made my hair glossy and silky', 'loved it – because it worked on my thin hair', 'smelt lovely'.

E'SPA Pink Hair and Scalp Mud

This clay-based mask is designed to help dry scalp problems as well as boost hair condition, without leaving hair in any way greasy.
COMMENTS: 'my hair felt soft and silky', 'this was a healing experience as well as soothing and cooling to the scalp', 'delicious to use, with good results...very pampering and treatful'.

Nu-Skin Hair Fitness Glacial Therapy

This product contains mud, as a deep treatment, together with botanical ingredients. Don't be put off by the slightly unappealing grey colour!
COMMENTS: 'my hair instantly felt silkier and fuller', 'lovely product – my hair felt thick, looked shiny and wasn't full of static, which it normally is'.

Best Budget Buys

Pantène Intensives Conditioner

This product features Pro-Vitamin B5, a vitamin that can actually be absorbed into the hair shaft.
COMMENTS: 'I'd recommend this to my friends', 'brilliant', 'made my hair really shiny, but I probably only need it for the ends'.

St Ives Swiss Formula Mud Miracle

Although this is mud-based, it looks and feels much like a normal conditioner, and is easy to use.
COMMENTS: 'the fact that it only takes two minutes is a major plus', 'it really invigorated my scalp and made my hair feel soft and manageable', 'I liked this almost as much as the Estée Lauder Herbal Hair Pack!'

Special Mention

Origins Happy Endings Conditioner

COMMENTS: 'a brilliant product – my hair looked and felt perfect, body-wise', 'delicious citrussy smell'.

GETTING THE PERFECT HAIRCUT

World famous hair stylist John Frieda spells out the vital guildelines.

There is a moment when you know you are ready for a new look. Logic seldom plays a part in this life-changing decision; more often it's a subconscious bid for freedom. You may not be able to leave your safe job, with mortgage and pension rights, or your nice but uninspiring man, or even buy a new wardrobe, but no one can stop you going for a new hairstyle.

Practically speaking, shearing off your mane has a lot going for it. It boosts the hair's condition, whatever type you have, gives movement and bounce (once it hits your shoulders, hair lies stock still) and makes hair easier to maintain. Most importantly, a flattering cut can enhance every face shape.

Satisfaction, however, is not guaranteed. Most of us have gone into a salon buoyed up with the hope that we will be transformed by Mr Golden Scissorhands, then slunk out afterwards longing for an all-concealing cloche hat. So what goes wrong? Quite simply, G. Scissorhands, who may actually be a megastar in the styling world, decides to plonk a hairstyle on your head which does not suit you. Even more astonishingly, you let him.

'There are a lot of good hairdressers, but there's always some risk in having your hair cut, and many people have had distressing experiences,' acknowledges John Frieda. He advises: 'Never ever have your hair cut the day before something important – get it done a week or two before so that if something goes wrong you have a chance to do something about it.' Personal fashion consultant Amanda Platt advises you to take charge yourself: 'Be mistress of your own hairstyle.' Remember, you want a hairstyle, not necessarily the latest fashion cut. 'If a cut is right for you, it's right absolutely,' points out John Frieda. 'After all, your face shape doesn't change with the seasons.'

For many women, the ideal hairdresser is as much, if not more, of a prize than the most engaging escort. Be prepared to put in time (see opposite). At a consultation, thoroughly discuss what the stylist proposes doing, suggests John Frieda. (The consultation should be free but be prepared to fit in with his or her schedule.) If you don't like the stylist or the salon, don't go back.

If the worst happens and you hate your shorn mane, it's not a life sentence. Hair grows at the rate of 15cm (6in) a year, so it will take two years maximum to get it back to shoulder length. But, however desperate you are for it to grow, do have it trimmed regularly. Most hairdressers suggest a trim every four weeks for short hair, four to six weeks for medium-length hair and up to eight weeks for long hair.

BEFORE YOU CUT

◆ Schedule time for a consultation before you commit yourself. Most stylists work to a tight schedule, and can't always take the time they should to discuss what you want for your hair. Salons should be able to book you in for a ten-minute (free) chat to talk things over before the appointment (maybe even several days before).

◆ Make sure you choose a supportive stylist. It's worth shopping around – and having more than one consultation if necessary – to discover someone who sincerely listens to you and is on your side. You shouldn't feel shy or uncomfortable about showing them a photo that's dramatically different from your current look; it may be just what's needed to pep up your appearance. They should also be able to give you sound advice on any hair problems, such as condition. If ever you sense that your stylist's ego is getting between them and the best interests of your hair, it's time to move on.

HOW TO LOOK AT YOUR HAIR

It's not creativity you need when assessing what hairstyle will suit you, explains John Frieda, but the ability to see yourself as you really are. First of all, tie your hair back so that you can study the shape of your face. Then, if possible, he advises standing in between two long mirrors placed at a 45° angle from each other: 'Look at the reflection of your image in the second mirror so that you see yourself as others see you. You can be more objective like this.'

WHAT TO LOOK FOR

When thinking about different styles, consider three criteria, says Frieda. Any hairstyle problem you have will fall into these.

1) Face Shape

This is defined by your hairline, by the width and length of your face and by its proportions (how features relate to each other). Remember also to look at your face and neck from the side. The basic face shapes are:

A CLASSIC OVAL FACE: this can take any style: with the other face shapes, the aim should be to create the illusion of an oval shape for the face and head silhouette.

A ROUND FACE: the hair should be cut onto the cheeks to shade them and narrow down the sides. A soft feathery look is the most flattering – you don't want a flat sleek look.

A LONG FACE: this can be made to look less long with a fringe and a chin-length cut which is fuller at the bottom to add width. Anything but a long straight bob, which will make you appear even more long-faced (and maybe even miserable).

A SQUARE FACE: avoid symmetry, short crops or anything geometric and go for soft curves which will hide the jaw.

HEART-SHAPED FACES: these look good with a kicking-out bob, which gives volume round the bottom of the face.

> **TIP** The way to disguise a high, low or uneven hairline is to have a fringe. Nicky Clarke, the man who famously de-frumped Fergie, points out there are 'At least 50 ways of cutting fringes, from the Cleopatra block to Claudia Schiffer's wisps...so don't decide a fringe won't suit you.'

The Crucial Jawline

The distance and angle between your earlobe and your chin is the defining factor in deciding the length of your hair, according to John Frieda. 'It's the most important proportion,' he believes.

'If that distance is short and you've got a sharp angle where the jaw turns and goes almost horizontal, like Audrey Hepburn or Isabella Rossellini, you can wear virtually any length hair or have it swept up.'

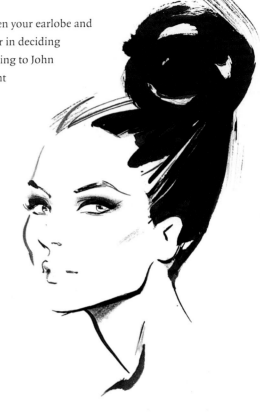

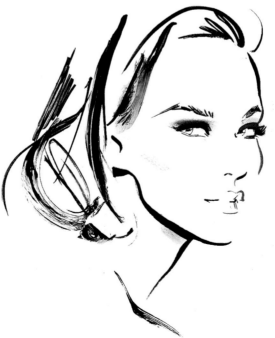

'If your jaw is long and sloping like, say, Jerry Hall, you can't wear *really* short hair – it exposes your jaw and is unflattering, whether it's a cheek-length Chanel bob or drawn back into a very severe style,' says John Frieda.

TIP Fringes can disguise patches of thinning hair at the temples. Grading the sides of longer hair from the fringe downwards can be very flattering – it's the gentle, casual look you get when you are growing out a fringe.

2) Head Shape

Look at yourself full on and sideways, and at the relation of your head to your body.

Ask yourself: what is the shape of my head? Do I need more height or less? A little more or a little less width across my face? What does my head look like in proportion to my body?

A good haircut doesn't start and end above your neck. The ratio of your head to your body is vital. The classic example of what can go wrong was Charlene Tilton in *Dallas*, whose long wavy hair romped around a head that disappeared almost straight into her elevated bosom and short body. You also need to consider head size, neck length and width of shoulders. A close-cut Eton crop on a small head with long neck and wide shoulders is unlikely to look balanced. Examine your clothes too: a big winter coat may look great with a swinging page-boy bob, but will hopelessly overwhelm a much shorter-layered urchin cut.

TIP Michael Rasser of Michaeljohn recommends slimming down a thick neck by taking the hair behind the ears, then bringing it forward to curve softly onto the neck.

TIP For the longer jaw, Frieda recommends an adaptable chin-length cut: 'Though it could be slightly shorter, say, level with the crease between your mouth and the bottom of the chin. It's worth scrutinising your chin; if it sticks out you may need an extra half inch in length as well as volume at the bottom; try also drying the ends under to soften the jawline.'

3) Surface and Texture of Hair

What styles should you consider to make the best of your hair type?

For instance, if your hair is FINE AND FLYAWAY, think about having a short, layered cut – it's easier to manage and will give your hair body. Talk to your hairdresser about how he/she will layer your hair. 'The layers shouldn't be of equal length,' says John Frieda. 'The problem areas are in a circle going from your forehead right round your head, where the head is sloping down and the hair grows in a downwards direction so there is no natural lift. So it's vital the layers there should be shorter to give you height and volume, gradually getting longer all the way down – unless you want it very wispy at the bottom.'

If you have THICK, UNCONTROLLABLY FRIZZY OR CURLY HAIR, the number one rule according to John Frieda is to avoid extreme layering. This type of hair expands upwards and outwards at every opportunity, and needs its own weight to stay down. However, gradual layers may be desirable around the hairline (to soften it) and at the bottom of the hair (to stop it flying out). Whether you cut it short or long depends primarily on the face shape, but a very short style, if it suits you, may make life easier. Maintaining good condition is essential for all frizzy hair, particularly if you have long pre-Raphaelite tresses. Since this type of hair tends to dry and split at the ends, John Frieda recommends trimming it every month; this is even more important, he insists, if it is very long.

TO BRUSH OR NOT TO BRUSH?

Our grandmothers would argue that brushing hair was its best beauty treatment. But that was when brushing was hair's only conditioner. Now that we have a galaxy of products to stimulate shine, brushing has come under fire for damaging hair, with some experts saying brushes should only be used as styling tools.

Top colourist Jo Hansford, however, protests that she, like many of us, would miss tipping her head upside down and giving her hair a good brush. She prefers a wooden brush with a cushion base and soft, flexible wooden bristles. A good solution, according to Dr Hugh Rushton, is always to detangle your hair before brushing by combing it, from the ends up, with a wide tooth comb. Hard rubber (vulcanite) combs, such as the range by Kent, are anti-static, easy to clean and moderately priced.

HOW TO SPEAK YOUR HAIRDRESSER'S LANGUAGE – IN PICTURES

Pictures taken from a magazine can be a great way of communicating with your stylist. Trying to describe the look you want can be tough because words such as 'feathering', 'wispy', 'layers', 'fringe' can mean a different look to you and a stylist. Think what happens, for instance, when you ask for only 'half an inch off'; it can show all too disastrously how your mental tape measure differs from your hairdresser's. A picture can give vital clues. Here are a few tips to making it work best for you.

◆ Before you go to the stylist, consider whether it is in fact the mood of the picture and the overall look that has seduced you. Separate the model's clothes and face from the haircut, and see if it still seems as appealing. (Having your hair cut like Catherine Deneuve's won't turn you into her – besides, we've heard that she goes to the hairdresser's once a day, sometimes twice.)

◆ Using the guides we have given, work out whether the model's cut will suit your face shape, hairline, bone structure and neck length. Discuss these points with the stylist at the consultation.

◆ When you do talk to the stylist, also ask if that cut will suit your hair texture. We always want the kind of hair we haven't got – but even Nicky Clarke can't turn fine, limp hair into a Farrah-esque mane. It may be that you could achieve the look in the picture but it would take 45 minutes of daily styling. Remember, the model probably has great hair naturally – apart from the fact that it was twirled and tweaked for hours to look that way for the shoot. Just outside the frame of the picture is the hairdresser with comb and spray can at the ready.

JOHN FRIEDA'S BLOWDRYING TIPS

◆ Get your hair to the point of being almost dry before you start styling. The critical time is when it's turning from wet to dry – whatever you do then will get locked into the hair.

◆ Start with your hairline; that's the bit that shows.

◆ Do the hair on top of your head before the underneath. Imagine looking down on your head and see it as a big diamond shape. Again, it's the important part that everyone·will see.

◆ If you've got time, then dry the underneath.

JOHN FRIEDA'S STYLING TIPS

◆ Pump up the volume on DEAD STRAIGHT HAIR by applying thickening lotion near to the roots and dry with your head upside down. Avoid using too many styling products.

◆ Use a thickening spray at the roots and a finishing spray to control FINE, FLYAWAY HAIR. You need to avoid static, so don't brush excessively or blowdry on a hot setting. Also try washing your brush or comb before use, then shaking dry.

◆ De-frizz BUSHY HAIR with serum products that coat the hair in a fine, light film (Frizz-Ease is the bestselling product in America). Don't towel dry and avoid heated styling tools. Once you've styled your hair, keep out of steamy bathrooms.

◆ As there are very few truly efficient styling brushes available to private customers, ask your hairdresser to get professional brushes for you: he/she will know exactly which ones you need.

TIPS Use a brush with a rounded cushion, which stops hair being tugged by the bristles ◆ Brush tangled hair from the ends; if you start at the top, you'll just pull the tangles into a clump ◆ Always use your brush gently; try not to pull or twist the hair too much, especially when blowdrying.

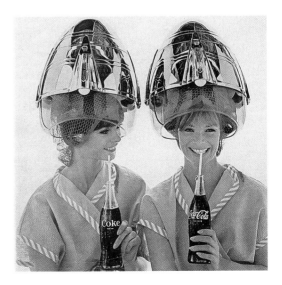

THE SECRETS OF THE HAIR STARS

The world's top hairdressers are able to make cover girls look like goddesses – and ordinary women look simply sensational. What they don't know about how to work wonders with difficult hair could be enscribed on the back of a Kirby-grip. They possess the secrets of a great cut (and how to keep it that way), and are masters of the art of blowdrying. Here is what some of them have to say on achieving high-style, low-maintenance, head-turning hair...

NICKY CLARKE

Nicky Clarke has clients who travel from Sydney to London twice a year for one of his haircuts. One regular jets in every six weeks from Barbados, and at any time there may be 100 clients on his waiting list, hoping for a cancellation so they, too, can experience the Clarke magic. Famous clients include Queen Noor of Jordan, Jerry Hall, Paula Yates and Yasmin Le Bon.

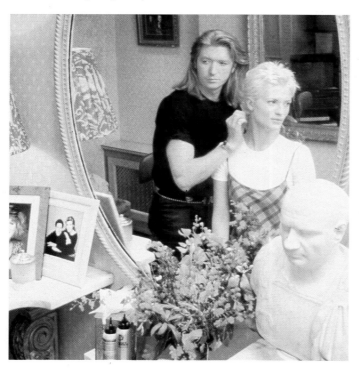

Unlike some stylists, whose trademark is hair that looks seriously 'done' (and won't move in a Force Ten gale), Nicky prefers a natural, casual look. 'A great haircut should look like you haven't tried too hard,' he believes.

Of course, it's easy for women who can afford the time and money for weekly blowdrys to have hair that looks a million dollars. But, assures Nicky, there are tricks of the trade which every hairdryer-owner could learn from.

✂ 'The right tools are essential – starting with the dryer. Most importantly, don't go for anything under 1500 watts. You're onto a winner if it has two air speeds and two heat settings. And if it's got a "cold" button for the last blast, even better.'

✂ 'A must for home styling is a "vent" brush, which is used to lift the roots or brush hair through. Then you need round boar-bristle brushes for styling. I've got a dozen – but only a hairdresser needs that many. If your hair's long, go for a large one; the shorter the hair, the smaller your brush should be. If you've got different lengths – maybe a fringe, or layers – you'll need more than one brush. Generally speaking, the brush should be just big enough to get it into the hair without wrapping the hair round and round it.'

✂ 'One good way to get body into your hair – especially if it's long – is to hang your head and dry your hair upside down. But it's much better to lean your head to one side, and, using the vent brush, lift the roots, putting a slight curve into them. Drying it in a gravity-defying position gives hair body. And after a certain age, all women need some volume; it's more flattering to the face. You have to be young to get away with that flat-against-the-head look.'

✂ 'Don't start styling your hair until it's 80 per cent dry – towel-dried or dryer-dried. That's the right time to apply styling products, too. If you use a styling brush before then, while you're getting rid of the moisture, you'll knock all the natural body out of your hair. This is probably the commonest mistake women – and plenty of hairdressers – make. If you've got frizzy hair, though, you can afford to have it a little damper before you start styling.'

✂ 'The big debate is whether you should use mousse, gel or lotion. I always prefer a lotion, because it's lighter, but it's basically a matter of personal preference. Gels do tend to give a stronger hold, so they may be the best choice if you really want your hair to stay put.'

✂ 'Styling's all in the wrist action. But try switching the hand you hold the dryer in; you'll find it easier to make both sides look symmetrical, if that's what you're after. It feels tricky at first but practice soon makes perfect.'

✂ 'I often prescribe a sixties-style hood dryer – like Braun's – and Velcro rollers. People reel in horror, but it's actually time-saving, provided you start when your hair's already 80 per cent dry. Take big sections, stick in big Velcro rollers and sit under it for ten minutes while you do your make-up. The final effect may be too much body, but it's always easier to take volume out, with a big brush, than put it in.'

✂ 'If you've got the kind of hair that's fine and delicate and tends to blow around, then a light holding of spray is fine. The problem with many sprays is that, in order to do the job, they dull the hair. What you want is a spray that holds and shines. And don't ever brush it through afterwards – you're just brushing the spray right out again.'

ORLANDO PITA

Fashion starts on the catwalk – and so, too, does hair style, and for the last few years the influence of New Yorker Orlando Pita – recently appointed as International Artistic Director of John Frieda – has been visible everywhere. Orlando has created hairstyles for designer shows at Chanel, Dolce & Gabanna, Jean-Paul Gaultier and Donna Karan. When you first see them on the catwalk, they can look outrageous. But within months, wearable versions of those styles are invariably seen on women in the street.

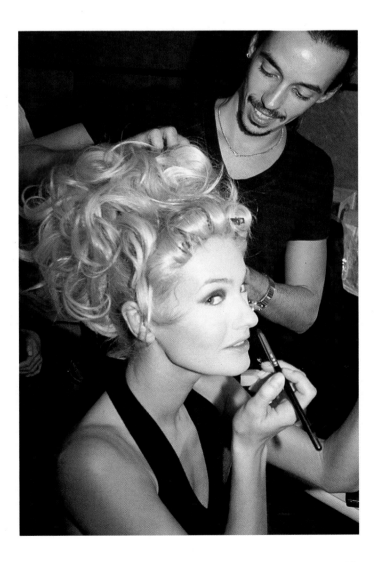

Orlando is a real favourite both with supermodels (**Naomi Campbell**, **Amber Valletta**, **Shalom Harlow**) and superstars (**Madonna** – even she has learned to book Orlando months in advance – describes him as 'an angel sent down from heaven to do my hair'). But while he may be the ultimate showman, Orlando has something to teach those of us who need wash-and-go styles.

✂ Great looks on anyone must start with hair that is in optimum condition. Orlando's prescription is 'regular deep-conditioning treatments or hair masks, preferably once a week. Leave-in conditioners are a help – and silicone-based hair "serums".' The silicone has an almost miraculous effect, re-glossing and sleeking hair. The best serum, in Orlando's opinion, is Frizz-Ease, the number one styling product in the US.

✂ He often uses leave-in conditioner as a pre-styling hair re-moisturiser, too, working it into hair that's been dried, 'because it gets rid of that just-washed, floppy look.'

✂ Orlando explains that models are also super-careful with their scalps, not just the hair itself; regular head massages (with or without aromatherapy oils) keep the scalp healthy and can help prevent dandruff.

✂ Despite the fact that bleaching and perming are notorious for damaging hair, Orlando likes to work with hair that's been chemically 'processed'. 'When hair has been permed or dyed, it is much easier to style. It's porous, so it absorbs styling products better, and holds a style longer.'

> ✂ Orlando truly believes it's a shame to cover up grey hair. 'I love grey hair; I don't think it makes women look old unless they start behaving like a grey-haired old woman. You don't have to colour it: maybe just put in a bold streak of what used to be your real hair colour at the front. Team that with a nifty navy suit – rather than your favourite old cardigan – and the result is head-turningly stylish.'

Orlando's Essentials
- ◆ J.F. Lazartigue boar-bristle brushes
- ◆ John Frieda's Photo Session thickening lotion
- ◆ Velcro rollers
- ◆ Frizz-Ease hair serum
- ◆ Denman styling brush
- ◆ Kiehl's leave-in conditioner
- ◆ Aveda paddle brush
- ◆ BaByliss curling tongs

✂ 'When women get to 50, they seem to think they have to have their hair cut short and permed,' Orlando observes. 'Because their hair gets thin as they get older, they think it'll give the impression of having more hair. But it's a look that's instantly ageing.' He prefers to see stylish bobs, ultra-short pixie cuts – even steel-grey plaits...

✂ Hair colour has to be either very natural or very obvious. 'I prefer great sun-bleached surfer-style streaks to those teeny little highlights,' says Orlando.

✂ Orlando is also a big fan of fake hair – wigs and extensions – because it helps prevent 'style stagnation'. 'A wig is a great way of playing with a different look.' And a better way to build volume in thinning hair than perming, he believes, is to use tiny clip-in clip-out hair extensions, which can be colour-matched to hair or provide low- or highlights, then cut and styled with your own hair, in-salon. (For more details, see page 113.)

✂ If you like a 'big hair' look, with flattering oomph at the roots, Orlando knows a fail-safe technique. 'Some women – **Cindy Crawford**, for instance – are blessed with the kind of hair which acquires volume if you just dry it upside down.' But the rest of us, advises Orlando, should invest in some thickening lotion and a set of large Velcro rollers. 'Then blowdry your hair till it's nearly dry and wind it, in big chunks, around six or eight Velcro rollers. Leave it while you finish getting ready. Then take out the rollers and – if your hair still needs it – tease it gently at the roots with a brush.'

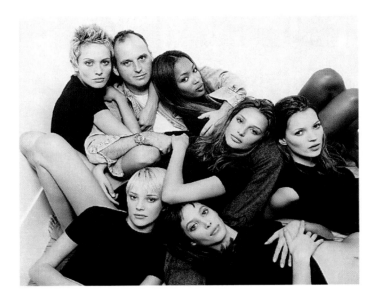

SAM McKNIGHT

Think of a beautiful fashion photo in the last decade and Sam McKnight probably had something to do with it. As *Vogue* put it: 'Sam McKnight doesn't look much like a supermodel – but he's the nearest thing the hairdressing industry has to one.' (He also just happens to be personal hairdresser to Diana, Princess of Wales.)

✂ Sam believes that we can all make more of our hair. 'Most women go to the hairdresser to have it trimmed, but that's wasting a fantastic opportunity to learn more about how to curl it, flip it or pin it up, to get a whole new look from the same haircut. You can learn far more from your hairdresser, face to face, than from any glossy magazine picture in the world. It's the best place to learn to use rollers or a blowdryer.'

✂ 'It's amazing what you can do with your hair if you just try,' he says. 'You just need someone – preferably your hairdresser – to show you how. I think it's wonderful to reinvent yourself, like **Linda Evangelista** constantly does. People should do that more in real life: try a colour, buy a can of gel, grease your hair back. Put a parting in your hair and scrape it back severely, put on a fake ponytail or build up big, big hair for the night. It's not permanent, it's a moment. I'm all for people being more adventurous.'

Sam McKnight has created his own signature styling range, which is well and truly 'supermodel-tested' (see Directory). But to stock up on hair accessories, he heads for a beauty supplies store in New York called Ricky's, on 4th Street. 'It's an absolute treasure trove for anyone who's interested in hair and beauty.'

✂ Your bank manager may not be thrilled to hear this but Sam believes that we don't go to the hairdresser enough. 'It takes a third party to look in the mirror and know what you ought to do next. We all have fixed ideas about our looks, and get stuck. I think you're lucky if you know yourself when it's time for a change. Someone else can look at your hair, however, and say, "You should cut some layers, or maybe make it blonde at the front," and it can make all the difference in the world.'

✂ If you haven't found one salon you're happy with, he advises you to experiment with having your hair blowdried in different salons before risking a cut. Settle on a place that feels comfortable and – crucially – friendly. 'A lot of salons are pretty scary and need to lighten up. I can't stand those "how would Modom like her hair?" kinds of places.'

✂ Sam is a big fan of back-combing to give hair more body – which has always been considered bad for hair. Sam says the way to avoid hair damage is, 'once you've teased it into bigness, to tease it out again with a big, soft brush such as a Mason Pearson. That way hair won't break off.'

Sam McKnight's Essentials
◆ Velcro rollers
◆ Denman styling brush
◆ Mason Pearson extra-firm bristle brush
◆ Clairol Set-To-Go travel hot rollers
◆ Braun cordless curling iron
◆ Vidal Sassoon 3-in-1 styling iron

CRACKING THE HAIR COLOUR CODE

A few decades ago, saying a woman dyed her hair was equivalent to calling her a painted hussy. Today, changing your hair colour is as acceptable as changing lipsticks.

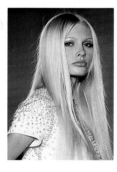

Modern products are brilliant both for colour and condition and a far cry from the dead peroxide blonde, garish red or matt flat black that used to be our only options. The right hair colour can flatter your skin tone, make your eyes sparkle and your whole face come alive.

Unfortunately, satisfaction is not guaranteed and, unlike your new lipstick, you can't just wipe off the colour and start again. A good number of the women we know who colour their hair have had some sort of disappointment or disaster. We asked Britain's leading colour expert Jo Hansford to give us the lowdown on getting results, both at home and in the salon, to lift looks and spirit.

JO HANSFORD'S GUIDELINES

◆ Your hair is the frame around your face, so the tone is really important. Sit yourself in front of a good mirror in a good clear light, with no make-up. Really study yourself and say, 'I'm going to be totally truthful.' Take your hair, hold it against your face and analyse what colour skin you have: is it pale; do you have high colour with broken veins; is it basically pink or are there yellow or sallow tones; do you have olive skin? What colour are your eyes and how does your hair look with them? How dark are your brows? (Remember you can lighten or darken them as well.) Finally, ask yourself, 'Does the colour I have now actually suit me?'

◆ If the answer is yes, forget all about hair colour. If the answer is no, or if you are bored with your existing colour, go on to the next stage.

◆ Now consider what hair colour would enhance your skin tone. Don't forget to bear in mind the texture of your hair as well. Is it thin and fine or thick and coarse? Thin hair is usually better with an overall colour, which will need to be retouched every four weeks on average; thick hair suits highlights or lowlights, which don't need so much attention.

◆ Colour is flexible but, generally, very short straight or straightish hair doesn't suit highlights because they look almost leopard-like; lights are perfect, however, on short wavy or curly hair. All-over colour looks good on practically any style.

◆ Now is the time to go on to seek some objective advice about changing the colour. Even if you don't end up having your colour done by a professional, it is worth consulting several for advice.

◆ When choosing a colourist, go for an expert who specialises in colour, not a hairdresser and permer who also colours.

◆ Interview several (most will give you a free five-minute consultation, but aim to book in at a time they're not rushed off their feet); mull over their ideas carefully before deciding.

◆ Take along pictures of colours and effects you have in mind; descriptions are notoriously imprecise – what's red to you may be deep auburn to a colourist.

◆ Be honest with the colourist about what you've done to your hair previously, e.g. colour, perm, successes, failures.

◆ Check how much maintenance their recommendations will need, how much time it will take, and how much it will cost.

◆ Also check what happens if you don't like the new colour. Will the salon tone it down or change it after you have had a few days to get used to your new self? How much will the charge be?

◆ Ask to try on wigs and hairpieces, if available. They may not be the right fit or style, but you can see the general effect.

◆ Before you leave the consultation, look around at the staff: if you like their hair colours, chances are you'll like what happens to you; if not, wave them goodbye.

COVERING UP GREY HAIR

Half the population is grey by about 50, when the production of melanin (the pigment that gives hair its natural colour) stops. Some women look wonderful with grey hair but, if you feel less happy, you can successfully enhance, blend, disguise or cover your grey hair at home.

Up to 20 per cent grey: hide the first grey hairs with a vegetable or semi-permanent colour in the same shade as your natural hair. The result will last for six to eight shampoos, gradually washing out. Try Wella Colour Mousse, or have an individual veggie rinse prescription made up for you at Jo Hansford.

Up to 50 per cent grey: cover with a longer-lasting semi-permanent which stays for 12 to 20 shampoos. Try L'Oréal Casting, Wella Soft Color.

Up to 100 per cent grey: replace colour completely with a permanent chemical dye (remember roots will need retouching about every four weeks), which will last two to three months. Try Clairol Nice n' Easy, Poly Color Tint.

Don't forget you *can* go grey gracefully: there are now specialist products to enhance the silver in grey hair. Try Schwarzkopf Bonacure Silvergloss Shampoo (from salons only), Nexus Simply Silver Toning Shampoo, Phytangent Shampoo.

To keep the green out of grey – swimming in chlorinated water can result in chemical build-up and unsightly greenish tones – try Lamaur Nutra-Cleanz shampoo, Nexus Aloe Rid Clarifying Shampoo and Treatment.

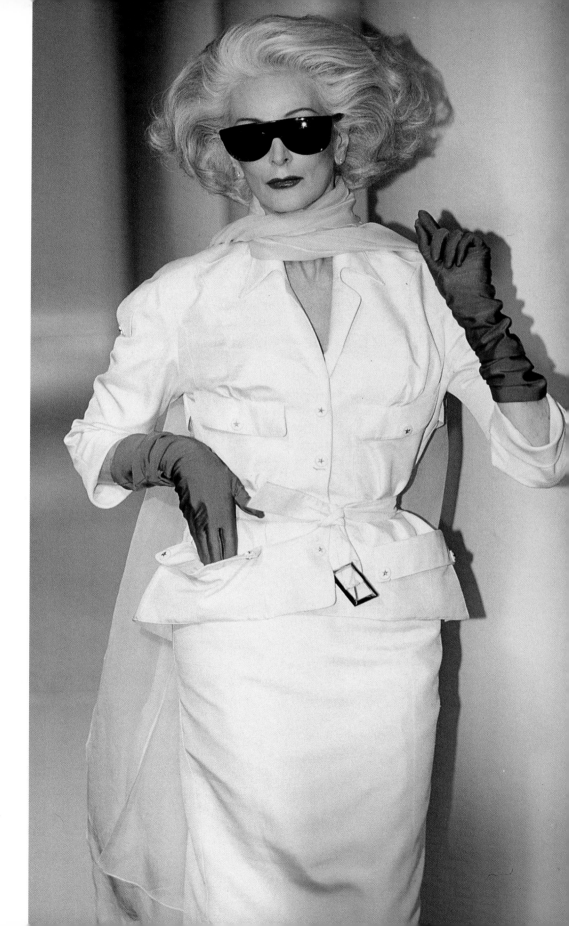

COLOUR CHART

Skin and Hair Colours

PINK SKIN: choose neutral tones: ash blonde, ash brown or dark brown. Red, blue/red or yellow blonde are usually a total disaster.

PALE WHITE, IVORY, CREAMY: the perfect skin for any hair colour. You can choose whatever you like – red, dark, pale – as your skin has no pink in it. Look at **Linda Evangelista**; she can be ash blonde one day and auburn the next because her skin and her eyes go with anything. Notice she also changes lip and eye colours to complement her hair.

YELLOW/SALLOW: go for dark rich tones with blue notes, such as burgundy or deep auburn, to counteract the sallowness in your skin.

OLIVE: stay dark – olive skin with dark hair is one of the most perfect combinations. To give interest, you could add a few rich lowlights in any of the red shades from burgundy to chestnut.

TIP FROM THE TOP

Traditionally, dark-haired women like to lighten their hair – but it sometimes happens the other way around. Hollywood actress **Winona Ryder** is actually bottle brunette. 'My hair colouring isn't just blonde, it's virtually white,' she reveals. 'I've got dark brown eyes and very pale skin so I look seriously weird unless I dye my hair and my eyebrows black. I also feel much more like a dark-haired person than a blonde. People expect you to be bubbly if you are blonde. I'm quite serious, so I feel this is my natural colour.'

Hair and Hair Colours

If your natural hair colour is ▼	So you want to go:		
	Blonde	Brunette	Red
Black	Don't even try it	Glossy black, blue black	Don't try it
Dark to light brown	Streaks: mid golden sunny or strawberry blonde	Black, dark chocolate auburn, dark honey	Auburn to fiery copper
Dark to light blonde	Warm shades: honey, copper, wheat, apricot, pale blonde	Milky brown, copper, honey, dark chestnut	Warmer shades: chestnut to apricot
Blonde to grey	Pale icy blonde or darker warm colours	Pale ash brown, copper brown, beige, milk chocolate	Don't try it
Red	Highlights: pale or bleached	Chestnut, auburn, dark brown	Leave it alone or add blonde

D-I-Y DYE: WHAT DOES IT ALL MEAN?

COLOUR-ENHANCING SHAMPOOS: wonderful conditioners with a hint of colour. Good for maintaining previously coloured hair.

TEMPORARY COLOURS: colourants held in styling products such as mousse. Will last one to three washes on virgin (uncoloured) hair. Don't use on permed or coloured hair.

HENNA: unlike modern vegetable rinses, henna is a permanent metallic stain; you can't lift it or put colour over it successfully. If you don't like it, you have to wait for it to grow out, which may take a year or more (hair grows at about half an inch a month). Nor can you perm hennaed hair.

CHEMICAL DYES: come in three types – semi-permanent, which last six to eight shampoos; longer-lasting semi-permanent, which last 12 to 20 shampoos; permanent, which last two to three months.

RETOUCHING ROOTS: vegetable dyes and semi-permanent colour fade without noticeable regrowth. Longer-lasting semi-permanents tend to leave a slight regrowth; permanent colour means that roots will need a fresh application every four weeks on average. Apply colour to new growth only; overlapping will produce a two-tone effect. Since retouching is tricky, it may help to get a friend or partner to do this for you.

NATURAL-V-CHEMICAL COLOUR: natural non-catalyst vegetable dyes (which are semi-permanent) coat the outer layer of hair with colour, whilst chemical dyes contain ammonia and peroxide which penetrate the hair shaft. Contrary to received wisdom, some modern chemical formulations are almost as gentle as their vegetable counterparts. However, a very small percentage of people are allergic to some chemicals, so it is vital to do a skin test on your inside arm before use.

TIPS If it's your first time, we suggest you don't go for drama. Choose a semi-permanent or vegetable rinse, a couple of shades lighter or darker than your natural colour. If you don't like it, wait for it to fade or wash it out with a shampoo labelled 'body building' or 'clarifying'. If you do like it and want a more definite change, then build up to it gradually. But however often you wash it, don't change your hair colour more than every three months at the very minimum; there may be residual colour lurking which could give you unexpected results. Whichever product you use, always follow the instructions carefully.

HAIR COLOUR UPKEEP

◆ As a general rule, don't go into the sun, the sea, the shower or, most important of all, a chlorinated swimming pool for 48 hours after you've had your hair coloured. During the colouring process, your hair cuticles open and are vulnerable to damage until they close again.

◆ Use a shampoo and conditioner specially formulated for colour-treated hair. Deep-cleansing shampoos will lift tint faster. Look for shampoos with panthenol to strengthen the hair shaft.

◆ Always wear a hat when sunbathing.

◆ Remember blonde highlights will go lighter in the sun, so warn your colourist if you are going off on a beach holiday.

◆ When swimming use a Speedo head-hugging cap, or protective cream. Find Speedo products at good sports shops and an increasing range of hair protective creams at chemists.

◆ UV light may also fade colour faster, so wash hair daily with a shampoo containing UV protectants.

CURL TALK – THE SECRETS OF PERFECT PERMING

Perming is the hairdressing process that there's (almost) no turning back from. Although there is no magic way to ensure perm perfection, following expert advice will at least give you a head start.

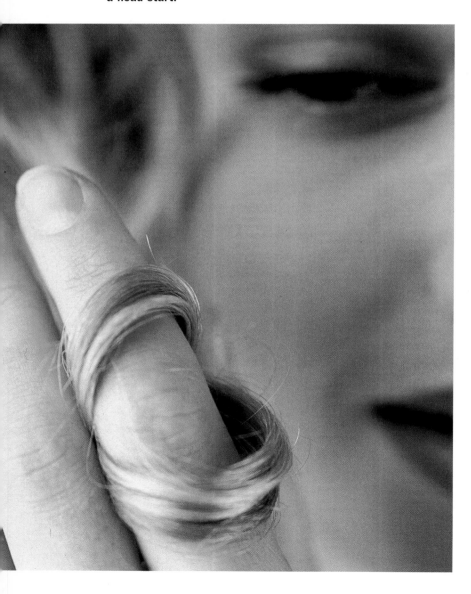

Perming technology hasn't advanced much in 50 years – though we can't wait to hear more about a top secret technique, supposedly in the pipeline, which curls hair with an electro-magnetic process.

Perming is a chemical process that breaks down and rearranges the internal structure of hair – if it didn't, it wouldn't do the job. There is no gentle way to achieve a perm; so-called 'body waves' or 'body curls' suggest a kinder process, but the chemicals used are similar to those in a regular perm. Perming solution is applied to hair, which is then wound around rollers. As the solution penetrates the hair shaft, the hair softens; the solution chemically realigns the hair's protein links, bending them into the shape of the rollers. When the right degree of curl has been achieved, a 'neutralising' agent – another chemical – is applied, which hardens the hair and fixes the curl.

The commonest downside of a perm is frizziness. And, additionally, because there's no miracle pill that stops hair growing, the perm will grow out at around half an inch (13mm) a month and eventually flop at the roots, giving a curious spaniel-like effect on long hair. At this point, the woman with the perm has two options: go for the chop or get a 'root perm', which covers the already-permed hair with a cellophane wrap so the perming lotion penetrates just at the roots. As an alternative to cellophane wrapping, Wella produce a special protective product called Stop & Wind (available in salons only), which also coats the hair to prevent absorption of the perming lotion. It's vital that one of these hair-shielding techniques is used, because putting one perm on top of an existing perm is a recipe for brittle and broken hair.

'Perming coloured hair – or colouring permed hair – should only be done after very careful consultation,' warns leading hairdresser Paul Edmonds. 'It's risky, particularly with bleached or highlighted hair. But in some cases it is possible, if the hair undergoes a series of deep conditioning treatments to improve its strength.' If you're considering a perm, his advice is to: 'Think carefully, consult carefully – and condition, condition, condition. Remember: it's not called a permanent for nothing.'

PERM GUIDELINES

◆ If you want a perm, go to an expert; ask around for personal recommendations.

◆ Perming is a tricky technique and not every salon has adequate expertise. When you do find a recommended stylist, ask to see pictures of his or her handiwork.

◆ Discuss the condition and type of your hair with the perm stylist to ensure it's suitable for perming: healthy hair is elastic enough to stretch without breaking.

◆ To improve elasticity and strength, deep-condition hair with intensive hair masks for a few weeks before you go for a perm. (See *Tried & Tested Hair Masks*.) 'People worry that if they use conditioner, the perm won't "take",'says top hairdresser Paul Edmonds. 'That's a myth; it won't interfere with the perm's action at all.'

◆ Illustrate the kind of curl you are seeking with pictures; it's easy to end up with a too tight or too loose perm because you didn't communicate well enough. Perm stylists can vary the size of curls by using different perming rods. But, says Paul Edmonds, 'The look which most women want – loose curls – is almost impossible to achieve with a perm. Every time you see a picture in a magazine of a model with loose curls, it's almost always been tonged or curlered to get it looking that way.'

◆ Be aware that pregnancy, breast-feeding and other hormonal and physical conditions (even a recent anaesthetic) can all have an impact on the effectiveness of a perm.

◆ 'Get a trim afterwards rather than before,' advises Paul Edmonds. 'That way any damaged ends can just be snipped off.'

◆ Lavish TLC on your permed hair. Look for haircare products targeted at permed hair. Give it frequent deep conditioning treatments to restore shine and keep it out of the sun at all times.

◆ Frizz control is crucial. You'll find John Frieda's bestselling Frizz-Ease Hair Serum (widely available), and Kiehl's Creme with Silk Groom (see DIRECTORY) in most photo-session hairdressers' kit bags.

◆ You can relax a disastrous perm by piling in conditioners to soften the frizz. Olive oil massaged through the hair before shampooing helps bring back flexibility and shine, and buffers against over-cleansing.

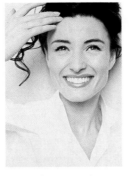

RELAX... (SHOULD YOU?)

Hair straightening, a.k.a. 'relaxing', is another chemical process, particularly popular with black women who have very tight curls or frizzy hair. Biologically, there is no such thing as 'black hair', but curly hair does have a unique texture that includes a flattened twist every half inch (13mm) or so down each strand. Curls often wrap themselves around each other, leading to tangles. To straighten curly hair without chemicals requires elbow grease, laborious setting on rollers, blowdrying or hot-combing.

The time-saving solution – chemical straightening – works like this. Instead of winding the hair on curlers, the hair is combed out straight from the root to the tip; chemicals are once again applied to soften the hair – so the straightness will 'take' – and a neutralising agent is applied once the desired look is achieved.

Potentially, this is even more damaging to hair than perming, because pulling hair tight to straighten it can cause it to break – or even yank it out, resulting in traction alopecia, or baldness around the margins of the scalp (fortunately, usually only temporary). The chemicals themselves are high in alkalinity, which can leave hair dry and brittle if the relaxing solution is left on too long.

Relaxed or straightened hair should ideally be given regular deep-moisturising treatments as often as twice a week. You should use a wide tooth comb, rather than a brush. Hair re-moisturising ingredients that women with black hair or frizzy curls should look for include jojoba oil, silk protein, chamomile, panthenol, aloe vera and rosewater – but not alcohol (which is too drying) or balsams (which don't provide enough moisture for black hair). For suppliers of haircare products specially tailored for black women, see DIRECTORY. Paul Mitchell and Sebastian market their all-hair types products to all different nationalities; look for their Laminates range. Aveda Anti-Humectant Pomade is another useful styling product.

NB: The strong solutions used for straightening and perming can damage the scalp. That's why going to a reputable salon, where they take great care to avoid the scalp while applying the chemicals, is a must. Relaxing can also be done on hair that has been over-permed, to reduce the curl, but this double-whammy of chemicals should be avoided unless your perm is truly tragic. (Remember: with time, perms 'drop' of their own accord.)

HAIR STYLING

Evening Hair
– in a Hurry

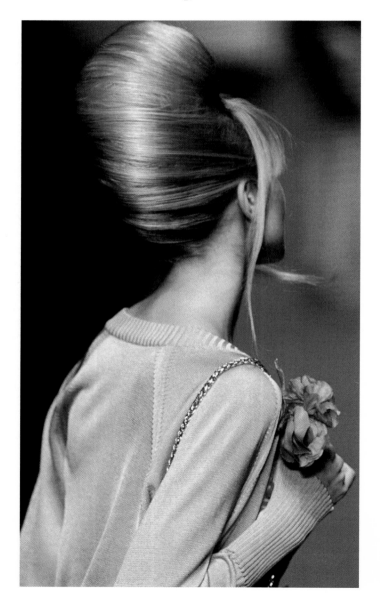

We all know that Cinderella had a Fairy Godmother to turn her rags into a ball gown and her flip-flops into glass slippers, but legend has never explained what happened to her hair. Since modern-day Cinders invariably need quick solutions, we've asked leading hairdressers to tell us what to do when we're going straight to the ball – whether from the kitchen or the office – and there isn't a moment to wash and style our hair. (You could, of course, adapt all these ideas for freshly washed hair too.)

FOR FLAT HAIR

✿ If hair has become flat during the day, spritz with water to dampen it slightly, then use your palms to work over the head in rotating movements. This will lift the roots and provide instant volume and body. For added height, gently back-comb the crown area, smooth and spray lightly with setting spray.

With a hairdryer:
✿ For short hair that has become flat, apply mousse all over the hair and power dry using the fast setting of the hairdryer to give instant volume and natural movement. Leave it ruffled or smooth back into the original style.

✿ If you have a fringe, apply a small amount of mousse around the hairline, then blowdry hair, pushing the fringe in the opposite direction to the way it grows, then back on itself. This will produce lift and a slight quiff. Give hair a sleek 1920s look by smoothing the rest with a tiny amount of wax warmed in your hands first. But don't overload the hair with mousse or wax.

✿ Apply a strong styling spray, lifting hair away from the head, and blast the roots with a fast-flow-hairdryer. Rub a small amount of shine gel through the fingertips and touch the ends of the hair, pushing it away from the scalp. Don't brush through, leave it tousled-looking.

Hairstyling suggestions from Denise McAdam, Ian Henry Team, Dom Migele, Alan Edwards, Eamonn Boreham, Jon Pereira-Santos.

FOR CURLY OR WAVY HAIR

✿ Remember that hair which isn't squeaky clean is easier to handle. With curly hair that has become frizzy, work with one inch sections, adding a tiny amount of serum to each one, encouraging the curl by using finger twirls. Don't brush or use a hairdryer.

✿ To revitalise naturally curly or wavy hair, tip your head upside down and pump hairspray into the hair roots. Repeat with side sections for all-over volume. Finish by dipping your fingertips into pomade or wax and lightly running through the hair.

✿ Take random sections of hair, twist them loosely along the lengths, and secure close to the scalp with a grip. The secret is to leave tendrils loose and not fasten the coils too tightly.

With a hairdryer:
✿ Spray your hair with a light mist of water, then dry with a diffuser attachment to encourage and revitalise curl. Catch it back into a low ponytail, allowing side sections to fall loose. Dress with hair accessories if you wish.

FOR MID TO LONG HAIR

✿ Gather your hair tightly at the back of your head, fold it over into a pleat, twisting and tightening from crown to nape. Secure it with grips and hide with accessories, such as big combs.

✿ To give wave and body, use large heated rollers. When you take them out, don't brush out the waves, just gently ruffle your hair with your fingers.

FOR LONG HAIR

✿ Pull your hair back into a high ponytail and wear a velvet Alice band across the front section for real fifties retro-glamour.

✿ Don't overwork hair, or it will become more greasy. Using a bristle brush, take it back onto the nape of the neck and make a low ponytail, securing with a scarf, ribbon or slide.

FAST FIXES FOR BAD HAIR DAYS...

When it's raining
◆ Use gel to slick your hair back behind your ears – that way it'll look the same wet or dry.

When it's humid
◆ If your hair gets too wild, spray it with hairspray and hold it flat against your scalp with your hands until it's under control.
◆ Or, instead of trying to flatten your hair – which may be a losing battle – wet it and scrunch it with styling mousse, for a casual look.
◆ If it's very humid, pull your hair back into a low ponytail and tuck it under a hat. When you get to work, let the ponytail loose and brush your hair.

No time to blowdry?
◆ Comb through a touch of gel, slick it back and let it air dry.
◆ Do the 'sunglasses' trick – fashion and beauty editors everywhere swear by it. While your hair's still damp, put on a pair of sunglasses as if they were a hairband. You can wear them there all day. (They'll also be handy for blasts of bright sunshine.)

Your hair's flat and won't cooperate?
◆ At Philip B.'s salon in Los Angeles, they tease hair with a toothbrush. 'The tiny bristles give you much more control because you can work on smaller areas. A firm-bristled toothbrush also lets you get at the roots, which really lifts hair and gives it volume, without making it big.' This is best for spot-teasing, for instance a fringe, because it takes too long all over.

Your grey roots are showing through?
◆ In an emergency, Bobbi Brown has been known to use an eyeliner pencil – in dark brown – to touch up roots, as a short-term fix while waiting for a colouring appointment. (Be sure to choose a colour that matches your hair.)

The ultimate cure for a Bad Hair Day
◆ Provided your hair is long enough, put it in a top-knot. (According to New York stylist Gil Gamlieli, it's actually better if hair is unwashed and slightly messy.)

SUN, SEA – AND SHINE

The recipe for a great holiday – sun, sea and sand – is also the perfect recipe for ruining the condition of your hair. Just like skin, hair will burn if exposed to strong sunshine. But, unlike skin, it can't signal it's suffering; by the time you notice the damage, it will be too late. So to avoid a case of the sun-baked frizzies, it's vital to treat your hair with the same consideration as you do your skin.

◆ Give hair a head start: make an intensive conditioning treatment once a week part of your regime, especially in the run-up to a holiday. (See *Tried & Tested Hair Masks*, page 117.)

◆ For hair to be soft and easy to style, it must retain moisture, which is especially difficult in summer heat. All hair types are vulnerable to damage, but some more so than others. If your hair is chemically processed – permed or coloured – it will lose moisture faster rate than untreated hair. Similarly, black hair – which is more porous and so prone to drying out – needs maximum protection. Long hair – especially beyond shoulder-length – is also fragile because the hair ends are that much older. Give the ends an intensive moisturising treatment whenever you wash your hair.

◆ Optimum protection is a hat, rather than a visor which exposes the delicate parting area and roots. Don't forget to tuck up the vulnerable ends under the hat.

◆ You can also give hair a veil of specially designed sunscreen. (Try J.H. Lazartigue's Protective Hair Milk or Protective Hair Cream, and Molton Brown's Parasol – which was withdrawn from the market a couple of years ago, until they got so many pleas from distraught customers that they reintroduced it.) Less expensive ranges are also bringing out hair protection lotions intended to be left on the hair: look for Parsol MCX – a UV filter – on the label.

◆ Apply hair protection as often as you'd slather on sun lotion.

◆ Chlorine is disastrous for lightened hair as it's another form of bleach – and not one your colourist would recommend. **Claudia Schiffer** says her hair once went green after swimming in chlorinated water, although the chances of that happening are fairly remote. However, hair that gets wet – in a pool or seawater – should be washed again fast.

◆ Avoid the double threat of chlorine plus strong sunlight; try not to swim during prime sun hours.

◆ If you want to keep your hair in good condition, forget the old tip about putting fresh lemon juice on your hair to bleach it in the sun. (Or – in supermodel Eva Herzigova's case – neat vodka!) It may work, but, in tandem with the sun's rays, it can be extremely drying and may leave your scalp light-sensitive and temporarily sore.

◆ Coarse hair should be treated with a leave-in conditioner or serum to fight the frizzies.

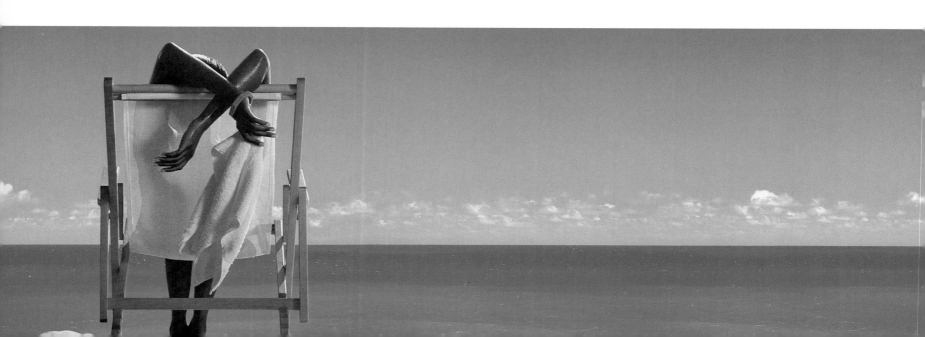

BOTANICAL HAIR BEAUTY SECRETS

❀ A rinse of mint tea after conditioning helps oily hair shine, without being greasy.

❀ For dandruff control, massage a cupful of fresh apple juice from hair roots through to ends. Follow conditioning with a rinse of two teaspoons of apple cider vinegar, diluted in a cup of water. Expect to see results after two or three applications.

❀ The enzymes and proteins in natural yoghurt soften and purify, making a low-cost hair pack.

❀ According to Philip Berkowitz, creator of the Philip B. Botanical Hair and Treatment range (see DIRECTORY), oregano makes a brilliant hair detangler: mix half a cup of chopped fresh oregano leaves with a teaspoonful of pure vanilla extract and one cup of water; place over a low heat and simmer for 30 minutes. Strain to filter out particles. Once cooled, pour into a spray bottle and spray directly onto hair, saturating the strands and scalp. This keeps for three days in the fridge.

❀ Eggs are renowned for making hair shine. Hair guru Philip Kingsley suggests a basic egg shampoo: take two eggs, crack them in a bowl, fill the empty shells with olive oil, pour into the eggs and mix. Massage into hair and scalp; rinse thoroughly.

❀ Believe it or not: an ancient Himalayan remedy for stress-induced dry scalp problems, says London hairdresser Zah, is to mix a finely-chopped chilli pepper with three teaspoons of olive oil, heat gently, then massage into the scalp for five minutes. Rinse well. (For other natural secrets, see page 97.)

STAR HAIR TIPS

◆ **Paula Abdul**: 'My hair is just as curly as Mariah Carey's if I let it go. Holding back the frizziness is really difficult under the lights, with the moisture and the humidity. So I buy every product that is anti-frizz or hair gloss. Currently I'm using frizz-tamers by Sebastian, Phyto and John Frieda.' ◆ **Steve Martin**, **Sharon Stone** and **Madonna** are all fans of Aveda's Purefume Brilliant Spray-On, which adds sheen without stickiness – and smells fantastic.

◆ Redken's CAT conditioning haircare line is a favourite with **Cher**, **Mel Gibson** and **Michelle Pfeiffer**. Its amino acid-based, hair-strengthening formula helps repair the damage done by hot studio lights (and sun). ◆ **Janet Jackson** loves the Sebastian Laminates range, and also uses Sebastian's Molding Mud to keep her hair firmly under control. ◆ **Elle MacPherson** likes the Phyto products and the Biotherm range (which is available in France). 'Personally, I find my hair is more manageable if I wash it every two or three days.' ◆ **Keanu Reeves** has been spotted stocking up with The Body Shop's Ice Blue Shampoo, which fights oil, and contains scalp-tingling menthol. ◆ **Jerry Hall** (and **Mick Jagger**) are fans of Philip Kingsley's signature range of haircare.

TIP FROM THE TOP

International model agent Laraine Ashton advises girls to take extra care of their hair when going on shoots in sunny locations. 'We advise them to wear hats between sessions to protect the hair, and when they have a day off, to apply intensive conditioner and leave it on all day, if possible.'

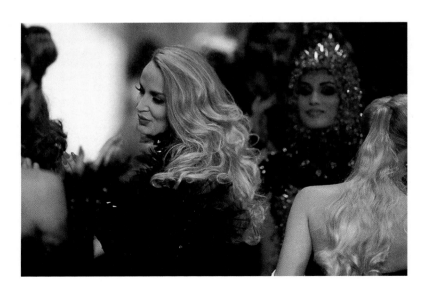

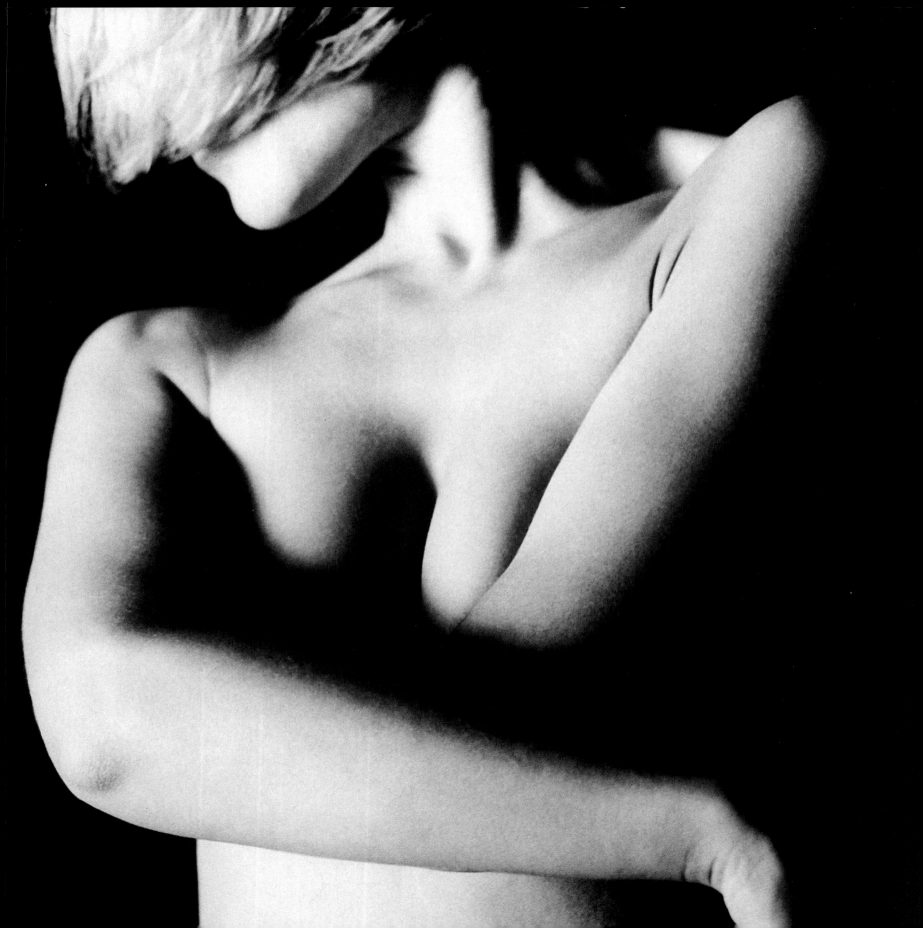

5

Helping
Nature

Sometimes it takes more than sensible eating, exercise, a new hairdo or expertly applied make-up to convince you that you look great – whatever others say. Some people live peacefully with the marks of time; 'I'm used to my face travelling south', one 50-something beauty told us. Others feel that improving on the effects of ageing, an accident or simply altering a long-disliked feature will boost their self-confidence. **Here is the lowdown on cosmetic surgery and cosmetic dentistry, plus our tips for gentler, non-surgical ways to delay the march of time.**

CHOOSING A SURGEON

No one goes in for cosmetic surgery for fun – so read the hard facts first, and only then make a decision.

We've seen wonderful results from cosmetic surgery, and we've seen dreadful ones. We've heard stories from patients who are delighted and we've talked to those whose lives have been put in jeopardy. On the positive side, one recent British study revealed that cosmetic surgery improved the lives of a majority of those who had psychological problems, large or small, as a result of their appearance.

The most important factor you must bear in mind is this: whether you are contemplating skin peeling, a face lift, liposuction or having your teeth crowned, surgery is an invasive procedure which carries risks – some potentially life-threatening. No one will embark on it as if it were a hairdo, but do read our guidelines on choosing a surgeon, and when you go for an initial consultation, remember it's your face, your body, your life you are entrusting to this person. What's more, you are paying the piper – usually a lot since cosmetic surgery is almost always private – so make sure you call the tune: be thorough but not aggressive with the surgeon. Establishing a good rapport with him/her is essential.

There are three principal ways to find a surgeon:
1. Ask your doctor, but be aware that many won't know either the best person to go to or the most appropriate procedure.
2. Ask friends for recommendations.
3. Ask your doctor to get a list of consultant plastic surgeons from the British Association of Plastic Surgeons (BAPS). Or apply yourself to the British Association of Aesthetic Plastic Surgeons (BAAPS), which provides lists of members to the general public, and then make an appointment for an initial consultation. If you are not happy with the first surgeon, consult another surgeon before making a decision.

Make sure that whoever you choose is a fully accredited plastic surgeon and that they have experience and interest in cosmetic (as well as reconstructive) surgery. We do not recommend you approach the clinics who advertise in the back of magazines. However impressive they sound – and many may be – some have been exposed as having unqualified staff and/or poor facilities, which have had life-threatening consequences for some patients.

When you meet a surgeon, he or she will be interviewing you to see that you are in the right state of mind – too anxious and they may consider you unsuitable for surgery. It is also important for you to interview him or her, to see whether you get on, whether they listen and if they seem to understand you and your hopes. Find out your surgeon's qualifications and training, how long they have been practising and where, and exactly what can be done for you. Many surgeons say that the most important attribute is the ability to draw and model in clay. Groups of dedicated surgeons actually spend their spare time in art galleries and museums, studying the human face and body.

A surgeon may try to impress you with computer video-sculpting, showing what you could look like by computer mock-ups. It looks flashy but it's really only useful for the surgeon to play around on. Most condemn it as a selling technique when shown to patients. Some patients like to see before and after pictures of previous patients. These are fine as a point of comparison, but bear in mind that you will never be shown the ones that have gone wrong.

Although there are worthwhile new techniques, such as the endoscopic brow lift (see opposite), complex and/or innovative procedures are not necessarily the best. You want the surgeon to do what he/she is experienced at and what is appropriate for you, not something he/she is longing to try out. Remember that no wise surgeon can or should guarantee a specific result.

A thorough initial consultation (make sure to check the fee for this when you book) should include counselling to ensure you are really ready to go through surgery, and detailed information on the procedures, possible complications, pain relief and recovery times. Many surgeons now prefer to operate without a general anaesthetic, using instead deep sedation or local anaesthesia so that patients don't suffer grogginess or hangovers. In this way, you can be in and out in a day for some procedures.

Always confirm costs at this stage and see how many follow-up visits are included (some surgeons see you up to 12 months later; some even longer). If you decide to go ahead, you will be asked to sign an informed consent form; read it carefully. Make sure your chosen surgeon is comprehensively insured. (Roughly one in a thousand patients sue their surgeons, a BAPS source revealed.) The two leading UK insurers are the Medical Defence Union (MDU) and the Medical Protection Society (MPS).

(See DIRECTORY for qualified surgeons and professional bodies in the UK and worldwide.)

PROCEDURES

Medical terms

haemorrhage – bleeding

haematoma – blood clot

necrosis – delayed healing

Face Lifts and Other Facial Operations

Time was when a face lift meant such prolonged bruising, swelling and visible scarring that patients had to disappear for months. Today's medical advances mean much shorter in-patient and recovery times.

Endoscopic Face Lift and Brow Lift

Endoscopic or keyhole surgery for faces is a recent arrival. For the 'endoface', the surgeon inserts the endoscope (a surgical telescope) through five small cuts in the hairline and two inside the mouth, which heal rapidly, leaving virtually no visible scars. A minute camera on the endoscope allows the surgeon to reposition facial tissues and muscle inside the face and brow by watching progress on a large television screen.

The **'endoface'** has very limited application because it does not remove slack skin but relies on repositioning skin and anchoring it with a form of skin glue, so it's only suitable for mild cases in young-ish patients.

RECOVERY TIME: post-operative swelling should subside by 14 days, six weeks at worst. The 'endoface' should give a younger-looking upper face and jawline, plus tauter skin texture, but is not as effective as 'open' face lifts in patients with severe sagging.

RISKS: there is a greater risk of damage to facial nerves with this way of operating than with other types of face lift.

The **'endobrow'**, which can be combined with any type of face lift, involves just three small cuts on the scalp, unlike the traditional brow lift which necessitates an Alice-band cut from ear to ear. It can be done in a day and corrects furrows, lines and heavy brows.

Like any brow lift, it is not advised for those with a high forehead (as it will make it even higher), but is an ideal procedure to lift a heavy brow. As the incisions are so small, it is also useful for men who have gone thin on top, where an ear-to-ear brow lift would be impossible because the scars would show.

RECOVERY TIME: swift (about a week) – although one energetic patient was ballroom dancing four days afterwards.

RISKS: damage to sensory nerve with numbness in the forehead and the scalp; also damage to the motor (movement) nerve to the forehead.

Mask (or Sub-Periostal) Lift

The soft tissues of the face are detached from the bone and repositioned. Some of the facial bone structure can also be altered. Two small cuts are made inside the mouth; the other cut runs from ear to ear.

The mask lift is suitable for the same group of patients as the 'endoface'.

RECOVERY TIME: results are usually dramatic, although there is considerable swelling and most patients need six to eight weeks' recuperation.

RISKS: disadvantages are that this Alice-band cut will feel numb for two to three months after surgery and there is a five per cent risk of temporary injury to the facial nerve, particularly with surgeons less experienced in this technique.

Skin Lift with SMAS Lift

The most commonly performed lift is the skin lift, where the surgeon cuts around the ear, pulls up the skin, tightens the musculoaponeurotic fascia (the deeper layer of fibrous tissue and the sling muscle which embraces the jawline), and removes the excess skin. Most surgeons combine the skin lift with a SMAS lift: the skin is lifted from the SMAS (subcutaneous aponeurotic system – the layer where the muscles are attached to the skin) through a cut which runs around the ears and down into the hairline. The SMAS and the muscle are repositioned and excess skin removed. This corrects heavy cheeks, jowls and sagging necks in patients of any age.

This can give quite dramatic results in older patients and, as with the skin lift, usually lasts ten years, providing patients keep a constant weight. Some patients do have more than one operation.

RECOVERY TIME: patients are leading a normal life within two weeks.

RISKS: permanent damage is extremely rare; possible short-term problems include haemorrhage, haematoma, skin necrosis and temporary facial nerve damage.

Extended SMAS Lift

The extended SMAS, which needs a very experienced facial surgeon, penetrates further down to smooth out heavy lines between nose and mouth.

RECOVERY TIME: usually about two weeks.

RISKS: same as for skin lift.

Brow Smoothers

As well as the endoscopic brow lift, which removes the grooves by detaching the skin from the muscle, there are other methods, notably injections of a plant toxin called Botulinum (known as Botox). These have for years been used for blepharospasm (eyelid twitching) and squints and appear to be completely safe, with no side effects. Botox is ideal for vertical frown lines where collagen injections (another option, see *Lip Re-Shaping*, opposite) are usually inappropriate. Not only do you then lose the habit of frowning but, with the release of pressure, the lines start fading almost immediately. The initial effect lasts about three months but should become permanent after several injections and a year or two of frown line immobilisation.

RECOVERY TIME: none needed.

RISKS: safe in experienced hands but toxic if the wrong dose is given.

Arteplast (Artecol)

This combination of 40 per cent collagen and 60 per cent dental cement PPMA (polymermethylmethacrylate) is said by some surgeons to be effective on superficial facial lines.

RECOVERY TIME: none needed.

RISKS: irregularity of the treated area, allergy (prolonged swelling and redness).

Eyelid Surgery (Upper and/or Lower Blepharoplasty)

This removes the fatty tissue, extra skin and wrinkles which build up around the eyes. Scars, positioned in the upper eyelid groove just above the crease or under the lower eyelashes, should be virtually invisible. The most painful part is removing the stitches.

Operating inside the eye (trans-conjunctival surgery) avoids stitches but is only suitable for younger patients with minimal excess skin to remove.

RECOVERY TIME: seven to ten days.

RISKS: pulling down of the lower eyelid if too much skin is removed, excessive scar tissue formations, haematoma, dry eye syndrome.

Cheek Implants

These are traditionally made of silicone, but the cheek may also be built up with collagen or the patient's own (autologous) fat. The most recent advance is hydroxyapitite, a synthetic with the same composition as bone, which is mixed with the patient's blood to make a paste that can be moulded and applied directly to the bone.

This is recommended for cheeks or other bone-deficient sites, but not for chins where there is too much motion. The results should be permanent.

RECOVERY TIME: seven days.

RISKS: asymmetry, infection.

Ear Correction (Otoplasty)

Surgery to pin back protruding ears, an inherited condition, can be performed as early as five years old. Incisions are made in the groove behind the ears so that the scars are hidden from view. (N.B. babies may be able to have protruding ears corrected with a soft pliable splint called an Ear Buddy, which retrains the ear.)

RECOVERY TIME: seven days.

RISKS: incomplete correction, haemorrhage, infection.

Nose Re-shaping (Rhinoplasty)

Bumps can be removed, a broad nose slimmed down or the tip altered. Underlying excess bone and cartilage are usually removed from inside the nose, thus leaving no scars.

Noses can also be built up with cartilage, bone or, less commonly, with silicone.

RECOVERY TIME: mouth breathing is necessary for several days after surgery which can be uncomfortable. Ninety per cent of swelling and bruising should go down in two to three weeks, although the nose shape may take up to six months to settle down.

RISKS: haemorrhage, a poor result, asymmetry.

Lip Re-shaping

Temporary re-shapers include:

– injection of collagen. A patch test is necessary four weeks beforehand to test for possible allergy to the purified bovine collagen (now also caught up in the problem of BSE, 'Mad Cow Disease'). Results are only short term – lasting from two to six months.

– your own (autologous) fat, often taken from the stomach, being processed and injected into numbed lips. The supply is inexhaustible and your own fat won't set off a reaction. Results should last up to a year. (Hands can also be treated this way.)

More *permanent* methods include:

– injection of micro-droplets of silicone into the lip, although many surgeons reject this method because the silicone can cause skin ulceration.

– removal of skin from an over-long upper lip, or of skin and underlying tissue from over-thick lips.

RECOVERY TIME: two to seven days (for both).

Over-thin lips can be enhanced by:

– shaping and threading Gore-Tex (the biologically compatible membrane used in cold-weather clothes and equipment, including skiwear) into the lip;

– or by inserting a dermis (skin) graft.

RECOVERY TIME: two to seven days.

RISKS: with Gore-Tex, lip induration (abnormal hardening), possible rejection.

Chin Augmentation (Mentoplasty)

Permanent re-shaping of receding chins is sometimes performed at the same time as nose re-shaping to get a better profile. This uses an implant – traditionally silicone, although new materials including HTR polymers are starting to be used. The incision is usually made inside the mouth or under the chin. People with long jaws can also have bone removed to improve the shape of the jawline.

RECOVERY TIME: one week for implants, two weeks if bone is removed.

RISKS: infection, damage to the mental nerve (which controls sensation in the chin and lower lip) by anaesthetising the chin.

Skin Peeling, Dermabrasion and Laser Re-surfacing

These various techniques have revolutionised the treatment of fine lines, poor skin texture, brown spots, dark circles and even acne scars, but they must be performed by experts (dermatologists, cosmeto-dermatologists or aesthetic plastic surgeons) – never by the local beauty salon.

Skin Peels deep clean and soften skin. The mildest professional chemical peeling agents are high-concentration glycolic or lactic acid, followed by trichloroacetic acid, then phenol. Skin is often prepared with Retin-A, itself a peeling agent.

Dermabrasion uses an electrically-operated fine brush to remove scars and create a smoother surface.

RECOVERY TIME: both these treatments may be uncomfortable, although surgeons will take care to alleviate pain. Afterwards, the skin reddens, becomes itchy and dry and possibly painful for several days or even weeks before the new soft skin grows through. The new skin is also very sensitive to UV light and must be zealously protected with high factor sun preparations (SPF 25/30 or total block).

Laser Resurfacing Rapid shallow pulses of laser light burn away the top layer of skin, tightening skin and helping with acne scarring. There are several types of lasers used for different purposes. The Silk Touch laser is currently the most popular for skin rejuvenation, but some predict the new Ultra-Pulse CO_2 laser will replace it. The PhotoDerm laser is showing great promise with facial thread veins.

Experts claim that laser treatment is more predictable and safer than dermabrasion and chemical peels.

RECOVERY TIME: skin will be noticeably pink for a few weeks.

RISKS: the main danger of all the above lies in going too deep into the skin, so creating a lasting scar rather than removing problems. However, new laser technology, such as the Ultra-Pulse CO_2 laser, is computerised, making it easier for the surgeon to control.

Fat Removal

Liposuction

The removal of fat by suction means that most regions of the body can be re-contoured, including the face and neck (particularly double chins and back neck humps), breasts, arms, waist, abdomen, buttocks, inner and outer thighs and knees. This is suitable for removing stubborn localised areas of fat – it is not an alternative to exercise and sensible eating.

RECOVERY TIME: seven days, although bruising takes up to four weeks to fade.

RISKS: liposuction is more complex than it seems, and can cause nasty problems if not done by an expert (one woman ended up in intensive care after poor surgery and there have been deaths reported). If too much fat is removed, the skin will ripple or sag irreversibly. Poor liposuction can cause grooves and ruts which are difficult to put right. And if you put on weight again, the fat settles in a different area, which can lead to odd shape changes.

Liposculpture

This is another name for liposuction but sometimes also involves injecting fat into depressed areas to re-contour the body. It also includes superficial liposuction – the removal of fat just below the surface of the skin with a very fine cannula (syringe). Results can be excellent but you must go to an experienced surgeon.

RECOVERY TIME: as for liposuction.

RISKS: as for liposuction.

Ultrasonic Liposuction

With the patient under local anaesthetic, incisions are made in the skin and an ultrasound probe slid into the tissue. By using a specific frequency of ultrasound, surgeons claim fat can be dissolved, then suctioned off, so more can be removed. Skin is said to shrink better.

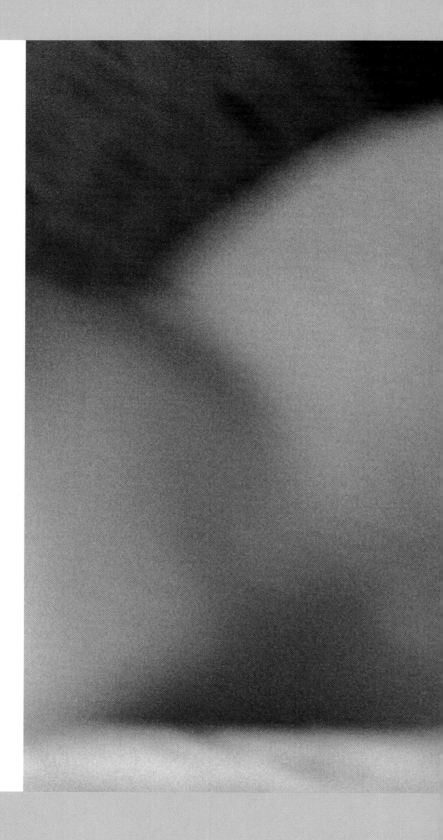

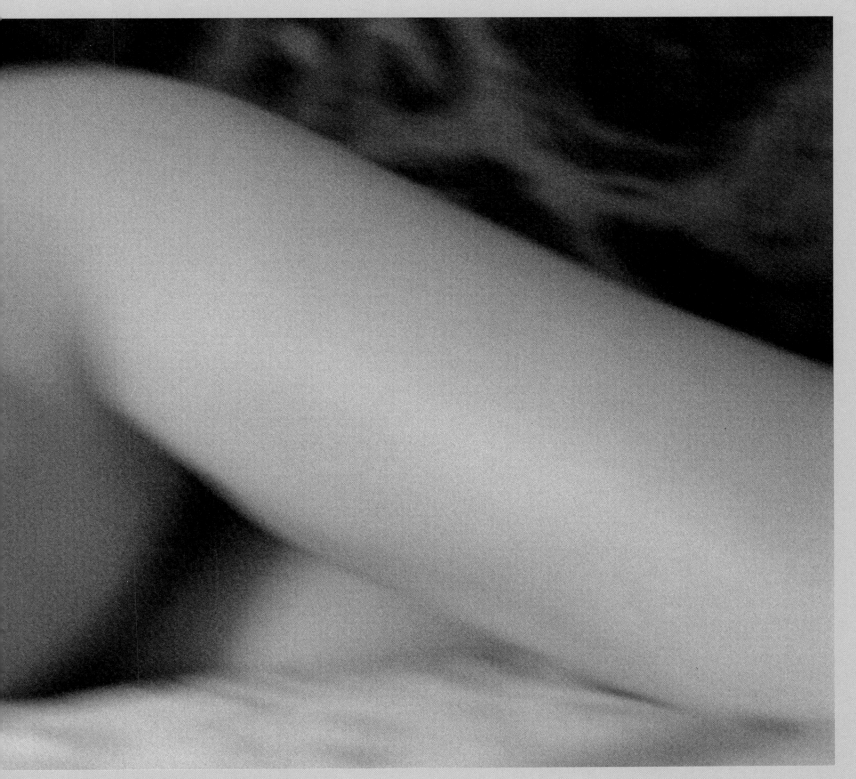

RECOVERY TIME: as for liposuction.

RISKS: as for liposuction, plus skin necrosis which can be a serious complication so, again, this should only be done by experts.

Abdominal Reduction (Abdominoplasty)

This 'tummy tuck' operation takes out the excess skin and fat which often affect women after pregnancy and which defy exercise. Tummy muscles can be tightened at the same time. Liposuction is often carried out simultaneously for best results.

RECOVERY TIME: three weeks.

RISKS: infection, haemorrhage, asymmetry, poor quality scars, skin necrosis.

Breast Reduction and Augmentation (Mastopexy)

Breast Reduction and Uplift

Over-large, pendulous breasts can be surgically reduced and uplifted. Breasts are marked with a special pen before the operation with the patient standing. Under general anaesthetic, the nipple is detached from the skin but left attached to the breast tissue, then an incision made vertically down and under the breast, skin and breast tissue are removed, the nipple replaced and the wounds sewn up. Scarring will fade but is permanent. More recent techniques avoid a scar under the breast, but leave a wrinkled vertical scar which takes a few months to become even.

Pregnancy must be avoided for one year to avoid stretching the scars.

RECOVERY TIME: two to three weeks.

RISKS: haemorrhage, infection, skin and nipple necrosis, asymmetry.

Breast Augmentation

Demand for this once common operation dropped off sharply after the eruption of the (ongoing) fear that silicone implants filled with silicone gel may lead to an increased risk of cancer or of auto-immune disease. Although subsequent medical research suggests that the risk is probably no greater for women with implants, they can form hard lump scar tissue; if so, one can either repeat the operation, or live with the lumps. Improved implants with a textured surface reduce this risk.

Patients now have a choice between saline-filled implants (which don't look or feel very natural and may leak), silicone gel-filled implants (which give the best shape and feel), or triluscent implants filled with soya bean oil (which have the advantage of being radiotranslucent so that they allow better imaging in mammography, and fall halfway between saline-filled implants in feel and shape).

RECOVERY TIME: two weeks. We don't recommend exposing delicate breast skin at any time, let alone after surgery.

RISKS: haemorrhage, infection, capsules contract and harden, asymmetry.

Varicose Veins

This common problem is best treated with a combination of surgery and sclerotherapy (injections of an irritant solution which shrinks the vein). An expert assessment with ultrasound scanning is vital, even if the only surface sign is a slight 'flare' of veins. A general (rather than cosmetic) surgeon with special expertise in veins may be your best bet for treatment (see DIRECTORY).

RECOVERY TIME: back at work in three to five days.

RISKS: the main risk lies in not removing all the affected veins (which can lead to further problems).

SUPPORT SYSTEMS

❏ Take a good multivitamin/multimineral supplement at least four weeks before and eight weeks after surgery to speed healing.

❏ Also take arnica (available from some chemists and homoeopathic pharmacies) before, during and after surgery.

❏ Avoid salt after surgery – it promotes fluid retention; alcohol and aspirin – they tend to increase bleeding and oozing; smoking – it slows down the rate of tissue repair.

❏ Apply ice packs or cold compresses with witch hazel continuously for the first 24 hours to lessen bruising.

❏ Use a good moisturiser.

❏ Vitamin E is believed to help healing so you could try applying natural vitamin E directly.

Detailed fact sheets on many of these procedures are available from the British Association of Aesthetic Plastic Surgeons, and some surgeons have also written their own information sheets for patients. The more information you can get, the better placed you are to make a decision.

NON-SURGICAL FACE AND BODY TREATMENTS

If you're waging war primarily against the ravages of time, there are plenty of ways to delay surgery – possibly for good.

As well as all the suggestions we have made in the rest of this book, there is now a range of non-invasive treatments which can make a short, and occasionally long-term difference.

These home and salon treatments can give you a marvellous temporary (one to two days) boost if used on a one-off basis. Some clients find that continuous use means more lasting results. Generally speaking, the most grateful are the 40-somethings (men as well as women – including **Mel Gibson**) whose skin has begun to sag slightly. Some dermatologists and cosmetic surgeons now recommend these types of treatment, which were originally developed from technology originating in hospitals.

There are many possibilities out there; the following methods are the ones we have researched and on which we have had the best feedback. (See DIRECTORY for contact details.)

Home

Eva Fraser's facial exercises (see page 92): our tip for the best one-off investment you can make for your face.

Amstrad Integra: electro-microcurrent therapy machine packaged in a small bleeping box which comes with a video and idiot-proof instructions. It is tiring because you have to push the probes all over your face in different directions.

Tester says: 'It gives the most incredible glow and plumps up your skin temporarily, like a fantastic facial.'

Isolift (also salon): electro-microcurrent therapy machine in small casing, half the size of a hairdryer, which lifts muscles and reduces puffiness.

Tester says: 'You can feel muscles lifting; gives a glow and tightens skin.'

Cleo: electro-microcurrent therapy, using suction pads applied to the face in different combinations. Easy instructions are given but it is time-intensive – 40 minutes daily for three months, then alternate days.

Tester says: 'I would recommend it to anyone…at 49 I don't need to wear make-up because my complexion is so good now.'

Salon

Bio-therapeutics: electro-therapy using water as a conductor. For lasting improvements, 12 60-minute sessions are recommended, plus top-ups. Bio-therapeutics is said to make the skin glow, help sagging and reduce lines.

Tester says: 'It can't make you look 19 when you're 40 something but it can make you look bloody good.'

CACI (Computer Aided Cosmetology Instrument): the original 'non-surgical face-lift' uses a low-frequency microcurrent to 'recharge' the muscle's own electrical currents, thus stimulating the fibres responsible for maintaining muscle tone, length and elasticity. The recommended number of sessions varies widely.

Tester says: 'Great short-term results with tiny overall improvement after fifteen sessions.'

Dibitron: an individually prescribed programme is fed into a computerised electro-stimulation machine. It is said to massage your 48 facial muscles 21,000 times in 30 minutes as well as speed up the elimination of toxins, improve tone and texture and smooth out fine lines. Plant-based lotions are usually applied before, during and after treatment.

Tester says: 'Restful, energising, skin looked radiant.'

Rejuvannessence: a specific form of facial massage which is likened to facial reflexology. This type of massage claims to stimulate tone and texture and 'lift' the face; testers found significant immediate and short- to medium-term results. A course of six is normally recommended with regular top-ups. Holistic as well as nutritional and lifestyle advice is given.

Tester says: 'Relaxing and enjoyable; a friend said I looked radiant.'

TEETH: A BRIGHTER SHADE OF WHITE

If you weren't lucky enough to be born with a set of Californian babe pearly whites, there's no need to despair. Practically any problem can be remedied by your cosmetic dentist – at a price.

As with every other part of your body, keeping your teeth healthy and bright and your breath fresh demands action on your part – before you even consider cosmetic dentistry. Brush your teeth properly (either with an electric toothbrush, or round and round gently with a soft toothbrush – not from side to side with a hard one); floss them regularly (try thick or waxed floss first if you're not yet a floss fan); and try to avoid letting citrus fruit or fruit juices linger in your mouth – they create an acid environment in your mouth which is now thought to be the biggest cause of tooth decay (even more so than sugar).

Surprisingly, stress is another important factor in the health of your teeth. Just like citrus fruit, stress brings acid into your mouth. So if you come under a lot of pressure, try to reduce it for your teeth's sake as much as anything else. (To beat stress, see *Instant Stress Busters*, page 185.)

As with every other facet of health and beauty, smoking is a villain: it stains teeth and causes bad breath. Many people, smokers and otherwise, are now turning to whitening toothpastes, but the big questions are: do they work? And if so, which ones?

'Whitening' is actually a misnomer; according to dentists, these toothpastes cannot whiten (to do so would require an oxidising agent) but they may clean more effectively, remove existing stains, prevent other stains building up and polish teeth to make them smoother and shinier. In a recent article in *The Daily Telegraph*, dentist Dr Edward Lynch, who has been studying the effects of tooth-whitening products for more than a decade, gave top marks to Ultrawhite Opal by Janina International because of its 16 active ingredients for improving oral health, whitening teeth and freshening breath.

WHAT YOUR DENTIST CAN DO FOR YOU

Cosmetic dentist Mr Stanley Kay in London has helped us compile the following list of procedures.

Scaling and polishing: make a regular six-monthly appointment with the dental hygienist to remove plaque and surface stains, and give teeth a brightening polish. Ultrasonic scalers are generally available; the latest technology is the air-abrader – an 'airgun' which fires high-speed abrasive powder at the teeth, giving excellent results in stain removal.

Bleaching: whitening teeth professionally with hydrogen peroxide is currently illegal in the UK – despite its use on hair, skin and nails - but the British Dental Association is trying to get the legislation changed and it is worth talking to your dentist about it.

Crowns: the traditional way to repair a broken or unsightly tooth is by grinding the tooth down to a peg and fitting a replica over the top. Leading dentists are now working in porcelains which are so hard that metal reinforcement is unnecessary – so crowns look better, last longer and never have a black line around the margin. With healthy gums, a porcelain crown will last 20 years.

Bonding: sticking tooth-coloured material to an existing tooth is an alternative to crowning. The tooth is etched using a weak acid which creates a rough surface on the tooth, to which composite or porcelain in-lays or on-lays are attached (see *Veneers*, below), depending on the problem. Bonding is far easier than other means of fixing. It's particularly helpful for filling gaps between widely spaced front teeth. Expect to need replacements every five years or so.

Veneers: a popular solution for badly discoloured or misshapen teeth – a very thin layer of porcelain, rather like a false fingernail, is bonded to the tooth. Increasingly, veneers are so super-thin that they can be applied without removing any of the tooth. Disadvantages are that veneers can chip and, in rare cases, they may fall off, usually because of poor technique. Since teeth darken with age, veneers will need to be re-done at intervals to match other teeth.

Implants: titanium screw implants have revolutionised the replacement of lost teeth; until recently their use was limited to places where there was sufficient bone to screw in the implants – otherwise false teeth was the only option. Now, however, advanced surgical procedures mean that surgeons can graft the patient's own bone from another part of the body into the mouth as a 'bed' for the implant.

Amalgams: removing amalgam (mercury) fillings and substituting composite (plastic and ceramic) or porcelain fillings will give you an all-white yawn instead of a mouth like the inside of an ironmonger's. For larger fillings, where shrinkage is a big problem, the dentist takes an impression and the filling is made in the laboratory and pre-shrunk before use. These fillings are also stronger and can be excellently colour-matched, but they are more expensive.

(Taking out amalgam fillings may help your general health too: there is considerable evidence that the neurotoxic mercury continuously released from amalgams can lead to a wide range of illness, including allergies, headaches, fatigue syndromes and skin conditions.)

Orthodontics: using fixed braces, a trained orthodontist can correct the alignment of teeth, adjust the relationship of teeth and jaw to give a better bite, improve the shape of a sticking out or receding jaw and correct congenital anomalies such as cleft lip and palate. In extreme cases, the upper and lower jaw are so poorly aligned that surgery is also necessary.

Adult orthodontic work, mainly private, is becoming more common. The latest ceramic technology means that fixed braces can be tooth-coloured rather than silver. Treatment may take 18 months to two years.

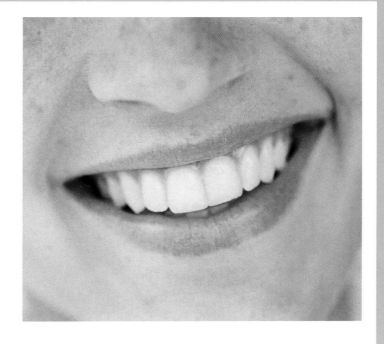

NATURAL WAYS TO HEALTHY TEETH

❒ Try to breathe through your nose: mouth breathing dries out protective saliva and may lead to teeth and gum problems.

❒ Boost gum health by massaging gums with your fingertips.

❒ Floss teeth before brushing: try naturally disinfecting teatree dental floss.

❒ Remove stains by rubbing teeth with slices of fresh strawberries or fresh sage leaves, or sprinkle $1/2$ teaspoon bicarbonate of soda on a damp toothbrush.

❒ Heal infected or inflamed gums with a golden seal mouthwash: mix $1/4$ teaspoon salt and $1/2$ teaspoon or one capsule of golden seal powder (available from health food stores or herbalists) in a cup of warm water and swill it round your mouth.

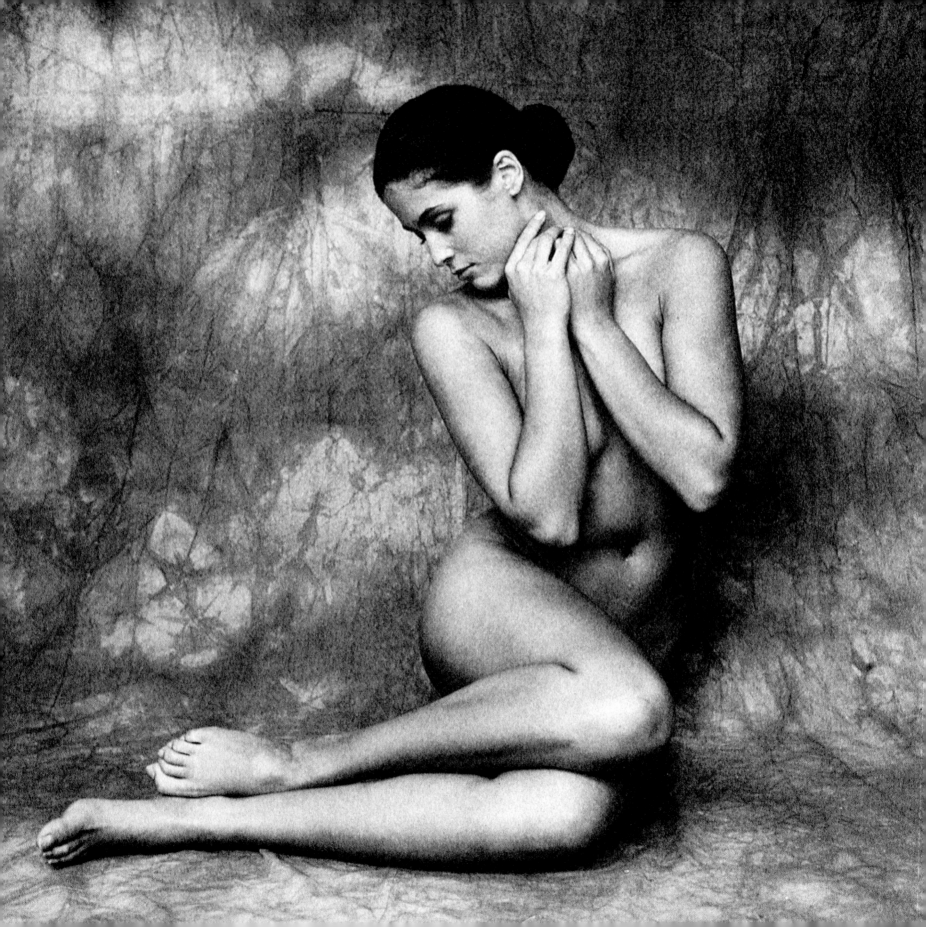

6

Body Beautiful

We don't believe there's a woman alive who is 100 per cent happy with her body. (Even supermodels complain endlessly about their flaws.) But what we need is not more impossible diets and exercise regimes you can only follow if you have iron discipline, time to spare and the cash for a personal trainer. **Instead, we need a new mind-set for the millennium, a re-think of what is and is not beautiful, plus acceptance of what we can and can't achieve or change.** We think the 'body beautiful' should be about much more than working towards a bikini-worthy bottom; it should mean smooth-skinned, fit and glowing with energy...

BODY AND MIND

Beautifying your body should be about relaxing, cherishing and making yourself feel special – because when you feel good in your own skin, that's what other people notice. Not a lumpy bum or Marilyn Monroe belly, or even knock knees...

There's no doubt that the greatest beautifiers in the world are happiness and health. A joyful smile and abundant energy are far more attractive, whatever the owner's physique, than the most perfectly made-up, flawlessly formed but miserable face above a droopy body.

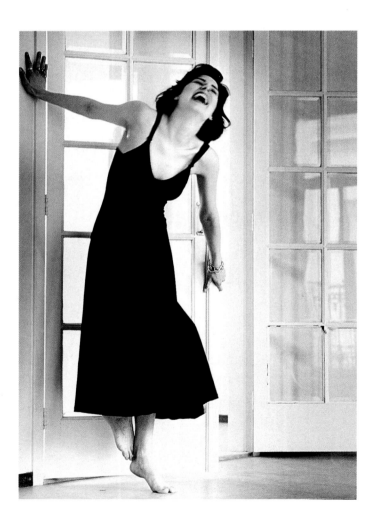

Easy to say, but if you aren't one of those lucky souls who were born under a laughing star, how do you get happy? Particularly if you have long-standing health or emotional problems to cope with. Happiness is a composite emotion. The French describe it as being 'comfortable in your skin' – in other words, liking yourself, feeling content with who you are and satisfied by what you do, feeling loved and loving. In a phrase, it is self-esteem. If you like or, if possible, love yourself unconditionally, you will like your face and body – no matter what Nature or Fate has given you. One of our best friends has scars from her severe cleft lip and is still self-conscious about them, but she is so enchanting as a person that no one else notices whether they are camouflaged or not.

It's true that some people seem to have an easier time finding joy and fun in life but each person's happiness quotient is, of course, also linked to their circumstances. Dr Clive Wood, author of *Say Yes To Life*, identifies seven key areas of your life which relate to happiness: love, work, family, children, friends, home life and surroundings, and time for yourself. Not all of these need be perfect for you to be happy, but it is useful to examine them if you persistently feel bad about yourself. You may find it helpful to do this with someone else, whether a friend, priest or professional therapist (see DIRECTORY).

Self-esteem is vital to your relationship with your body. Look after your body, respect it, enjoy it, listen to its needs – from food and drink to exercise or sleep – and it will reward you by working well. Many problems of the body are caused by the mind. This can be direct – anorexia, for instance – or indirect, when we simply aren't in tune with our body and its needs. British consultant psychiatrist Dr Jill Welbourne says the 'really dazzling common characteristic' among the increasing number of women with eating problems is that they do not communicate with their bodies below the neck. That applies to many of us in different ways; how often have you disregarded an aching neck or back, overtiredness or stress, and so made the problem infinitely worse?

It's quite clear that good health contributes to our feeling of well-being. Indeed, traditional Chinese medicine identifies the liver as the organ of happiness (or unhappiness) and treats it appropriately with herbal tonics. Activity of all sorts has been shown to raise your mood instantly and, as you get fitter, to improve your long-term sense of self-esteem. Relaxation is also vital to a sense of calm and of being at peace with yourself. It goes without saying that to be in harmony with your body you must clear up any long-standing physical problems, whether that's a sore neck or poor digestion.

There are many areas of our lives that we probably can't change – and certainly not at a moment's notice. But there are things that everyone can do to be happier *now*. Professor Michael Argyle, the author of *The Psychology of Happiness* (see BEAUTY BOOKSHELF) and many other works on the subject, compiled with us these ways of helping yourself to happiness:

Reel away the blues: dancing, whether it's Scottish reels, waltzing or doing the lambada, scores the highest points for making you feel joyful, followed by involvement in sport, music and drama.

Get closer to friends and people you love: being with old and new friends, expressing love and being told you are loved, and praising others make you feel better and warmer for the whole day.

Practise being a good talker and a good listener: the single most important factor in close relationships is communication. Learn to be open about your feelings and to listen to other people – without interrupting or judging them.

Don't live in the problem, live in the solution: think positive and bring problems out in the open. Then set about finding constructive ways to deal with them, with others' help if necessary. Solutions may be simple – such as letting time heal wounds or rebuilding bridges with other people – or more demanding – such as completing a task, attaining a goal, e.g. a work deadline, or consulting an expert for advice, whether the problem in emotional or practical.

Keep laughing: smiling and laughing – even if you fake them – and watching funny films and plays trigger the release of feel-good hormones from your brain, which improve your mood and help you sleep better.

Set attainable goals: make a list of goals you need to achieve, and those you want to achieve, and give yourself a realistic time frame, e.g. one goal a week. Don't overcommit yourself.

Be assertive: assertiveness on one day helps ensure a positive mood the next. Being assertive means asking for what you want, and sometimes saying 'no' to requests – clearly (but nicely). Practise saying 'no' in front of the mirror; it really does get easier.

Get close to nature: seeing beautiful scenery, breathing clean air, watching animals and birds in the outdoors, and sitting in the sun are all effective blues beaters, and help you sleep soundly.

Explore spirituality: a sense that life has meaning and direction, plus confidence in a set of guiding values, makes many people happier. Choose whatever spiritual path appeals. You could start by simply lighting a candle at home or in a holy place.

QUICK FIXES: Listen to music ✳ Pay someone a compliment ✳ Plan a trip or holiday ✳ Read a poem, short story or novel ✳ Eat a good meal ✳ Stroke an animal

FLOWER POWER

Bluebells for depression, holly for anger, chamomile/lavender/red clover and self heal for stress...

It may seem extraordinary that distillations of flowers can succeed where pharmaceutical drugs often fail (or leave you with horrible side effects) but we are firm believers in the power of flower essences to improve negative emotional states of mind. Amanda Cochrane, a devotee of flower remedies and co-author, with Clare Harvey, of *The Encyclopedia of Flower Remedies*, describes these homoeopathic drops as 'a type of liquid energy'. Best known is Dr Edward Bach's Rescue Remedy for stressful situations, but there are now hundreds of different essences from all corners of the globe; these can help you through all sorts of problems, from depression via procrastination to 'brain fog' and insomnia. (See DIRECTORY for full details of suppliers.)

GET MOVING

Our planet moves. So does the rest of the solar system. But, in the middle of it all, human beings are becoming more and more sedentary. Latest government figures show that nearly half the British nation is overweight, some to the point of obesity. And the main culprit is simply lack of exercise.

Our bodies are designed to take in energy through food and expend it by exercise. Surplus sits around, stored as fat. However much you cut calories and fat intake (and we don't think dieting is the best way of slimming, see page 162) you won't be able to lose weight efficiently and permanently unless you get moving.

Over the course of the 20th century, our patterns of exercise have changed dramatically. Although our mothers and grandmothers probably never went to the gym, they might well have taken a brisk walk every day, or gone riding and, since there were no washing machines or vacuum cleaners, most of them would have exerted a lot of energy doing the housework. The trouble now is that to deal with what most of us have to get through in a day, we have to cut corners – dash into the car, take a lift or escalator, tumble-dry washing rather than pegging it out and so on. Some days, we hardly move at all.

The solution, we are convinced, is to take exercise that you enjoy so that it becomes fun, combining fitness and relaxation. As well as making the body function better (from sending oxygen scudding to every part of your system to making your digestive system work more efficiently), exercise is a proven mood enhancer. It triggers the release of 'feel-good' hormones which whoosh round your body and give you a sense of well-being.

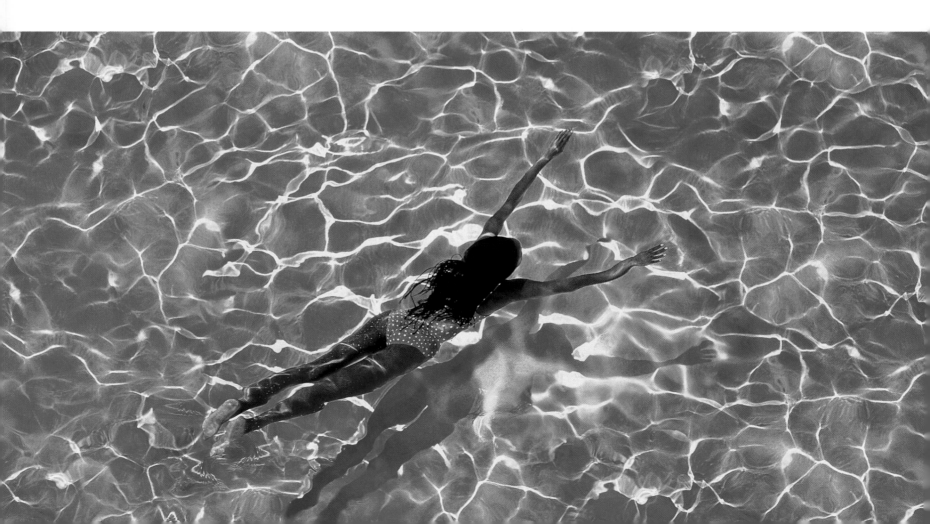

Working your body not only helps you lose weight and re-shapes it, it also boosts your energy levels, strengthens your heart and helps guard against all sorts of illness. We know too that it is vital in preventing osteoporosis, the loss of bone density which leads to brittle bones. And exercise is also pretty well guaranteed to improve your sex life.

How much and what sort of exercise do you need for general fitness?

In a perfect world, according to fitness expert Gloria Thomas, one of the star instructors of London's Harbour Club, we would exercise for at least 30 to 40 minutes six days a week, doing a combination of strength, aerobic and flexibility routines. But, she says, the main thing is to do what you can fit in and never feel guilty. 'Ten minutes every day is much better than nothing.'

You will notice some benefits immediately: the 'exercise glow', increased energy, improved spirits, fewer aches and pains (but don't overdo it at first if you're usually sedentary) and sounder sleep. Over three to six weeks, your body shape will start to change and firm up, but only if you eat a healthy diet as well. You may lose weight, but don't worry if you are working out diligently and yet *put on* weight – muscle weighs more than fat.

If you are not used to exercise, it's always a good idea to check with your doctor first, then start with a short time every day and build up gradually. Always start and finish exercise with some warm-up breathing and stretches, whether it's a full-blown workout, speed-walking (also known as power-walking) in the park, or even a wild solo dance around your kitchen.

A useful tip from pros is that, while working out, you should always be able to chat easily, without puffing or panting, whatever the exercise. And never forget to breathe deeply, slowly, rhythmically.

Finally, don't exercise if you have an injury or are ill in any way, and don't overtrain as it may leave you more vulnerable to infection. If you are feeling below par, take a gentle walk or do a short stretching session and leave the power stuff for a day or two.

TIP Make sure you have the right clothing, appropriate shoes (any sports shop will advise you) and a supportive bra.

Aim for a combination of these three types of exercise. Don't forget to warm up before and stretch after.

STRENGTH: helps tone and redefines body shape, boosts metabolic rate and burns calories, helps protect against osteoporosis, is good for posture, can help prevent bad backs. **Try:** weight training at home (add small dumbbells or ankle weights to your walk, jog, stretch routine) or at a local gym, but don't use large weights while walking, jogging or stretching – they may cause injury. Try using your own weight against your muscles – for instance with resistance bands. **Aim for:** ten to 20 minute sessions two to four times a week, on alternate days.

AEROBIC (cardiovascular): strengthens heart and lungs, improves circulation, excellent for burning calories and body fat. **Try:** brisk walking, walking up and down stairs or steps, dancing, swimming, water aerobics, running, cycling, jogging, rebounding (on a mini-trampoline), golf, tennis, aerobics or step classes, an exercise bike, treadmill, stair machines, kick boxing, squash (for advanced exercisers only). **Aim for:** three to five sessions weekly, each 15 to 60 minutes.

FLEXIBILITY (stretching): you need to stretch out all major muscle groups after any workout to keep you flexible and help prevent injuries to joints and muscles. Stretching also helps even out lumpiness. It's especially important for older people. **Try:** the warm up and stretch routine on page 158, yoga, any martial arts. **Aim for:** daily stretch sessions, of five to ten minutes or more, plus one to two classes weekly (yoga classes are often 90 minutes long).

TIP Facial exercise guru Eva Fraser (see page 92) recommends the long established and much respected Medau method of exercise, which combines strength, stamina, suppleness and stretch for all ages (see DIRECTORY).

Wake Up, Warm Up and Stretch

Take a tip from cats and start your day and any exercise with gentle breathing and warm-up stretches to invigorate you and help prevent joint or muscle injuries. Warming up is particularly important for anyone who is stiff or has limited mobility.

START BY CHECKING YOUR POSTURE

You can lose five pounds (2.27kg) instantly – or look as if you have – by the way you stand and sit and walk. Droopy bodies with hunched shoulders are not only unattractive – they are positively bad for you because they restrict your circulation.

Begin by looking at how you stand. Stand side on to a mirror with your feet a hip width apart, legs straight – but don't lock your knees. Pull your tummy in and check your spine. It should gently curve at your upper and lower back. There should be a straight line running down from your ears, through your shoulders, hips and knees to your ankles. Your arms should hang in the middle of your thighs as you look at them from the side.

If your shoulders are hunched, don't force them back – let your shoulder blades sink down to open your chest and shoulders. The brain has such remarkable powers that simply 'thinking' your body into this shape can encourage good posture. The Alexander Technique is also wonderful for bodies which store tension or are out of alignment.

If your tummy is sticking out, lift it gently towards your spine. Then tighten your buttock muscles and tuck your pelvis under your bottom. Think tall – imagine a string (or a golden silk thread if you're feeling romantic) lifting up your crown and pulling it towards the sky.

Now start walking gracefully around the room, concentrating on your posture. Think of how big cats move. Your feet should be facing forward with the second toe leading, heel first on the ground; let your hips and bottom move freely while you swing your arms back and forward.

Load-bearing exercise to beat brittle bones

This sort of exercise (also called weight-bearing) has been shown to protect against loss of bone density (osteoporosis) and is important for all women. Basically it includes every type of movement that puts weight on your muscles and bones, including running, walking, swimming, weight training, cycling, aerobics, dancing.

Music

Very often the key to making exercise joyful is music, whether it's pop, rock, jazz, classical or rhythmic drumming. In the cold western climate, most of us have forgotten the pleasure of moving to music. Yet you only have to go to a show like Riverdance to see how the toe-tapping rhythm uplifts the spirits of everyone there. So try exercising to your favourite music: dance wildly around your house, power-walk with a personal stereo, persuade the gym to play music with an appropriate beat as you pound the treadmill or stairmaster. (See DIRECTORY for details of where to get tapes with the right beat.)

Children love exercising to music so you could organise family fitness sessions while the beat goes on in the background.

TANIA ALEXANDER'S A.M. FITNESS ROUTINE

This simple routine, which takes about ten minutes altogether, was devised by UK fitness expert Tania Alexander, author of *No Sweat Fitness* (see BEAUTY BOOKSHELF), and is suitable for anyone, at any age and any level of fitness. However, you should always check with your doctor before embarking on any unaccustomed exercise, or if you are pregnant or have a bad back. Don't rush these exercises: do them slowly, preferably out of doors or by an open window.

Start with a breathing exercise

Stand with your feet forward, parallel and a hip width apart, tummy muscles gently drawn in, back and neck long as if a string is pulling you through the crown of your head. Let your shoulder blades relax and sink. Look ahead, then close your eyes, spread your toes and feel the ground. Stand in the same position throughout.

Breathe gently and rhythmically, in through your nose and out through your mouth. Take the same time inhaling as exhaling – count three or four beats on the in-breath, and on the out. As you get more practised, try holding your breath for a beat after inhaling and exhaling. If you enjoy visualisation, imagine your breathing pattern as a wave creeping up the beach, hovering for a moment, then flowing out. Once your breathing has settled, take five long slow breaths.

TIP: this is a wonderful exercise for calming yourself during the day.

Shake it all up

Shake your hands and one foot at a time, up and down, round and round, as vigorously as possible – if you can lie on the floor or some grass, even better, so you can shake hands and feet simultaneously.

TIP: shaking your hands briskly whenever you're worried or stiff can relieve tension and stress and re-energise you.

Get your body moving from top to toe

Breathe slowly and rhythmically through these exercises.

SHOULDERS: stand with feet a hip width apart, knees bent a little and tummy muscles drawn in. Rest your fingertips on the outside of your thighs. Using smooth controlled movements, slowly roll your shoulders backwards in a large circle. Keep your hips facing forward and your lower body still. Repeat five times backwards, five forwards.

Now place your right palm on the centre of your stomach and stretch up to the sky with the fingertips of your left hand. Then circle your left arm backwards from the shoulder five times in a wide movement as if you are swimming backstroke. Repeat forwards five times. Then repeat the routine the other side.

NECK: mobilise a stiff neck by turning your head slowly to the right, then tuck your chin down towards your shoulder and gently roll to the left. Repeat five times in each direction. This is a semi-circular movement; do not take your head back.

HIPS: with your feet still a hip width apart, upper body straight, tummy tucked in, put your hands on hips, and slowly circle them in a clockwise direction. Keep your upper body and feet still so your hips alone are moving. Repeat five times clockwise, five anti-clockwise.

Side Stretch

Standing as for your breathing exercise, place your right hand on your right thigh. On an exhalation, swing your left hand straight up to the sky so that you feel a mild stretch down the left side of your body. Keep your upper body straight. Breathe in, then, breathing out, swing the arm down to the starting point. Repeat twice on each side.

March on

Remembering to keep tummy and bottom tucked in and walking tall, march around, inside (include stairs) or outside (up and over obstacles if you can) for two to five minutes at least.

Hail the sun

On an out-breath, keep looking straight ahead and swing both arms in front of you up towards the sky, simultaneously lifting one knee as high as you comfortably can. Breathe in, then, as you breathe out, lower arms and leg. Repeat five times alternately on each leg.

Finish by breathing your mind clear

Place your right thumb lightly over your right nostril. Breathe in deeply through your left nostril. Now close your left nostril with your middle finger and, as you do so, release your thumb and exhale through your right nostril. Then reverse the process: keeping your left nostril closed, breathe in through your right nostril, then place your thumb over your right nostril again, release your middle finger and exhale through the left nostril. Continue for 30 to 60 seconds.

TIP: This technique is marvellous for clearing the mind at any time.

TIP Drink plenty of water: keep an unbreakable bottle handy.

TARGETED EXERCISES

Even if you are taking plenty of exercise, you may have particular problem areas which will respond well to a simple routine. The culprits for most of us are tummies and legs.

Fitness expert Tania Alexander has devised these easy exercises for *The Beauty Bible* to give you lean and lovely pins and a washboard stomach.

Instant Stomach Slimmers

As well as making you look good, strong muscle tone in your stomach will improve your posture and help prevent back problems. Start by doing five of each exercise daily and increase the number by five each week. With faithful practice, you should start to see results within a couple of weeks. These gentle exercises should be suitable for all ages and shapes, but consult your doctor first if you are pregnant or have any injuries or health complaints.

Breathe in through your nose to prepare for each exercise and out through your mouth as you do each one.

Curl ups

Lie on your back with your knees bent, feet flat on the floor. Concentrate on anchoring your lower back to the ground, then raise your head and shoulders slightly off the floor as you let your hips roll up and your body form a C-shape.

Rest your arms loosely on your stomach or, if you are more advanced, put them behind your head. (N.B. take care not to pull on the neck as you come forward.)

As with all these exercises, it's much more effective to do five controlled curl-ups than ten rushed ones. A common mistake is to curl up slowly then crash down. Curl up to the count of two, repeat on the way down. Check by placing one hand on your stomach as you curl up. If the muscles start to bulge, you are coming up too far or too fast.

Again, when you're more advanced, you can add in a twist to work the side stomach muscles and help create a slimmer waist: place your hands behind your head and curl towards each knee with the opposite elbow leading.

Pull your stomach in

Not only does this make you look better, it's good exercise for the stomach muscles. Make a conscious effort to do this as often as possible, even if you're just walking down the road or standing in a queue. Also pull your bottom in, clenching the muscles. Don't let your shoulders rise.

Walk tall

While you are pulling your tummy and bottom in, imagine you are being pulled upwards by a string at the top of your head. Remember to keep your shoulders and upper body relaxed all the time; it helps to imagine your shoulder blades sinking down.

Breathe and tone

Visualise your stomach as a balloon. When you breathe in, imagine it inflating. As you breathe out, let the air out like a balloon deflating. Your stomach will flatten almost miraculously. It's easier to do this when standing, lying or sitting rather than walking.

Exercise your pelvic floor muscles

The lower part of your stomach, known as the 'double belly', is the hardest to tone, particularly if you have had children. Strong pelvic floor muscles act as an internal corset supporting your lower stomach muscles. The muscles on your pelvic floor form a figure of eight, from the pubic bones in the front to the coccyx at the back, and are the ones used to control the flow of urine. To exercise them, draw them all up internally and tighten. You can do this when you're stuck in a traffic jam, at a bus stop or working at your desk.

Perfect Pins

The following exercises should produce mild tension in the muscles.
Practise diligently and you should see an improvement in two weeks.

Walking

Stride out briskly for 20 minutes at least every other day. It works all
the muscles from the top of the thighs to the feet.

Toning inner thighs

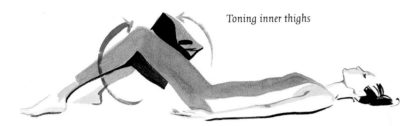

To tone inner thighs, swim breaststroke, go skating or take slide
classes. Or try this easy exercise (above). Lie on your back, legs bent,
feet flat on the floor. Place a large cushion between your knees.
Breathe in, then exhale, squeezing
the cushion as hard as possible.
Hold for a count of two, then
slowly release. Repeat ten
times.

Toning outer thighs
To tone outer thighs, do
leg raisers. Hold on to a
table or draining board,
and stand on your left
leg, bending it slightly.
Lift your right leg out to the side
and, from the relaxed position
shown (left) flex your right foot
(flexing is the opposite of
pointing) until you feel tension in
the outer thigh. Keep your hips
square and facing forwards. Repeat
ten to 15 times each side.

Toning fronts and backs of thighs

First, to get a stretch down the
front of your thighs, stand facing
the table or draining board
(right), keeping your knees soft,
not locked. Flex one foot and curl
it up to your bottom. Repeat ten
to 15 times on either side.
 To exercise the back of
your thighs, from the
same standing position,
shuffle your feet backwards
so that you are at least an arm's
length away and your back is as flat as
possible. Hold on if necessary. Repeat
the exercise, as above.

Slimming ankles

Slim puffy ankles with ankle circles. Circle
five times slowly in each direction, keeping the rest of
your leg still.

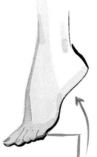

Shaping up calves

Shape up calves on the
staircase. Hold on to the rail
for balance.

Place your heels over the
edge of the step, then rise
on your toes and slowly down
again so that your heels drop
beneath the step. Repeat ten
to 20 times daily.

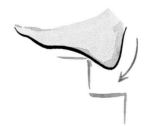

FOOD

For most women from their early teens on, food means dieting. Ninety-five per cent of women are said to diet at some point in their lives and virtually all put back the weight they lose. And more.

Yoyo diets, especially diet drinks which replace meals, are probably the most futile. Amphetamines are usually a waste of time and may also prove dangerous. Almost any attempt to lose a lot of weight very quickly is doomed and extremely bad for your health. (Although there may be exceptions to this when diets are carried out under *strict* medical supervision.) Your body doesn't understand that what you want to do is get into that slinky little black dress; all it comprehends is famine. So it pulls out all the stops to deal with the looming food shortage, shutting down your body systems to save energy and, as it perceives itself under threat, making you search ravenously for food.

We're not saying 'don't slim'. We are saying 'don't diet'. If you want to lose weight permanently, you can. Aim to do so slowly and safely, with a combination of well-chosen, delicious food (which puts you in harmony with your body rather than at war with it), plus exercise (which is vital to help tone and reshape your body and keep it functioning at peak level).

If you were brought up being told that the food you couldn't stand was the one which did you the most good, forget it. Dietbreakers, the effective self-help organisation which has enabled many women and some men to kick the dieting habit, suggests always choosing food you fancy, which you can really taste and enjoy. Depriving yourself is a short cut to bingeing.

Many people also find it useful to de-tox once in a while; some practitioners of traditional medicine suggest fasting as often as once a week. This doesn't mean eating nothing, unless you are resting in bed and expending no energy (which we positively enjoy from time to time), but, instead, giving your digestive system a rest by eating lots of fruit, salads and vegetables and drinking pure water and herbal teas. (See *Go Into De-Tox*, page 196.)

If you have a real problem with food, whether it's overeating, under-eating or bingeing, feeling ashamed or frightened won't make it go away. Many of us have been in exactly the same situation, not knowing where to turn or what to do. There are good sources of help, including the international self-help organisation Overeaters Anonymous. Nutritionists and naturopaths, amongst other complementary therapists, can suggest sensible eating plans. Counselling or psychotherapy can help with low self-esteem. The Eating Disorders Association also provides excellent information packs for the estimated one in ten people with serious problems.

Learning to eat well and enjoy your food will give you health, prevent illness and provide you with that energy and *joie de vivre* which are essential to beauty.

GUIDELINES FOR HEALTHY EATING

The joy of eating well is that putting good food into your body gives you more energy, which in turn means you rush around more, boost your metabolism (the rate at which you burn up food energy). Then you can eat more than many of us would ever dream of allowing on our plates.

Nutritionists Gillian Hamer and Kathryn Marsden suggest the following:

✦ **Each day, aim to eat:**
one serving of PROTEIN (eggs, cheese, soya, meat, fish)
at least five servings of VEGETABLES and FRUIT (preferably more vegetables than fruit)
at least 1 tsp of good quality OIL (extra virgin cold-pressed olive oil, sesame, flax)
at least one serving of CARBOHYDRATES (large jacket potato; cupful of cooked rice, pulses or cereals; up to four slices of bread, made with stoneground, unrefined flour, preferably rye rather than wheat)

(Further guidelines continued on page 164.)

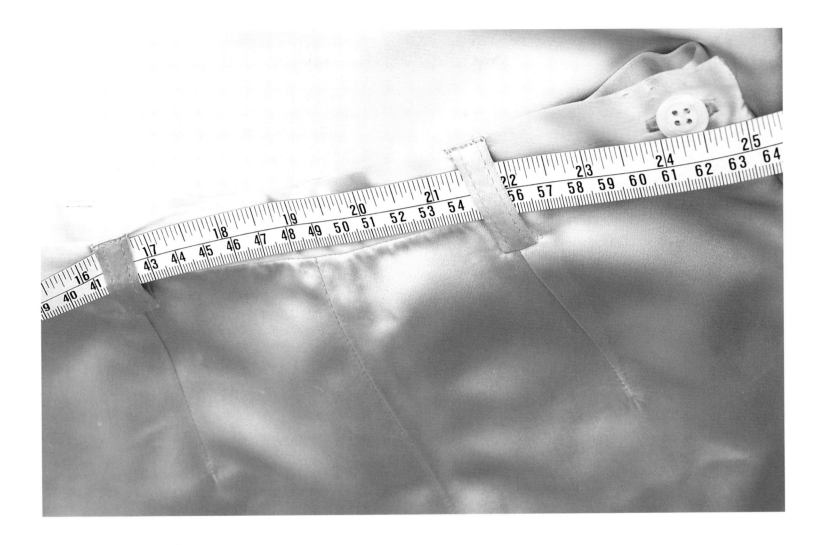

QUICK WEIGHT LOSS

Although we think diets are the work of the devil, there are times when women feel desperately unhappy if they do not lose some weight quickly. If you only have a few pounds to lose, try food combining or the light de-tox outlined on page 196, but if all else fails, don't stop eating. This high-protein eating plan, recommended by London doctor Dr Richard Petty, can be safely followed for a week or, at most, two.

✦ Avoid dairy produce, sugar, caffeine, alcohol, root vegetables, wheat and fruit.

✦ Four times a day, eat 2–3oz (56–85g) of protein (tofu, egg, fish, chicken) with as much salad or vegetables (not root) as you like, and any sort of dressing (yes, that does include mayonnaise).

✦ Drink at least 2 litres of water (you will feel ill if you don't) and take a good multivitamin and mineral supplement daily.

GUIDELINES FOR HEALTHY EATING, contd.

✦ **Drink lots of** WATER to keep your kidneys working well, de-tox your system and improve your complexion (see SKIN). Start by drinking a litre of pure, still water at room temperature throughout the day and work up to 2 litres. If you like, a glass of good wine a day is fine.

✦ **Cut down on** FAT but don't count fat grammes or go on a fat-free diet. Your body needs natural poly- and mono-unsaturated fats to work properly (try vegetable oils and seeds or oily fish such as mackerel, trout, sardines and salmon) as well as sensible amounts of saturated fats (butter and cream). So kick the cakes, biscuits, take-aways, chips and hydrogenated margarine spreads. Use olive oil for cooking and salad dressings, and small amounts of butter, not hydrogenated margarine for spreading. Never deep-fry food – instead, grill, steam, sauté, stew or stir-fry in a wok.

✦ **Eat more** FIBRE but banish wheat bran – it can actually irritate your colon. Go for brown rice, pulses, rye bread instead. Grind linseed, pumpkin and sunflower seeds in a coffee grinder and sprinkle onto salads or on your breakfast, which could be either non-wheat cereal, porridge or sheep or goat's milk yoghurt.

✦ **Wash all** vegetables and fruits thoroughly. Supermarket apples have probably been sprayed about 18 times with chemical pesticides. Fruit, vegetables, meat and fish may contain antibiotics, hormones and other chemicals, so buy ORGANIC produce wherever possible.

✦ **Begin with** a good breakfast and eat four or five smaller meals a day. Grazing on nutritious foods and snacking are now believed to be good for you.

✦ **Eat slowly** until you are comfortably full. Then stop.

✦ **Prepare meals** in good time: don't leave it until you're so starving you'll hoover up anything to quell the pangs of hunger. If you do come home ravenous, drink a home-juiced vegetable or fruit cocktail (or commercial fruit juices with no added sugar) – this will keep you going for at least 40 minutes while you prepare your meal.

FOOD COMBINING

Although many doctors are reluctant to support it, food combining (also known as the Hay Diet) has helped millions overcome health problems, from migraine and skin problems to aching joints and irritable bowel syndrome (which affects about one person in four). Lately a gourmet gloss was put on this approach by Michel Montignac, whose bestselling slimming books adopt virtually the same theory in a rather more sophisticated form.

The basis of food combining is knowing which foods you should – or shouldn't – eat at the same time. Fruit is eaten on its own (i.e. at least 30 minutes apart from other foods), while protein and starch are eaten separately from each other with vegetables and salads. For instance, you wouldn't eat roast chicken with bread sauce and roast potatoes; instead you would combine it with vegetables or salad and a thin gravy. Food combining is therefore easier if you are vegetarian.

Food combining has the wonderful bonus of being a very effective slimming plan. Whether this is because you eat much less (as sceptical doctors insist but food combiners dispute) or whether it is because your body functions better and stores less fat (as Hay Diet followers believe) is not clear.

FOOD CRAVINGS

If you suffer from wild cravings for chocolates or jam sandwiches, don't feel guilty – there may be underlying physical factors. The most likely are candida (the yeast-like fungus linked to thrush and to what's charmingly called leaky gut) and food allergies or intolerances which can, paradoxically, cause cravings. Wheat allergy, for instance, which is very common, often triggers an apparent addiction to the substance in sufferers. Blood sugar imbalance is another condition which can trigger people to binge, almost invariably on sweet, fatty foods.

Food cravings are often combined with flatulence, bloating, constipation, diarrhoea, lethargy, tiredness, depression, fuzzy-headedness, PMS and painful periods. Sufferers of vaginal thrush may also have itching and the typical white curdy discharge. There are several useful books (see DIRECTORY) and we recommend you consider consulting a reputable nutritionist or naturopath.

CAN SUPPLEMENTS HELP?

The argument about whether or not to take supplements has raged for a number of years. Many doctors and dieticians have maintained that a good balanced western diet supplies all the nutrients you need. Now research is coming down firmly on the side of sensible supplementation, confirming what many of us have found from personal experience.

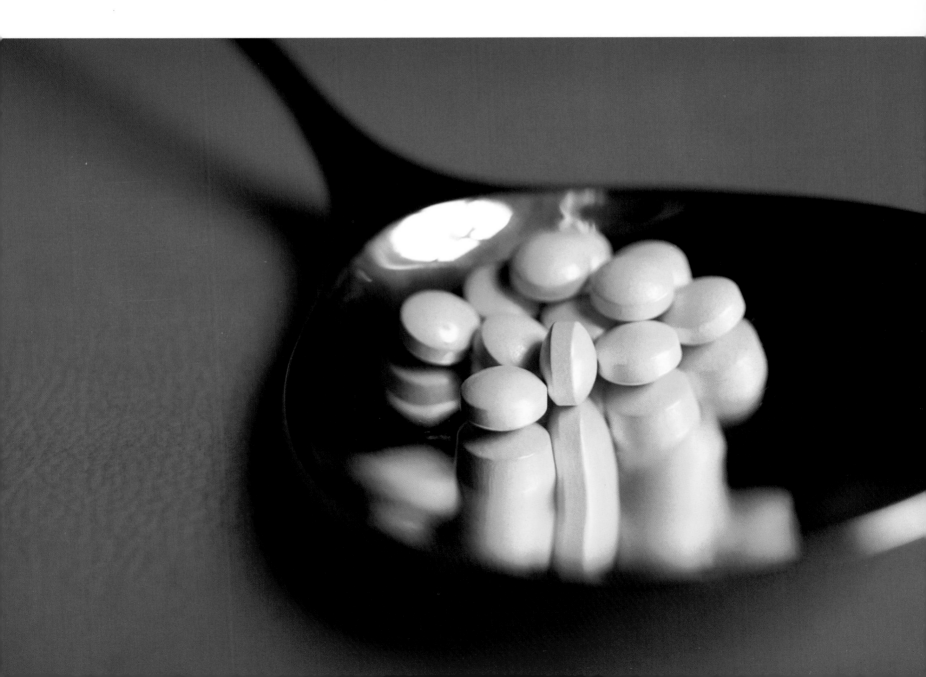

The National Food Survey, based on food diaries kept by 8,043 households during 1993, revealed that the average person in Britain is deficient in eight out of 13 vitamins and minerals, compared with the new European recommended daily levels. An American government study of 20,000 people found that every single subject was deficient in one or other of ten essential nutrients.

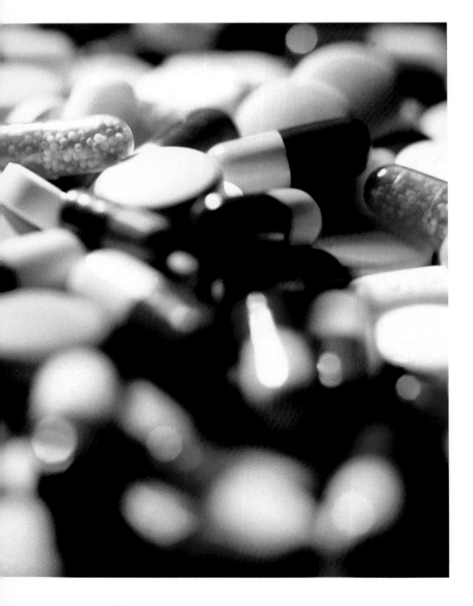

Research also suggests that the way we live now – stressed out, smoking and drinking, bombarded by UV rays, petrol fumes and, often, radiation from office equipment – can deplete our bodies' stores of essential nutrients. At the same time, modern farming techniques, food processing technology and the way we cook our meals mean that actual foodstuffs are not as nutritious as they used to be.

We are not suggesting that you become supplement junkies. It's vital to eat the best possible diet, preferably organic, but we would have to sit and chew from dawn to dusk to get the levels of some vitamins and minerals now recommended by eminent researchers worldwide. Both of us firmly believe in the value of well-formulated supplements to prevent illness and keep us functioning at peak energy and fitness – and that, of course, means looking good, too.

Supplements are virtually non-toxic, so there is no real issue about safety. If in doubt about quantities it's best to stick to the manufacturer's dosage instructions. Very occasionally someone discovers they are allergic to an ingredient in a supplement. If you find you have, say, a rash stop all your supplements, then start adding them back at the rate of one every three days to find the culprit.

We think it is worth buying the best brands you can afford because more expensive ones are invariably better formulated and so more effectively absorbed into your system. Our preferred brands are Biocare, Blackmore's, Higher Nature, Missing Link, Natural Flow, Pharma Nord, Quest, Scotia Pharmaceuticals and Solgar. (See Directory for where to buy and mail order.)

If the supplement is doing you good, you should feel noticeably better at the end of four weeks.

IF SO, WHICH?

The difficulty is choosing which supplements to take. Gazing at rows of bottles with complicated names is not enlightening. We asked nutritionist Patrick Holford of the Institute for Optimum Nutrition to suggest supplements for this book. Here are his guidelines:

Every day

✦ At a minimum, take a good multivitamin and multimineral supplement.

✦ If possible, also take a 'super' antioxidant formula, containing vitamins beta carotene, C and E, minerals including selenium, plus amino acids.

◆ Essential fatty acids are vital and most people don't get enough. Look for gamma linolenic acid (GLA; Omega-6), which is found in evening primrose, starflower or borage oils. You should have 150mg of actual GLA daily so read the label carefully. You also need linolenic acid (Omega-3), which comes from flax seed oil – try taking one dessertspoonful daily in soup, or on cereal or salad. (But don't take flax on its own long term; you need to combine it with Omega-6.)

◆ Take 1g of vitamin C daily, with 3g if you're under stress. If a cold threatens, take 3g every four hours.

◆ Women aged 45 upwards should consider taking a supplement to help prevent bone density loss, particularly if they have osteoporosis (brittle bones) in the family. The most important nutrients are calcium, magnesium, zinc, vitamin D and boron. Aim for a product containing a ratio of 400mg of calcium to 200mg of magnesium.

IF YOU'RE FEELING POORLY

◆ Boost your immune system with echinacaea (try Echinaforce by Bioforce) and an infusion of the rain forest herb Cat's Claw, in addition to your vitamin C.

FOR TUMMY TROUBLE AND OTHER ILLNESS

◆ Grape seed extract (also called citricidal) is a natural anti-fungal, anti-viral, anti-bacterial and anti-parasitical. It's marvellous for anything from food poisoning and cystitis to ear infections and sore throats. Take ten drops twice daily whilst infection lasts.

◆ For any sort of digestive upset, and always following a course of antibiotics, probiotics (which replace the friendly gut bacteria) are invaluable. Look for capsules or pills containing strains of lactobacillus and bifidus, which naturally populate the human gut.

FOR A HEALTHY BABY

Patrick suggests taking 400mg of folic acid before conception and during the first three months of pregnancy. Zinc, vitamin B6, essential fatty acids and selenium are also very important. It's always wise to get specific advice from organisations such as Foresight (see DIRECTORY).

FOR ENERGY

◆ When you exert a lot of energy, you often crave sweet foods and caffeine for a quick energy fix. This is the time to take chromium, which stabilises your blood sugar levels. Try it as chromium polynicotinate, which contains vitamin B3 (200mg daily).

◆ Support the adrenal gland, which controls your reactions to stress of all kinds, with pantothenic acid (500mg daily).

WHEN SHOULD YOU TAKE SUPPLEMENTS?

Here are Patrick's guidelines for supplementation:

❖ Take most of your supplements with your first meal of the day

❖ Take vitamins and minerals 15 minutes before or after, or during a meal

❖ If you're taking two or more B Complex or vitamin C tablets, take one at each meal

❖ Don't take B vitamins at night if you have difficulty sleeping

❖ Don't take individual B vitamins unless you are also taking a general B Complex, perhaps in a multivitamin

❖ Take multiminerals in the evening to help you sleep

❖ Don't take individual minerals unless you are also taking a general multimineral

❖ Take your supplements every day. Irregular supplementation doesn't work

OUR SUGGESTIONS

In addition to Patrick's suggestions we wouldn't be without:

Galium Complex by Blackmore's – for a booster after bacterial or viral infections

Blue green algae – a general nutritional supplement

Ginseng – a wonderful tonic and energiser

Co-enzyme Q-10 – hailed by some experts as the most exciting antioxidant of all

CELLULITE

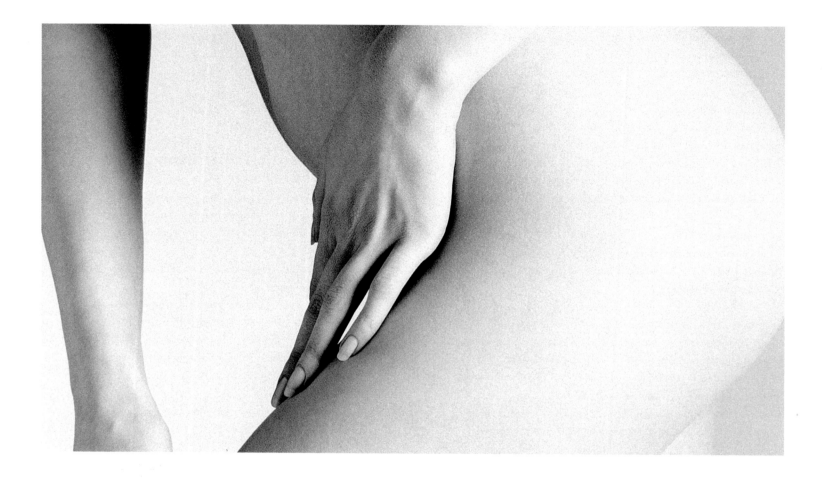

Until recently, most doctors denied the existence of cellulite – that squishy, dimply orange peel look which decorates the thighs and bottoms of about 95 per cent of women to a greater or lesser extent. 'It's what middle-aged women's thighs look like, isn't it?' one expert told us dismissively. That may be so but, increasingly, doctors – particularly in mainland Europe – are admitting that cellulite is not just a beauty whim but a medical condition which can respond to appropriate treatment.

Why and how cellulite forms is the topic of endless theories. It is fat, no doubt about it, but it doesn't look like other fat and it doesn't always behave in the same way. Show us another area of fat which may look smoothish on the surface but dimples like a button-back chair when pressed or squeezed. What's more, a fat woman may not necessarily have cellulite, while a rake-thin, superfit athlete may.

Many doctors, as we have said, still adopt a dismissive approach. Two women doctors, however, have spearheaded a counter attack, Dr Karen Burke, a New York dermatologist, author of *Thin Thighs for Life* and Dr Elizabeth Dancey, a London-based Europe-trained doctor and author of *The Cellulite Solution*. Not only do they validate cellulite medically, but they offer sensible guidelines to holistic treatment.

Dr Burke gives an interesting explanation for the structure of these particular fat cells. Firstly, she emphasises, cellulite is a *natural female condition*, just like having breasts and no facial hair. Like most experts, Dr Burke believes that the fundamental basis of cellulite is related to the female hormone oestrogen. This swings into action at puberty, creating feminine curves by enlarging fat cells, particularly on hips and thighs. From then on, women live in a flurry of natural hormonal activity, which is exacerbated by taking synthetic hormones in the form of the Pill or HRT. (The male hormone, testosterone, actually induces fat *loss* on hips and thighs, and men also tend to store fat at a deeper level in the liver and intestines.)

More curiously, Dr Burke says the appearance of cellulite is caused by the way women's fat cells are *packaged* under the skin. The fat cells themselves are the same in men and women, and both sexes store fat in sacs divided by connective tissue. In women, however, the sacs are *standing* chambers of fat – tall, thin and arched like Gothic windows, with the points attached deep in the skin. From these points, ropes of fibre project up towards the surface, creating the dimpled or button-back chair effect. On men's thighs, though, not only is the skin thicker and the fat sacs smaller but the connective tissue anchors are in a *horizontal* lattice-like pattern which does not show on the surface.

As women grow older, those connective tissue anchors thicken and create the mattress effect. Surface skin becomes thinner, showing all too clearly the bulging fat sacs beneath. Most of us also put on weight, which reduces both blood flow and drainage of the lymphatic system, so the cellulite becomes difficult to budge. The combination of all these factors can result in big blobby lumps of cellulite.

Whatever the state of your cellulite, it can be vastly improved upon – as we can testify. Cellulite is a sign of long-term imbalance in the body, and is largely a result of lifestyle, not genes. The key to treatment is to bring the body back to a state where it is functioning smoothly. You *can* beat your cellulite – but be prepared for it to take time and dedication. It didn't come in a week, and it won't go in one.

THE BOTTOM LINE
Where does it affect you?
Principally on bottom, thighs and knees, but it can also appear on tummy, back of neck and backs of arms.
What does it look like?
Anything from the first stages of faint dimpling when the skin is pressed or gathered up, to the final stages where you see large pasty blobs on the surface, 'tethered' like a mattress to the deeper layers of skin. Early signs of cellulite are bruises and cuts which are slow to heal, easy bruising, broken veins, discoloured thick or tender skin.
What is happening medically?
Cells and tissues need an effective blood transport and waste-removal system to function well. In areas of cellulite, this system is impaired, leaving the fat trapped in webs of fibre. This can mean that:
❖ the blood supply is not delivering sufficient oxygen and vital nutrients;
❖ the venous system is not removing carbon dioxide and toxins;
❖ and/or the lymphatic drainage system is not draining the lymph fluid.

Once one of these is under way, the others are likely to follow suit, mounting a three-pronged attack on your body.

What causes cellulite?
❶ **Your diet** – in short, anything which deposits fat on your bottom half. This includes:
❖ too much fat and sugar: these are stored as fat, principally around your thighs and bottom. Particular villains include sugary, fatty treats and skipping meals (your body is then forced to store fat).
❖ yoyo dieting: women store fat six times more readily on their lower body than the upper. What's worse, the lower body is six times less keen on releasing its fat. So if we gain 7lb (3.2kg) in weight, 6lb (2.7kg) go on our bottom half. If we lose 7lb, 6lb go from the top and only one from the bottom. If we continually yoyo diet, the pattern intensifies (try the maths – it's mind-boggling). You can change your body shape permanently – for the worse.
❖ blood sugar imbalance (see *Food Cravings*, page 164).
❖ insufficient trace elements (mainly zinc, chromium, nickel and cobalt); this is usually due to too many processed, ready-made,

pre-packed foods and not enough fresh fruit, vegetables, nuts, pulses, fish and meat (for non-vegetarians). Symptoms of this deficiency include general fatigue and lack of energy, and may lead to a sugar craving, particularly before menstruation. Lack of fresh fruit and vegetables can also upset the sodium-potassium balance and contribute to cellulite. Other causes are:

❖ not drinking enough water.
❖ diuretics: these ultimately cause more water retention.
❖ slimming pills: these lead to water retention, plus fatigue and irritability.
❖ too little protein.
❖ artificial additives: pesticides, colouring, flavourings, sweeteners.

❷ Food allergies and intolerance

Many popular foods can trigger reactions ranging from mild intolerance to full-blown allergy. The most extreme (and rare) examples include some types of nuts or fish, which can send sufferers into possibly fatal anaphylactic shock, where the respiratory system shuts down. About one in two thousand people in the UK are estimated to suffer from a severe food allergy. Many others are believed to suffer from some less dramatic form of reaction to food.

The most common trigger foods are: wheat, milk (particularly cow's), eggs, coffee and tea, tomatoes, oranges, chocolate, fish and shellfish.

Although it's not a view that is popular amongst many conventional doctors, those who have studied the subject say that food reactivity can lead to a gamut of physical symptoms in addition to weight gain: migraine, aching joints, water retention, bloating and other symptoms of candida albicans and Irritable Bowel Syndrome, including constipation, diarrhoea and flatulence. (IBS symptoms can directly affect cellulite by hampering essential body functions.) Food reactivity can also induce mental symptoms, notably mood swings and depression, which can be severe, and is implicated in other allergic conditions such as asthma, eczema and hay fever.

❸ Hormones

As we have said, natural female hormones are the basis of cellulite, but many experts believe that prescribed hormones can exacerbate the problem. Any hormonal disruption from puberty through pregnancy to menopause can affect cellulite.

❹ Pelvic surgery

This disrupts the lymph system.

❺ Stress

This can alter body chemistry and prompt the storage of fat.

❻ Free radical damage

We need some free radical molecules for our bodies to function (see page 70), but an excess leads to a range of problems which almost certainly include heart disease and cancer. Free radicals can also contribute to cellulite by damaging the circulation. An excess of them is principally caused by smoking, pollution of all kinds and UV light.

Then comes the big question:

How do you get rid of it?

Given what we now know about cellulite, you need to attack it on two fronts; firstly, by losing weight and firming flesh, and, secondly, by liberating fat from the cellulite deposits. Treatment divides into what you can do for yourself, at low cost, and what you can have done for you, which may be expensive. In our experience, which chimes with the experts, the following are the staples of successful cellulite treatment. They are also, incidentally, the bases of good health – so you can achieve a double whammy.

Diet
❖ eat little and often
❖ minimise intake of dairy products, alcohol, caffeine and sugar and, if you're not vegetarian, red meat
❖ avoid solid animal fat
❖ avoid fat/sugar and fat/salt combinations
❖ feast on high-fibre fruit and vegetables: current medical thinking in the US dictates six to ten portions of vegetables daily (poach or steam vegetables if you have digestive problems)
❖ reduce your protein intake to 1–3oz (28kg–85g) of egg, fish or chicken daily
❖ buy organic produce if possible
❖ drink 1 or 2 litres daily of still, pure water at room temperature, and herbal teas

Supplements

Vitamins C and E may directly help to reduce cellulite, according to Dr Burke. She recommends taking 1g to 6g of vitamin C daily, 400 international units of natural vitamin E in capsule form, and supplementing with calcium to make up for the reduction in dairy foods. (Take calcium with magnesium in a ratio of 2:1, a useful dose is 400mg calcium to 200mg magnesium.) See page 165.

Exercise

This is simply essential (see page 156 for our exercise suggestions). Dr Burke recommends yoga and dance which stretch and tone rather than bodybuilding. Swimming is universally applauded, and don't dismiss a brisk daily walk, swinging your arms as you go. Aim to stretch daily and walk if you can, with up to four sessions of swimming, dancing or yoga each week.

Dry skin brushing

This is one of the cheapest and most effective methods of stimulating your circulation. With a small, stiff brush or massage glove (preferably made with natural bristles or fibres), start with your feet and brush in long strokes all over your body towards the heart. Brush firmly enough to induce a pink glow, concentrating on the worst patches of cellulite. (Be careful if you have any problem skin conditions, or healing wounds.) It may sound – and feel – like masochism at first, but it is the most wonderfully invigorating treatment. You can do it before or after a shower or bath. If you shower, try skin brushing before taking a hot shower followed by a cool or cold one; the effect is electrifying.

Massage

Again, be wary of optimistic claims. The only safe and effective massage for cellulite is manual lymphatic drainage massage. Gentle self-massage with anti-cellulite oil can also help. Too violent massage may damage the lymph system and cause more problems.

Stress reduction

It's vital to reduce unmanageable stress. (This applies of course to all parts of your life, not just your cellulite.) The quickest thing you can do, right now, is to start breathing better – see page 159. Then turn to our suggestions for stress-busting techniques on page 185.

OTHER PROFESSIONAL THERAPIES

(For contact details, see DIRECTORY)

IONITHERMIE: A method of combining plant and mineral preparation with a gentle electric current. Good for tone and texture. May be useful in combination with our basic home treatment (above) and other professional treatments.

MESOTHERAPY: A technique respected in mainland Europe, where minute quantities of pharmacological drugs are injected into the cellulite deposits to boost circulation, stimulate drainage and digest hard lump tissues around cells. Must be administered by a medical practitioner and should be done in conjunction with the home techniques given above. Patients usually need 15 sessions.

CELLULOLIPOLYSIS: An invasive medical technique usually carried out at cosmetic surgery clinics, where electrodes encased in long needles are inserted into the cellulite. Claimed to be a long-lasting method of burning up fat by forcing cells to fight against the current, thus stimulating cellular activity. It is painful and, in a small unpublished study by a leading British surgeon, only half of the patients said they saw any improvement.

SURGERY: Surgical interventions in the form of liposuction, liposculpture and ultrasonic liposuction (see HELPING NATURE) have been touted as the answer to cellulite. In fact, they remove fat, not actual cellulite. Neither do they repair the damaged micro-circulation and lymph system. Surgery is likely to inflict further damage on these, leading to more cellulite.

SKIN CREAMS AND GELS

Massaging in creams or gels after brushing will improve texture and tone, and some products may actually help disperse cellulite. Dr Dancey recommends two products – Cellulène by Carilène and Madacason by Laroche Naveron, available in French pharmacies or by mail order (see DIRECTORY). Try a cream for dry skin, gel for oily.

Beware: regardless of claims, cellulite preparation alone will never produce lasting results. Some creams may even invite more problems than they solve (apart from the problem with your bank manager). Liz Earle, author of *The Quick Guide to Beating Cellulite* (see BEAUTY BOOKSHELF), says her testers both developed a rash after using a cream containing aminophylline, and they saw no improvement in their cellulite. Aminophylline is unstable in cream form and may break down after as little as three weeks in a hot salon and become ineffective.

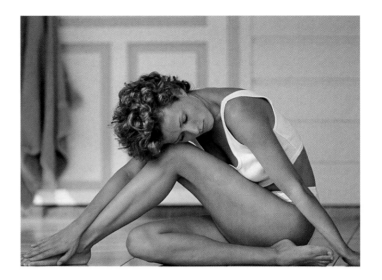

TRIED & TESTED

CELLULITE CREAMS

This is a booming industry with promises that can be wild – and with hefty price tags to match. We asked testers whether they reduced cellulite – both dimpling and quantity – and whether they improved tone and texture. Somewhat to our surprise, several of these products scored extremely highly – although no product scored unanimously good results with all of the panel.

Top Treats

Clarins Body Lift

A thigh-chilling gel which everyone agreed had a noticeable effect.
COMMENTS: 'revitalising and energising...feels like it's really doing something', 'smoothing and tautening', 'my skirts slipped on more easily'.

Juvena Body Results Styling Gel

This 'jelly-textured' formulation – which received all-round good marks – has a cooling effect on the areas it's massaged into.
COMMENTS: 'legs felt a lot firmer and smoother', 'I loved using this product – especially the cool sensation after a few minutes', 'my thighs felt firmer and smoother – although this wasn't permanent'.

Gatineau Body Contour Gel

This scored well for its easy-to-use dispenser and quick absorption, as well as for the results.

COMMENTS: 'cellulite seemed less noticeable', 'made my skin feel more taut'.

Best Budget Buy

Boots Grapefruit Massage Oil

Although this is an oil, our testers found it was easily rubbed in and great for skin texture.
COMMENTS: 'a dramatic difference that I didn't expect', 'a lovely smell', 'my skin was beautifully soft afterwards'.

Honourable Mentions

Anne-Marie Börlind Body-Lind Cellulite Cream

This is an all-natural option which earned rave reviews from some testers.

Neal's Yard Cellulite Oil

Another natural choice which had a particularly appealing smell, according to testers.

Inchwrap Cellulite Programme

This three-step programme – Gel Exfoliant, Firming Gel and Firming Moisturiser – received some very good marks, particularly from one woman who used it on her upper arms.

HOW TO HAVE FABULOUS FEET

Happy feet make for a happy woman. When your feet are killing you, it shows on your face very quickly. With every step you take, your feet have to absorb the stress of up to twice your body weight – so no wonder eight out of ten people suffer from foot problems.

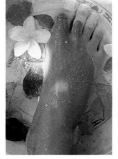

Except for the strappy sandal season, we tend to neglect feet because they're under wraps. But a regular pedicure isn't just a beauty indulgence; it can keep foot troubles at bay. In winter, you can of course skip colourful varnish and leave nails naked, or with a coat of clear polish.

TEN STEPS TO SEXY FEET

1 Cut nails straight across; shaping can result in ingrown nails. (Some people find it easier to do this after soaking feet, see step 3.)

2 Apply cuticle oil or lotion to soften them; any product designed for manicures is fine for feet, too.

3 Soak your feet in a washing-up bowl of lukewarm water, with a few drops of essential oils well blended into the water. Peppermint cools, chamomile softens and lavender heals.

4 Rub in cuticle remover; wait a minute, then push back cuticles with a rubber 'hoof' stick or orange stick wrapped in cotton wool. Don't cut cuticle skin: leave that to professionals. Don't be tempted to push back cuticles so far the little 'moon' shows; cuticles protect the nail bed, which is a mass of blood vessels and damages easily.

5 Slough off dead skin with a pumice stone or foot exfoliant.

6 Using sweeping movements from the toes to the ankle, massage the feet with a rich cream to stimulate, relax and help flexibility. According to dermatologists, kneading and rubbing the feet not only relieves aches but also helps relax the mind.

7 Before you varnish, clean nails with soapy water. Dry thoroughly.

8 If you don't have any 'toe-separators', which salons use for pedicures, cheat by separating toes with rolled up tissues or cotton wool balls. Otherwise it's easy to smudge polish.

9 Apply base coat, varnish and then top coat. Work from little toe to big toe to avoid smudging, varnishing from the bottom of nails to tips. Then brush on two coats of colour, waiting a minute for each one to dry.

10 If you're in a hurry, when your varnish is no longer tacky, very gently massage in a tiny drop of baby oil or jojoba oil, which will set the polish fast. If not, enjoy the opportunity to put your feet up while your nails dry.

TIPS FROM THE TOP

Coco Chanel never painted her fingernails but always wore toenail polish, working on the theory that feet were a dreary business and needed every help possible.

Follow the advice of that great style-setter **The Duke of Windsor**, who said: 'Only two rules really count: never miss an opportunity to relieve yourself, and never miss an opportunity to rest your feet.'

Explorer **Monica Kristensen** not only massages Elizabeth Arden's Eight-hour Cream into her own feet but also those of her sled dogs, to prevent cracking. (This works just as well outside Antarctica.)

Chiropodists can instantly diagnose a cigarette smoker by their dry, rather cold feet as smoking inhibits the delivery of oxygen to the extremities.

PUTTING YOUR BEST FOOT FORWARD

✦ A good salon pedicure should include a soak in an antiseptic foot bath, removal of calluses or thickened skin on the foot's pressure points, a foot and lower leg massage, and varnish.

✦ If you have your toenails painted in a salon, take strappy shoes of flip flops along and wear them afterwards – or schedule another treatment before you get dressed to give polish time to dry. Otherwise your varnish will acquire the imprint of your tights on the way home.

✦ High heels not only throw you off balance, putting you at risk of back trouble; they can also cause painful bunions and ankle problems. Buying shoes that are too small makes the situation worse. Shop for shoes in the afternoon, when feet are slightly swollen, to avoid buying a size too small.

✦ Change your shoes and, if you like to wear high heels, vary your heel height every day.

✦ If you can't wean yourself off high heels, do what you can to help circulation by massaging calves and feet regularly, which will stop them from swelling.

✦ Carry a foot spray in your handbag. (See *Tried & Tested Foot Revivers*.)

✦ Whenever your feet are tired, revive them with a refreshing soak. Leading aromatherapist Clare Maxwell-Hudson recommends five drops of lavender essential oil mixed in 10ml jojoba oil, diffused in a warm (but not too hot) footbath. Soak your feet for ten minutes.

✦ Apart from incorrect nail cutting, ingrown toenails can be caused by tights or stockings that are too small.

✦ Each morning, give feet a dollop of moisturiser, a dusting of powder and a spray of eau de Cologne. Walk out light-footed and light-headed.

During the average lifetime, we will walk 70,000 miles (112,630km), or four times around the earth.

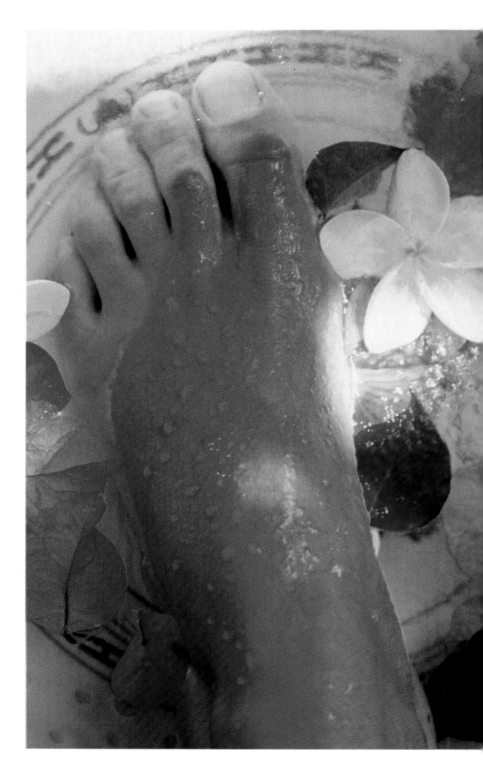

TRIED & TESTED

FOOT REVIVERS

The ones that scored highest with our testers are mostly moderately priced. The **Institut des Jambes Repair Cream** and **Clarins Les Jambes Lourdes** (see *Tried & Tested Foot Creams*, below) also work well as foot refreshers, too.

Best Budget Buys

Avon Foot Works Foot Spray

This is a fine mist spray that can even be used through tights.
COMMENTS: 'After walking miles, it was paradise for my feet', 'immediately revived and refreshed aching feet'.

Body Shop Refreshing Foot Spray

Our testers loved this and shop workers are said to swear by it. It has the advantage that you can spritz it through your tights.
COMMENTS: 'brilliant', 'in summer this would be a godsend and I will also take it on shopping expeditions'.

Body Shop Peppermint Foot Lotion

Diana, Princess of Wales' favourite and also a hit with fashion editors during the rigours of the designer collections.
COMMENTS: 'the all-time greatest', 'far outstripped any other product'.

Natural Choice

Jurlique Foot and Leg Care Lotion

This is potently scented with essential oils of menthol and camphor.
COMMENTS: 'the best product of all', 'immediately refreshing', 'reduced swelling and puffiness on a long plane ride'.

Special Mention

Avon Foot Works Foot File

This wooden tool with a sandpapery finish also got rave reviews.
COMMENTS: 'my feet felt and looked like a baby's'.

FOOT CREAMS

Rough dry feet can be uncomfortable as well as unsightly, and even snag tights. Feet, however, do respond quickly to TLC with rich creams, which are best used nightly, if not twice daily. The mint and menthol-based creams (below) also do double duty as foot revivers, and scored well in that category, too.

Top Treats

Institut des Jambes Repair Cream

This is from a Paris Institute which is specially devoted to leg and foot care, and lived up to its great reputation.
COMMENTS: 'excellent at getting rid of very dry skin on legs and feet', 'much smoother skin immediately', 'nice minty smell'.

Clarins Lait Jambes Lourdes

This cooling blue lotion, strongly scented with menthol, is great for feet and legs and can, at a pinch, be applied through tights.

COMMENTS: 'I would definitely buy this to use during flights and after long walks', 'it got the circulation going and cooled down my feet', 'very refreshing'.

Best Budget Buys

Crabtree & Evelyn Aloe Foot Lotion

This plant-based foot lotion incorporates aloe vera, renowned for its healing and softening powers.
COMMENTS: 'a great pick-me-up after the gym', 'very refreshing and moisturising', 'feet felt softer and more supple'.

Boots Spearmint Soothing Foot Lotion

Spearmint is another weapon in the herbal armoury for reviving tired feet.
COMMENTS: 'cooling and softening', 'refreshing tingle', 'softer skin, more relaxed feet'.

HELPING HANDS

The great thing about hands is that – unlike cats and small children – they respond gratefully to short bursts of undivided attention, and then you can leave them alone. Fingertips can go from grubby to groomed in just half an hour, and stay that way with a weekly manicure.

Hand care should be a vital part of any woman's beauty regime. But even women who invest fortunes in age-retarding face creams have a tendency to be cavalier about looking after their hands. Yet, since they don't have the benefit of make-up camouflage, hands never lie. At forty, your face can appear ten years younger, but one glance at your hands will give the game away: age spots begin to make their appearance, and one of the first signals of departing youth is loose and wrinkled skin on the back of the hands.

Nails suffer too. According to Howard Murad, M.D., Assistant Clinical Professor of Dermatology at UCLA (and founder of Murad, Inc, a skincare line): 'The older you get, the more your nails are like your skin; they become thinner and rougher.' They may also develop ridges, the result of natural changes in the nail matrix, the half-moon at the nail's base responsible for new growth. But, as Goro Uesugi, Hollywood manicurist to the stars, points out: 'Nails are like hair. If you keep them healthy and clean, they'll look better.'

For a successful home manicure, preparation is essential – like priming a wall before you decorate it with a beautiful colour paint. Christian Dior, who are famous not only for their range of rainbow shades but for the durability of their polishes, have a step-by-step programme for the perfect manicure:

CHRISTIAN DIOR'S TEN STEPS TO ELEGANT NAILS

1 Remove polish in upward strokes from base to tip of nail, using several new cotton wool balls for dark shades of enamel.
2 Begin with the little finger of the right hand; it's easier to start outside and work in. To shape a nail, take the wide ends of an emery board between thumb and index finger and file in one direction only, from outer corner to centre, never backwards and forwards. To shorten a nail, use the board's coarser side; finish with the finer side.

3 Lightly rub in a rich, nail-strengthening cream (such as Christian Dior's *Crème Abricot*) into the surface of the nail and surrounding skin.
4 Soak fingertips in a bowl of warm water. Alternatively, try an oil bath, using gently heated jojoba oil.
5 Apply cuticle remover with a brush around the edges of the nail and, with a cotton bud, gently push back the cuticle. Remove dead skin with circular movements, tissuing off the cuticle remover.
6 When the nails are completely clean and dry, apply a base coat. (We have had excellent results with Christian Dior *Diorlisse*, a ridge-filling, strengthening base which is pretty enough to use on its own.)
7 Put a little enamel on the brush and apply a fine coat from base to tip. After a few minutes, apply a second coat. Light or frosted enamels may need a third. Stephanie Hayano, of the nail-care company Sally Hansen, recommends the three-stroke method: which delivers exactly the right amount of lacquer to the nail.
8 Then try a clear top coat, which gives protective shine and significantly extends the life of a manicure.
9 Leave nails to dry naturally, if you can; trying to speed up the process can spoil the appearance and quality of the manicure. And don't wave your hands in the air; this creates an uneven texture.
10 When nails are dry, rub in hand cream lavishly.

TIPS FROM THE TOP

Top London restaurateur **Sally Clarke**'s hands are in and out of hot and cold water 50 times a day. She uses a gentle soap such as Neutrogena: 'And I lavish my hands with E45 before I go to sleep, in the hope they'll be restored by morning.'

Etiquette expert **Drusilla Beyfus** swears by Clarins Hand and Nail Treatment Cream, 'Which is the only cream I've ever found that helps get rid of age spots.'

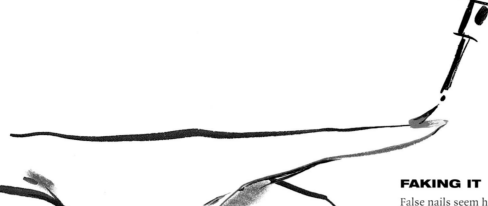

NAIL TIPS

Goro Uesugi, who gives **Angelica Huston**, **Winona Ryder**, **Bonnie Raitt**, even **Jack Nicholson** that 'star polish', has been booked up two months ahead for the last 15 years. To save you the wait (not to mention the airfare) here are some of the finger-and-toe guru's tips for the ultimate manicure:

✦ Always use acetone-free varnish remover, which won't strip vital oils from nails. (Dried out nails soon become cracked nails.) Look for 'gentle' or 'non-drying' on the label, or ask at a cosmetics counter.

✦ Rather than soaking nails in soapy water, Goro suggests adding a few drops of bath oil to very hot water to soften hands and cuticles.

✦ Remove excess cuticle using an orange stick with the tip wrapped in cotton wool, dipped in cuticle remover. Never work on a dry nail.

✦ Just before you varnish, wash nails thoroughly with soapy water. Some manicurists like to do this with polish remover, but, explains Goro, 'It's too drying so the polish won't go on smoothly.'

✦ For long-lasting colour, it is better to let nails dry naturally. Quick-dry sprays will deliver, but can mean your polish chips in double-quick time too.

NAIL FACTS ✦ Nails grow about 1mm (0.0394in) each week ✦ It takes three to four months for a nail to renew itself from base to tip, and six to seven months for the entire nail (both visible parts and under the skin) to regrow ✦ Growth can be slowed by illness or dieting ✦ Stress can speed up growth to such an extent that nails literally outgrow their strength

---

FAKING IT

False nails seem heaven-sent for any woman who has trouble growing her own. There are now several techniques to make up for unsightly or nibbled nails.

Acrylic tips: these don't cover the entire nail but are fixed mid-way up the natural nail, with the surface pared down to hide the join.

Built-up tips: oval paper or metal is inserted under the nail, acrylic is painted on and allowed to set. The tip is then filed to your chosen shape.

Silk wrapping: this is a strengthening treatment for nails that split easily. A layer of silk is glued to the nail and the raw edges buffed away. (This can also be done to rescue a single broken nail.)

False nails: these can be applied in a salon or at home, using an inexpensive acrylic kit. The nails come with their own adhesive and can be cut and filed to a shape and size that suits you.

Patching: if you split or break a nail, it's now possible to repair it with a patch that works on the same principle as a sticking plaster on skin. Inexpensive Repair-a-Nail kits are available for D-I-Y repairs, or they can be applied professionally in a salon. (See DIRECTORY.)

If you keep your nails permanently under wraps, it can lead to problems such as cracking, splitting, discolouration – or, at the worst, infections. If you do decide false nails or tips are for you, here are some nail-saving tactics.

✦ Don't wear false nails for more than two weeks at a time, and give your own nails at least two days to rest between applications.

✦ Replenish lost moisture by giving nails an oil bath in warmed jojoba oil, between applications.

✦ Be careful cleaning under nails; use a brush and soapy water or a Q-tip, never an orange stick.

✦ If you notice any green or yellow-ish discolourations of the nail bed, consult your GP or a dermatologist; it could signify a fungal or bacterial infection.

S.O.S. FOR NAILS IN TROUBLE

Who is Jessica? Jessica is what – or who – **Hillary Clinton**, **Diana, Princess of Wales**, **Jamie Lee Curtis** and **Jodie Foster** (aside from practically every Hollywood star) have, literally, at their immaculate fingertips. A Romanian emigrée from the Communist regime, Jessica Vartoughian is *the* Los Angeles manicurist and nail consultant. In 1965 she founded the world's first Nails Only Clinic, and since then there's been no stopping her meteoric progress worldwide.

Jessica insists: 'Every woman can have beautiful and healthy nails.' There are four nail types, she says: dry, brittle, normal and damaged, and each needs a different treatment and specialised products. If you follow her regime, and use her range of Home Care Kits, Jessica promises that beautiful nails are just a few weeks away.

Does Jessica's much-vaunted system work? Well, look at the many women who swear by it. However, some manicurists are trying out another therapeutic manicure system, Nailtiques, which claims it is 'proven to help nails that are inclined to peel, break or split...with a unique combination of proteins and conditioners'. (See DIRECTORY.)

We think that the real point in salon treatments lies in helping get your hands and nails in tip-top condition, and then – because you've invested time and money in them – you will be encouraged to keep up the good work at home.

TIP To avoid damaged nails, keep them short and away from water (wear rubber and gardening gloves). Eat a good diet with plenty of calcium-rich foods and consider calcium and magnesium supplements. Supplements of Evening Primrose Oil and Kervrans Silica (3g daily) strengthen nails. Clients of hair colourist Jo Hansford reported developing rock-hard nails from taking Nourkrin supplement for their hair. N.B.Results can take months.

FAST NAIL MAKEOVER

Polish pens – such as Stylo Guerlain Instant Nail Polish – are the new, quick, no-spill alternative to brush-on polish, and an easy way to touch up colour between manicures. If you only have ten minutes before an important appointment and your hands look dreadful, that's still enough for a manicure metamorphosis. First, clip or file nails so they're an even length. Then scrub hands and nails with a nail brush, warm water and soap until they gleam. Shake the polish pen for 20 seconds to blend the colour, then saturate the pen's tip by pressing it down on a piece of paper until you've made a blot of colour. Apply the polish, with a light touch, to your nails. Wait two minutes for the polish to dry hard and drench your hands in hand cream. That's it.

TRIED & TESTED

NAIL STRENGTHENERS

The secret of success with these products is that they have to be used diligently; it's not enough to apply once a week and hope for the best. They won't overcome nutritional deficiencies or hormonal problems, both of which contribute to poor nail quality, but they may be valuable as part of a general nail-strengthening programme. (Anything you take internally to improve your hair quality, e.g. Evening Primrose Oil and silica or fish oil will also boost your nails.)

Barielle Night Time Nail Renewal

This did very well in a difficult category – perhaps partly because it's easier to remember to use nail strengtheners as part of a bedtime ritual, just like brushing your teeth.

COMMENTS: 'brilliant – easy to use, I applied it last thing at night while reading or watching TV', 'made my nails very glossy', 'smelled great and did soften cuticles'.

Barielle Nail Strengthener Cream

Another product from Barielle – whose range was originally formulated for horses' hooves, before being applied to humans...
COMMENTS: 'after four weeks' use, my brittle nails became more flexible and only one broke, which was a great improvement'.

Nailtiques Kit

Although the instructions for this programme were difficult to follow, all our testers agreed that they would buy this product.
COMMENTS: 'my nails were softer and less likely to split', 'all the products smelt delicious', 'nails felt stronger'.

THE NAKED NAIL

If you don't like the look of polish, you can always buff nails to a pearly gleam. This steps up blood flow, leading to healthier nails over time. Buff nails rapidly in one direction. Don't be afraid to exert a little elbow grease – but if you feel a burning sensation, stop at once. A weekly buffing session should be enough to keep nails strong and healthy.

NAIL TIPS ✦ Apply a fresh layer to your varnish nightly, or at least every other night, to extend the life of your manicure. Do this just before bedtime and sleep with your hands outside the sheets ✦ Don't try to match lipstick or clothes to nail colour exactly ✦ Top US manicurist Sheril Bailey places her clients' fingers under cold running water to harden polish once applied ✦ Supernail of Los Angeles told us: 'Any cosmetic oil – even baby oil – works as a polish quick-dryer in an emergency'

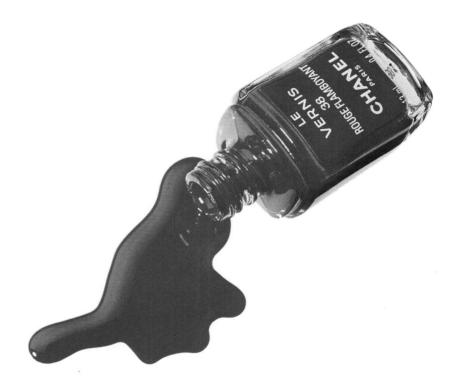

TRIED & TESTED

LONG-LASTING NAIL POLISH

For many women, there's something undeniably sensuous about polished nails. But it's a time-consuming task and you want the hard-won results to last. Of course, applying both base coats and top coats will help pretty well every nail varnish to last without chipping, but we wanted to find out which, if any, did it on their own – and looked good at the same time. Generally, the more expensive ranges performed better.

Top Treats

Helena Rubinstein Glorious Nail Colour
And glorious it proved. This was the winner, earning universally rave reviews.
COMMENTS: 'lasted three to four days without chipping', 'top marks for ease of application', 'loved the packaging'.

Lancôme Vernis Triple Tenue
A close second, with very high marks from most testers.
COMMENTS: 'very easy to apply', 'it went three to five days without chipping', 'excellent'.

Chanel Le Vernis
This lasted well and was generally liked, although one tester had reservations about the coverage.
COMMENTS: 'lasted three days on average', 'went on easily and smoothly', 'dried quickly'.

Best Budget Buy

Max Factor Diamond Hard
This performed well for the price, and several testers said they would buy it.
COMMENTS: 'lasted two to three days', 'took about 12 minutes to dry', 'good range of colours'.

Honourable Mention

Christian Dior Nail Enamel
This was the favourite for appearance – lustre, colour, coverage – but the tips did need topping up daily.
COMMENTS: 'wonderful colours', 'marvellously smooth coverage'.

MORE HANDY HINTS

✦ Beautiful hands start with hygiene: use a nail brush every day to scrub the underside of nails.

✦ Exfoliate hands once a week using your own home-made scrub: mix together crushed almonds, honey and lemon juice to slough off dead skin and moisturise.

✦ Make a 'salad dressing' for hands and nails of lemon juice and jojoba or even corn oil; pour into a shallow bowl and bathe hands in the mixture for 15 minutes. The lemon will bleach hands clean, and the oil will feed hands and nails.

✦ Rather than leaving leftover sun products to overwinter in the bathroom cabinet, use SPF creams as a ray-deflecting alternative to hand cream, particularly for gardening/sports/long-distance driving. (According to dermatologists, UV rays can actually penetrate windscreens.) But beware of high factors as they can discolour pale polish, turning it yellow.

✦ Keep hand cream – or sunscreen – by every single set of taps in your house, so you've no excuse for not using it.

✦ For a pampering boost, use a face mask on hands once weekly.

✦ If you are sleeping on your own, wear gloves to bed once a week. Heat your hands in warm water, dry, rub in some ultra-rich cream, then put the gloves on. You will wake up with amazingly silky hands.

TRIED & TESTED

HAND CREAMS

Virtually all women get through vats of hand cream every year. Our testers found many excellent hand-savers across the price range.

Top Treats

Clarins Jeunesse des Mains

COMMENTS: 'superb for day or night use', 'improved cuticles and made my hands more beautiful', 'I was impressed from the first application'.

Annick Goutal Hand Cream

COMMENTS: 'my hands felt softer and smoother instantly', 'unbelievably beautiful fragrance', 'I got a lot of compliments after using this'.

I Coloniali Velvet Hand Cream

This is a rich product from a new company whose products feature active botanical ingredients.

COMMENTS: 'instantly softening and soothing', 'overall effective product', 'I'd buy it for myself – and as a present'.

Best Budget Buys

Crabtree & Evelyn Jojoba Oil Barrier Hand Cream

This is especially effective if applied before gardening or cleaning.

COMMENTS: 'my hands felt silky and the nails looked as if they'd just been buffed', 'excellent product with a lovely refreshing smell'.

Superdrug Vitamin E Hand and Nail Treatment

COMMENTS: 'ten out of ten for texture and absorption', 'worth buying'.

Marks & Spencer Body Formula Hand & Nail Treatment Cream

COMMENTS: 'a superb hand cream', 'great to use before bedtime'.

Avon Naturals Hand Cream with Chamomile

COMMENTS: 'my hands felt hydrated and comfortable', 'my hands always felt soothed and my nails looked healthier and smoother'.

Natural Choice

Jurlique Hand Care Cream

A rich, swiftly absorbed cream from this Australian skincare company.

COMMENTS: 'the best hand cream I've ever used', 'feels wonderful, smells great and really works', 'my hands looked younger'.

Double Whammy

Estée Lauder Revelation Retexturing Complex For Hands & Chest

Although it didn't fit into a specific category, we thought you should know about this revolutionary gel/cream for areas which suffer sun-related ageing. Definitely an expensive top treat, but we're both fans.

COMMENTS: 'great texture and an immediate difference in softness and smoothness', 'I loved the smell and texture'.

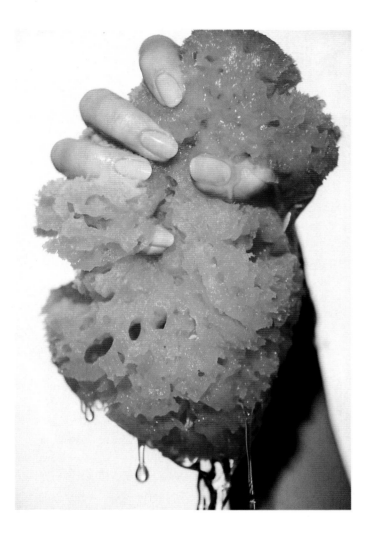

THE SECRETS OF A HAND MODEL

Amanda Wright is one of the world's top hand models. She has exquisite, pale, long-fingered hands and immaculate nails which are, of course, hangnail-free. She was the ideal person to share the secrets of achieving smooth, youthful hands and perfect nails.

✦ Rubber gloves for every household task are rule number one. 'I put them on every time I want to wipe the table or wash up a single cup, and I often put on hand cream first – although you have to be careful not to keep the gloves on for too long, or your hands get sweaty and dehydrated. Then for dusting, I have little cotton housework gloves that you can get in most pharmacies. They're real hand-savers.'

✦ All day long, regular as clockwork, Amanda makes a point of keeping her hands' moisture level topped up. 'Every time I wash my hands, I moisturise them immediately – while they're still slightly damp, which seems to "lock in" the moisture.' She spurns expensive hand creams – 'I've tried them all, and I'm allergic to most of them!' – in favour of Vaseline Derma Care. 'It's extremely rich, and very cheap. Which is just as well because I go through at least a bottle a week.' Cuticles get plenty of tender loving care, too, with Christian Dior's Crème Abricot. 'Worth every penny. I don't eat anything special to keep my nails healthy, but I do believe that massaging the nail bed regularly, to improve blood flow, stops nails from breaking, and prevents those little pieces of skin that "catch". I rub in Crème Abricot at least twice, maybe three times a day, and always last thing at night before I go to sleep.'

✦ Whenever she goes out, Amanda protects her hands with an SPF25 sunscreen to prevent freckling or photo-ageing. (You could try Piz Buin or Estée Lauder sunscreens.)

✦ Surprisingly, Amanda works as her own manicurist on shoots, no matter how important the job. 'I've had more practice than most make-up artists,' she explains. She carries around a hefty make-up box filled with tried and tested hand- and nail-care goodies. To keep her nails perfect and break-proof, must-haves include Christian Dior's Gentle Polish Remover, Revlon's Epoxy 1000 Nail Treatment ('A nail strengthener which doubles as the world's greatest top coat', says Amanda), and Delore Organic Nail Hardener, a two-in-one treatment and polish dryer which sets enamel fast. She has a rainbow of nail varnishes, from palest pearl to deep red. Amanda's favourite? 'Lancôme 201 – a natural-looking pink.' (See DIRECTORY for sources.)

✦ Amanda also boasts an armoury of nail files and buffers, cotton buds (used for cleaning under the nail tip, 'Because you should never use an orange stick'), and a Daffy Duck nail brush. She never goes anywhere without her own soap (The Body Shop's Coconut): 'Because I might be allergic to what they've got in the studio loo, and this one's really gentle.'

✦ Avoiding nail nightmares means using the side of the fingers for pulling up zips. 'And I'd never, ever plunge my hand into my bag to get my keys – nor should any woman who cares about her hands. It's all trial and error: I once did that and grazed myself on a Visa card!'

HOW TO TAKE WELL-BEING INTO YOUR OWN HANDS

You don't have to book a professional or even enlist a friend's help to give yourself a wonderful, soothing massage. If you know the correct techniques, then it's possible to experience many of the benefits of a salon or health centre treatment any time you feel in need of a boost or want to wind down.

By unblocking energy in the meridian channels that run like invisible connective highways through the body, you can relieve many common problems. Origins, the aromatherapy-based natural beauty company whose fans include **Demi Moore**, **Daryl Hannah**, **Dustin Hoffman** and **Jane Fonda**, suggest a self-massage programme based on an eastern system called 'Do-In'. They also produce a range of carefully blended Origins Sensory Therapy Massaging Oils which are ideal for this massage. (See DIRECTORY.) You can massage without any oil or cream at all, but they do make it easier and, we feel, give a more pleasurable sensory experience.

Before you begin, here are some important Dos and Don'ts on self-massage:

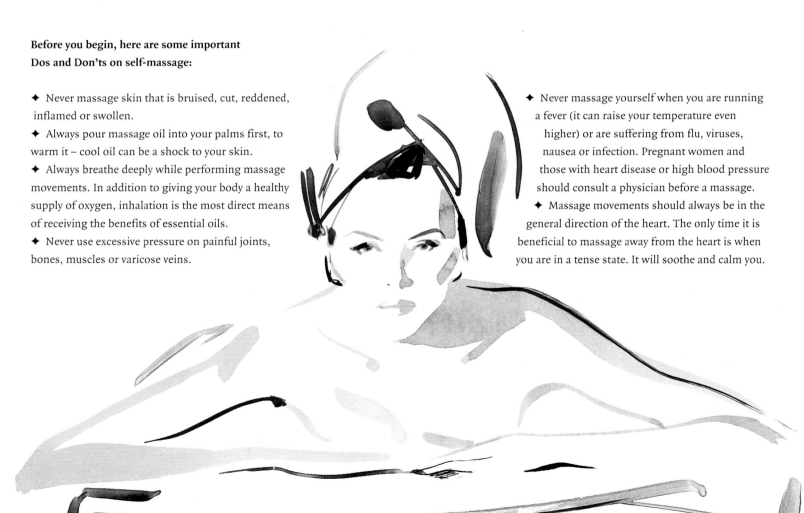

✦ Never massage skin that is bruised, cut, reddened, inflamed or swollen.

✦ Always pour massage oil into your palms first, to warm it – cool oil can be a shock to your skin.

✦ Always breathe deeply while performing massage movements. In addition to giving your body a healthy supply of oxygen, inhalation is the most direct means of receiving the benefits of essential oils.

✦ Never use excessive pressure on painful joints, bones, muscles or varicose veins.

✦ Never massage yourself when you are running a fever (it can raise your temperature even higher) or are suffering from flu, viruses, nausea or infection. Pregnant women and those with heart disease or high blood pressure should consult a physician before a massage.

✦ Massage movements should always be in the general direction of the heart. The only time it is beneficial to massage away from the heart is when you are in a tense state. It will soothe and calm you.

◆ To ensure full benefits of the essential oils, don't wash them off. So don't bathe or shower for several hours after treatment.

Once you're ready to begin your self-massage, here's how to go about it. (Of course, you can do this massage for other people, too.)

(a) Pour massage oil into the palms of your hands, rub together and then spread oil over the specific area you are working on.

(b) With your thumb, massage the soles of your feet using circular motions. Work your way from the heels to the toes.

(c) Alternately, take hold of fleshy areas of your leg, working upwards in sections from calves to thighs to buttocks. Gently and rhythmically squeeze them as if you were kneading dough. Use the heel of your hand to make repeated, firm, circular movements on areas of tension or cellulite. This friction creates intense heat which increases absorption of essential oils to relieve discomfort.

(d) Place your hands at the base of your back, on either side of your spine, with your four fingers pointing towards the centre of your spine. Stroke firmly upwards as far as you can comfortably reach. Repeat several times.

(e) Using clockwise motions, gently circle your abdomen with the palm of your hand. Abdominal massage is excellent for ensuring general well-being and relaxation.

(f) Repeat step **(c)** on your arms, from wrists upwards.

(g) Using your whole hand, grasp the flesh on either side of your neck and shoulder and, with firm pressure, start at the base of the skull and work down as far as possible until you reach the shoulder. Repeat until you reach the outside of the shoulder.

(h) Place your fingers on each side of your neck and, with firm pressure, start at the base of the skull and work down as far as possible until you reach the shoulders. Repeat three times.

(i) To end your massage, place the flat of your right hand on your left foot and your left hand on your right foot. This creates a positive-negative charge in the body, which is calming, releases stiff muscles and wakes up the nervous system. Count to 20, then slowly withdraw your hands. Relax for a few moments. Feel how your body absorbs your magnetic energy as it passes through your hands...

D-I-Y REFLEXOLOGY

There are various points on your feet which, when pressed, bring about physical and emotional changes in your body. Follow this diagram (which shows points on the *soles* of the feet) and experience the benefits of reflexology yourself.

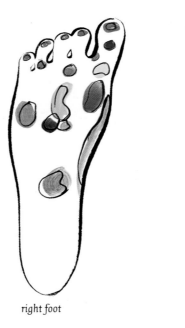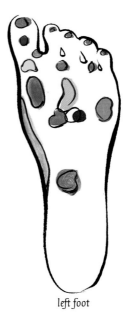

right foot   *left foot*

1 To breathe a sigh of relief
2 To get you back under control
3 To clear your troubled mind
4 To stop stress from being a pain in the neck
5 To open your eyes
6 To put you 'in the mood'
7 To take the weight of the world off your shoulders
8 To help you breathe easier
9 To take away tension
10 To keep your nerves from knotting
11 To get your system pumping up to speed
12 To de-tense your torso
13 To settle that sinking feeling (on the right foot only)
14 To banish the butterflies

HELP FOR BODY AND MIND

Today a marvellous range of therapies is available to help body and mind. Always be sure to consult a qualified practitioner whom you like and trust.

SELF-HELP

ALEXANDER TECHNIQUE: a course of lessons, usually one on one, which helps you to realign and balance your body; particularly good for bad backs.

AUTOGENIC TRAINING: a system of deep relaxation, recommended for stress management.

CREATIVE VISUALISATION: often used with meditation and breathing techniques; a way of leading your mind into positive, pleasurable or peaceful thoughts.

FLOWER REMEDIES: healing essences distilled from flowers; can be self-administered or prescribed (see page 155).

LIGHT THERAPY: a full spectrum light unit, delivering the equivalent of a bright spring day, can help a range of problems from Seasonal Affective Disorder and PMT to depression, jet lag and high blood pressure.

MARTIAL ARTS: a range of ancient body/mind techniques, including t'ai chi, qigong, karate, aikido, ju jitsu and kickboxing, focused on body movements which help centre physical, mental and physical energy.

MEDITATION: many different types, marvellous for stress relief, relaxing body and refreshing mind. Transcendental Meditation (TM) has been proven effective for a range of medical conditions and is easily learned from books or articles, or from good teachers.

YOGA: a form of body/mind workout which emphasises deep breathing.

THERAPIES

ACUPUNCTURE: fine needles are inserted (painlessly) into the meridians (energy channels) to balance energies and restore health and vitality.

APPLIED KINESIOLOGY: method of detecting physical imbalances such as food intolerance by testing muscle reactions.

BIODYNAMIC MASSAGE: combination of massage and psychotherapy.

BIOENERGETIC MEDICINE: combination of homoeopathy and acupuncture.

CHIROPRACTIC: hands-on manipulation aimed at diagnosing and treating disorders.

CHIROPODY AND PODIATRY: foot health and beauty.

COLONIC IRRIGATION: colon cleansing, which can be done by direct flushing out or over longer term, sometimes includes dietary therapy with specific supplements.

COLOUR THERAPY: system of helping mind/body health by the choice of certain colours individually prescribed to wear in your environment.

COUNSELLING: short- and long-term methods of easing emotional problems.

CRANIO-SACRAL THERAPY: a method of manually releasing tension.

CRYSTAL THERAPY: therapists, invariably healers, believe that crystals both receive and transmit energy signals. The energy generated by the healer is vested in the crystal which can then be used without the healer present.

ELECTRO-CRYSTAL THERAPY: is also becoming popular (see above).

FENG SHUI: a way of enhancing your home/work environment to promote harmony and good luck.

HEALING: transfer of healing energy from the healer to the client; has been demonstrated scientifically.

HOMOEOPATHY: use of microscopic amounts of natural substances to cure body and mind imbalances.

HYDROTHERAPY: intensive water therapy for skeletal problems; wonderful for bad backs.

HYPNOTHERAPY: clients are put into a trance-like state (this can also be self-induced) for therapeutic purposes.

IRIDOLOGY: a technique of analysing the iris of the eye to diagnose physical problems.

McTIMONEY CHIROPRACTIC: the most gentle form of chiropractic therapy.

MEDICAL HERBALISM: use of traditional western herbs to treat ill health.

NATUROPATHY: use of diet, osteopathy and hydrotherapy to treat illness and boost health; good results in chronic illness, including PMT and IBS.

NUTRITIONAL THERAPY: individually prescribed diet and supplement programmes to correct ill health and enhance energy.

OSTEOPATHY: manipulation of the skeleton, which can feel aggressive; sometimes combined with acupuncture.

POLARITY THERAPY: system of bodywork, mind awareness, diet and stretching exercises to promote self-healing of body and mind.

PSYCHOTHERAPY: short- and long-term aid to uncovering and solving emotional traumas.

STRESS MANAGEMENT: a combination of techniques (breathing, relaxation, cognitive behavioural therapy, etc) to alleviate unhealthy stress.

BODY AND MIND TREATS

AROMATHERAPY: heavenly massage with sweet-smelling essential oils; now used in NHS hospitals and other medical institutions (one of our great favourites).

FLOATATION: deep relaxation in an enclosed tank full of water with added salts (not for the claustrophobic).

MASSAGE (Shiatsu, Thai, manual lymphatic drainage, Swedish, Tuina, Ayurvedic): various methods of relaxing and therapeutic treatment which can greatly benefit both mind and body.

REFLEXOLOGY: therapists work on energy points in the feet which are related to organs in the body, uncannily accurate in diagnosing problems.

(See DIRECTORY for contact details.)

INSTANT STRESSBUSTERS

As well as using Tania Alexander's fitness routine (see page 159) and flower remedies (see page 155), try the following. (Remember to keep breathing gently, deeply and rhythmically, in through your nose and out through your mouth.)

✿ Unclench your fists, let your hands flop. Then shake them vigorously.

✿ Uncross arms and legs. Shake your feet, circle your ankles.

✿ Smile, or if you can remember a good joke, laugh out loud.

✿ Stroke away lines of tension: rest your fingers along your eyebrows then run them upwards, through your hair, down the back of the head to your nape. Repeat as often as possible.

✿ Starting with your face and jaw, mentally travel down your body, through shoulders, spine, pelvis, knees, ankles to your feet, relaxing each part. Imagine them as something soft, e.g. ice cream, unset jelly, a feather cushion.

✿ If you are angry, try mentally pushing out all the anger from your body and mind on the out-breath.

✿ If you are worried, lie on the floor if possible (if not, relax your body, as above), and imagine all your problems packed up into a balloon. Watch it floating away until it disappears.

✿ If work problems are bothering you at the end of the day, or before a meeting, visualise yourself filing them away and locking the cabinet. Undertake, however, to come back and sort them out at the soonest suitable time.

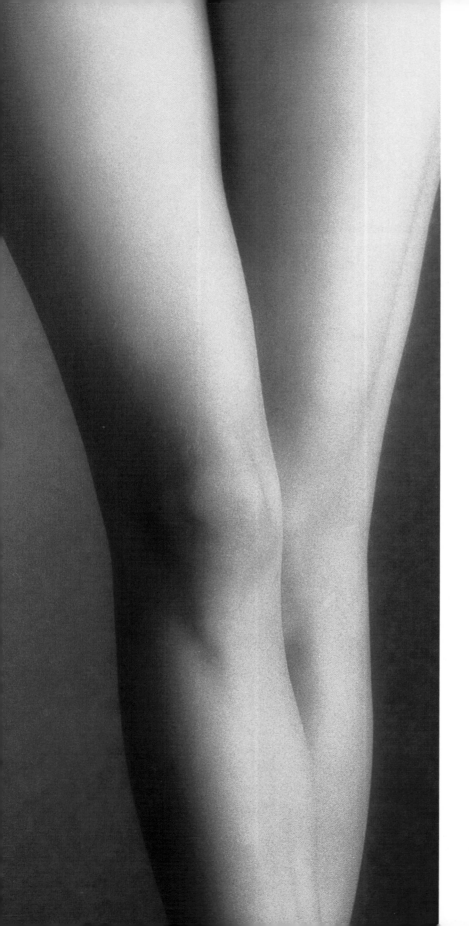

FUZZ BUSTING

Ever since Cleopatra's day, some women have been fighting Mother Nature in pursuit of smooth, baby-soft, hair-free skin. If you're happy with your body hair, lucky you. In Sikh circles, for instance, hair is regarded as a sacred gift, and depilation qualifies as a sin. Look up and down the sun-loungers on any Mediterranean beach and you'll see rows of furry armpits, aimed nonchalantly at the sun. Even Madonna apparently goes through phases of leaving her armpits fuzzy. But if you prefer smoother, fuzz-free skin, you'll find the answers here.

SHAVING

Where: at home

Best for: legs and underarms

Pros: quick, cheap (unless you use an electric razor), easily portable

Cons: occasional nicks, stubble, ingrown hairs, razor burn (on sensitive skins)

Pain factor: zero, unless you cut yourself

Growth factor: you'll have to do it daily if you want totally smooth skin

Tips: wait two to three minutes after getting into the shower or bath before shaving, to soften hairs. Apply steady, light pressure and change the blade every five to six shaves. Use water or oil rather than soap, which leaves skin unpleasantly dry and taut.

DEPILATORIES

Where: at home

Best for: legs, underarm, bikini area, facial hair (with specifically targeted products only)

Pros: inexpensive, long-lasting, no stubble; after you've used depilatories for a few months, hair grows back more slowly and sparsely

Cons: messy, sometimes smelly, time-consuming – usually takes ten minutes or more

Pain factor: none

Growth factor: between five to 20 days, depending on re-growth rate (but two weeks is about average)

Tips: always do a patch test first to make sure your skin isn't sensitive to the product; rinse off with cold water and avoid sunscreen, body lotions or self-tanners for at least two hours to prevent irritation

BLEACHING

Where: at home/in a salon

Best for: facial hair, dark hair on forearms, or shins if you're lucky enough never to have been seduced by shaving or other ways of hair removal!

Pros: no stubble or ingrown hairs

Cons: time-consuming, messy, impractical for large areas

Pain factor: none – unless you have sensitive skin, or make the mistake of leaving the bleach on for too long

Growth factor: usually needs re-bleaching after two to four weeks

Tips: always do a patch test first, and carefully time application

WAXING (hot or cold)

Where: at home/in a salon

Best for: legs, bikini area, upper lip, underarms

Pros: stubble-free, long-lasting, hair becomes finer with repeated use

Cons: expensive, messy, time-consuming – and painful! And you have to wait until there's a quarter to half an inch re-growth

Pain factor: off the top of the pain-o-meter

Growth factor: fine hairs reappear in around two weeks; thicker growth in four to six weeks

Tips: hold skin taut before the wax is pulled (you can also do this in a salon, clapping your palm on the area immediately to soothe); allow a few days between waxing and sun exposure, as newly exposed areas are more sensitive; if hair is long, trim it with scissors so waxing is faster and gentler. One expert we found told us to breathe in, then, on the out-breath, she pulled. Result: no pain at all

ELECTROLYSIS

Where: salon only

Best for: small areas (upper lip, brows, chin, nipples)

Pros: the only (almost) permanent method of hair removal

Cons: extremely expensive and time-consuming as only a few follicles can be treated per session – and it hurts

Pain factor: high – especially where skin is thin

Growth factor: some hairs need a few sessions before they disappear forever

GALVANIC TWEEZER HAIR REMOVAL

Where: salon only

Best for: face, arms, bikini area (like electrolysis)

Pros: considered by some to be a more permanent hair removal system as the root is destroyed (by a current, transmitted from the machine, which follows a gel electrode solution down to the follicle).

Cons: time-consuming and you have to make regular appointments because hair can only be 'zapped' at a precise time in its growth cycle; if you miss appointments, some of the hairs will be too late in their cycle to be removed, and you'll have to wait till the process repeats itself for the therapist to have another go.

Growth factor: provided a hair is removed at the right time in the growth cycle, there will be no regrowth.

SUGARING

Where: at home/in a salon

This 2,000-year-old Middle Eastern technique is similar to waxing, but because the paste sticks to the hair, rather than the skin, users say it's a less painful and more effective method of removal. Regrowth time is the same as for waxing.

TIPS FROM THE TOP

Actress **Heather Locklear** says: 'I can't live without waxing. I do it myself. Actually, I only wax my bikini area. I do it just for fun! You have to let the hairs grow to a certain length, and after you get those, two days later there are other ones that have grown long enough. You have to keep doing it until it evens out.'

TIPS At the Aida Thibiant salon in Beverly Hills (clients include supermodel **Rachel Hunter**), they teach women to avoid ingrowing hairs by gently massaging the area daily with a loofah or flannel, to keep pores open and prevent build-up of cellular debris. We love Decleor's *Épileor*, a spray-on herbal soother and antiseptic which also keeps ingrowing hairs at bay. ◆ Newly waxed skin is sensitive, but applying lotion straight away, even though it *feels* soothing, can block pores and encourage ingrowing hairs. Nina Novy, of top New York manicure salon Nails by Nina, shakes on baby powder instead.

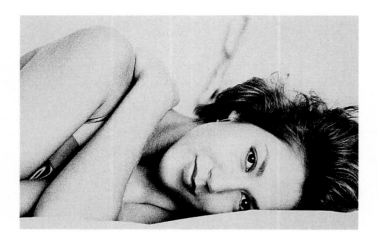

DO YOU NEED A DIFFERENT CREAM FOR EACH PART OF YOUR BODY?

Bathroom shelves can end up groaning with the variety of products designed for various bits of our bodies. There are products which can perform many different tasks – Vaseline, or Elizabeth Arden 8-Hour Cream, for instance (see *Double Duty Beauty*, page 50, for more suggestions) – but beauty companies would have us believe that we need something different for eyes, lips, face, chest, legs and feet.

Are they right? 'If you ask dermatologists, they'll say skin is skin, but there are certain differences in the skin of various body parts,' explains Gary L. Grove, PhD, Vice President of Research and Development at the Skin Study Centre in Philadelphia. 'Many of the skin's differences are to do with sensitivity and vulnerability,' he adds. For example, a high SPF product that stings on your face may feel worse on your chest – and not bother you at all on your legs.

Skin is thinner, he explains, near the eyes and on the lips, and thicker on ankles, knees and elbows. (Which is why these areas seem to drink up even the richest moisturiser in no time.) In recent tests, Dr Grove found even higher sensitivity levels to certain cosmetics ingredients on chest and neck skin than on facial skin. So if you are at all prone to irritation it is sensible to use a specific neck cream on your décolletage rather than sweep your face cream downwards.

Our rules are:

✦ You can use products that are safe for your face anywhere, but don't put products designed for your body on your face.

✦ Products created for eyes can be used on lips, but not vice versa.

✦ Hand creams work wonderfully on feet, but foot creams often contain menthol so it's safest to wash them off your hands after applying to feet; you may inadvertently touch your eyes and make them water.

✦ Keep bust and cellulite creams for areas they're designed for. If you stay within those guidelines, you can experiment all you like – and maybe even clear some of the clutter from the bathroom shelf...

T R I E D & T E S T E D

BUST CREAMS

The idea that a cream or a gel can reverse the effects of gravity, pregnancy and other hormonal changes almost defies belief. Our testers emerged sceptical about promises and generally not convinced by performance, although a few were immediate converts. We have come to the conclusion that these products are probably best for softening and smoothing, rather than toning and uplifting. And do you really need yet another jar on your bedside table?

Clarins Gel Buste

COMMENTS: 'I think my bust felt firmer and actually lifted a bit', 'dried fast and smelled nice', 'made little difference, but good for massage'.

Mary Cohr Bust Firming Cream

COMMENTS: 'breast tested was definitely softer and smoother but not firmer or more uplifted', 'this product is useful to encourage regular breast examination'.

Lancôme Energibuste

COMMENTS: 'I felt there was an improvement; my skin felt silky, smooth and better toned', 'softer and smoother', 'the only advantage I can think of is that it encouraged breast examination'.

Decleor Galbeor Harmonie

COMMENTS: 'I think there is a little more firmness, but needs long-term continuous use', 'I noticed a marginal difference'.

TRIED & TESTED

BODY LOTIONS

We separated body lotions into two groups because many women don't want to wear a highly perfumed cream or lotion every day. Here are the winners from the 'non-designer' scent category (for the signature scented creams, see page 209).

We asked testers to use the lotions for several days, but also to note any instant results – especially in such notoriously dry areas as elbows, heels and knees. We also asked them how quickly lotions were absorbed, since few of us have the leisure to wait several minutes to put on clothes these days. Because most of these body lotions aren't actually scent-*free*, we asked for their comments on the smell, too.

Top Treats

Mary Cohr Gentle Moisturising Body Lotion

This product scored extremely highly and was universally rated. Our testers also liked the easy-to-use, pump-action dispenser.
COMMENTS: 'skin felt smooth, soft and smelt lovely', 'really improved dryness', 'easily absorbed, with a nice light smell'.

Juvena Body Results Revitalising Cream

Another high scoring product, with a thick, creamy texture.
COMMENTS: 'lovely-feeling cream', 'made my skin feel smooth and soft all day', 'definite improvement to the dry bits'.

Clarins Lait Corps Soyeux

Within beauty circles, this is renowned as a highly effective body lotion, and our testers all confirmed its benefits.
COMMENTS: 'good overall moisturising effect, even on feet', 'smelled subtle but nice', 'absorbed quickly'.

Origins Precipitation

This lotion is another plant-based range available from Estée Lauuder.
COMMENTS: 'skin is smooth, non-flaky, no dry lines – and looks great', 'nice light feel and smell', 'love the design of the bottle'.

Best Budget Buys

Dead Sea Magik Body Lotion

This product incorporates into its formulation minerals from the Dead Sea, which doctors confirm are valuable for problem skins.
COMMENTS: 'immediately softened and hydrated tired skin', 'made my skin smooth for the whole day', 'a nice strong working cream'.

DSD Moisturising Lotion

Another product based on Dead Sea minerals, which also scored well with most testers.
COMMENTS: 'my skin has improved in look and texture', 'quite a strong but pleasant aroma', 'skin looked smooth and lustrous'.

Bath and Body Works Plumeria Body Cream

From a highly successful American company with a widening global network of outlets, this body product scored well for smell and creaminess.
COMMENTS: 'my skin looked and felt wonderful and velvety', 'soon started to dissolve tough skin', 'very good for sufferers of dry skin'.

Natural Choices

Australian Bodycare Treatment Lotion

This light lotion features tea tree oil, which is renowned for its skin-healing properties, and several testers mentioned that skin problems such as eczema and small abrasions improved after use.
COMMENTS: 'eucalyptus-smelling – strong but healthy', 'slight abrasions cleared up quickly – unheard of in a moisturiser', 'it was excellent for very dry areas'.

Elemis Body Moisturising Lotion

All our testers commented that this aromatherapy-based lotion sinks into the skin fast, without trace, while still moisturising.
COMMENTS: 'improved the look and feel of my very dry skin', 'very rich and moisturising', 'nice, old-fashioned smell'.

TURN YOUR HOME INTO A HEALTH SPA

Pamper yourself from top to toe with soothing, reviving spa treatments – without stepping out of your front door.

Most of us dream of getting away to a spa. Unfortunately, dreams don't always dovetail with reality. But there is a way you can enjoy the mind, body and spirit-soothing benefits of a spa trip in just a couple of days for a fraction of the cost. With a little know-how and preparation, you can create your own stay-home beauty sanctuary and give yourself an occasional weekend of pure escapism.

It's up to you whether you choose to be on your own or invite someone to share the experience with you – your best friend, husband or boyfriend, your daughter – so that you can take it in turns to be each other's beautician.

To keep the stressful world out, our advice is first to unplug the phone or switch on your answering machine (with the volume turned right down). Farm out any small children, if you possibly can. Shut the door on the world. Only then can you really start the body-perfecting, mood-shifting treatments that will take you from Friday evening through to Sunday evening, with time out for a Saturday rendez-vous, if you like.

Spa Homework

You will enjoy your weekend all the more if you prepare for it; you don't want to spend the weekend shopping or dashing around buying the beauty products that are supposed to be relaxing you. On Thursday night before your spa weekend, make sure you're stocked up with:

✦ a supply of freshly washed fluffy towels
✦ fresh sheets (always a treat)
✦ fresh fruit and vegetables, groceries – including any ingredients for masks you might make yourself, and lots of sea salt
✦ plenty of mineral water and fruit juices, herbal teas (during the weekend you should try to drink at least 2 litres of pure, still water each day)

✦ tapes and CDs that you might like to play over the weekend, piled up by your stereo
✦ cling-film (for beauty treatments)
✦ a mountaineer's blanket (if you're planning to give yourself a 'wrap')
✦ beauty products
✦ cotton wool, orange sticks, Q-tips
✦ tweezers
✦ casual clothes and sturdy walking shoes

Set the scene with mood music, on a battery-operated stereo which you can carry from room to room. (It isn't safe to plug in electric stereos in your bathroom.) Try some smoochy Sinatra or Vivaldi, medieval chants or relaxing New Age tapes. Turn up the heating if it's winter. Take no notice of the time, and put a blanket over the TV.

Friday Evening

Start your weekend on the right footing – with a smoothing shape-up for work-weary feet. Reflexologists believe that footcare can help maintain total body health, so begin with your feet, then work up the body.

For instance, if you have end-of-week tightness in the neck, firmly squeeze your big toe on the spot directly below the pad and towards the outside of the foot. Hold for 20 seconds; repeat five times.

Next, dissolve five soluble aspirin tablets in a plastic basin of warm water (the salicylic acid in the aspirin will soften callouses), or sprinkle in a handful of sea salt. Soak feet for 20 minutes to soften, then rub away hard skin with a stiff foot brush or a pumice stone – concentrate on making circular movements, especially on the heels.

Follow with an abrasive foot-and-leg scrub, made from $^1/_2$ cup finely chopped almonds or almond meal, 1 cup oatmeal, $^1/_2$ cup honey. Slather a quarter of the mixture over your soles, then rub with a circular motion, paying special attention to heels, toes and calloused areas.

Wrap your feet in cling-film and leave for five minutes. (It will rustle, but it does work.) Then remove the cling-film, rinse feet with warm water and smooth them with moisturiser.

Then, to exercise and deeply relax feet, put a rolling pin under a towel and move your feet backwards and forwards over it, while seated in a comfy chair.

Lastly, pedicure your feet (see *How to Have Fabulous Feet*, page 173), with the same care you would lavish on your hands.

Now that your feet feel fabulous, move upwards. Revitalise legs by whisking away dead skin cells with the remaining three-quarters of the scrub mixture, smoothing it into legs and the tops of your feet. Wrap your legs in cling-film.

Next, give your hands the kid glove treatment. Lydia Sarfati, owner of Manhattan's Repêchage salon, recommends heating your facial moisturiser in the top of a double boiler, until it's just warm. 'Then massage in thoroughly, working from the base of your palm to your fingertips – one at a time.' For maximum moisturising, you could even wear cotton gloves for the moisturiser to soak in overnight.

Saturday a.m.
First off, indulge in a deep-penetrating hair-conditioning treatment (for the brands our testers liked best, see *Tried & Tested Hair Masks*, page 117). For D-I-Y hair repair, take one egg white and beat until stiff, then stir in one teaspoon of honey. Massage into dry hair and comb through to distribute evenly. Then dab one teaspoon of sesame oil onto your hair. (Alternatively, apply one mashed banana mixed with one mashed avocado.) Cover hair with cling-film if you wish, or sit under a hood hairdryer (with or without cling-film), switched on low, for ten minutes, to turbo-charge the effects. Thoroughly wash hair after the treatment, then rinse, condition and style as usual.

Saturday p.m.
Give yourself a salon-perfect manicure. (See *Helping Hands*, page 176). Then, when your polish has dried completely, don sensible shoes and set off on a long, brisk walk – as far away from traffic fumes as possible. Try to walk fast enough to work up a sweat – that's the signal that your body is getting enough aerobic activity to improve cardio-vascular fitness and circulation, and to strengthen heart,

lungs, muscle and bones. Walk like a big cat – lithe, relaxed and graceful. Always walk with your second toe leading, rather than splay-footed or pigeon-toed.

Back home, run the taps, then sink into the tub as your soothing post-walk reward. To ease weary muscles, add up to one tablespoon of powdered ginger to the bath water, a cup of apple cider vinegar – which helps restore the skin's natural acid balance, so soothing itchiness, too – or a pound of Epsom salts. This treatment is said to help eliminate toxins through the skin, so should be indulged in only occasionally. Soak for 20 minutes. While you're lying back, close your eyes and apply two tea bags, cooled in the fridge – the chilling action constricts blood vessels, thereby reducing puffiness.

If you have a shower attachment, you can recreate a hydrotherapy jet massage: remove the nozzle, turn the taps on full and use short, stroking movements on fatty areas such as hips, thighs and bottom, working towards the lymphatic drainage points (in the groin and under-arm area).

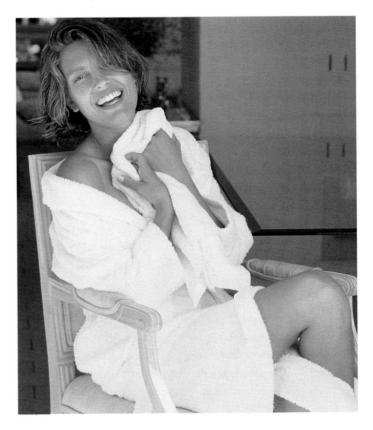

To revive yourself while you're in the tub, Luye Lui, creator of a NYC-based water aerobics programme, suggests trying:

Flutter kick: resting against the back of the tub, lift both legs slightly and flutter kick, first with toes pointed, then flexed.

Back stretch: sit up with both knees slightly bent, arms at your sides. Lean forward until you feel a slight stretch.

At the end of your bath, for smooth and glowing skin, try an invigorating exfoliating scrub. Wet your sponge or flannel, sprinkle some sea salt on it, and start rubbing gently, using a circular motion. Don't rub near cuts (salt stings) or your face.

When you get out of your bath, don't dry off completely; just pat yourself dry with a warm towel, then apply generous dollops of body lotion. (See *Tried & Tested Body Lotions*, page 189, for testers' favourites.)

Saturday Night

Cleanse your face, then give your skin a face mask for a radiant complexion (see *Maskmanship*, page 86). (If you're taking time off from your retreat to go out and socialise on Saturday night, you might prefer to do this tomorrow, as masks can sometimes leave you looking temporarily blotchy.)

The D-I-Y potential for making masks is limitless, see *Fridge Fresh and Fabulous*, page 96. If you're staying in and spending the weekend with a friend, one of you can give the other a relaxing aromatherapy massage, and vice versa the next night – see 'Sunday Night' (right) for suggestions of the best oils to use.

Sunday a.m.

Health farms and spas specialise in 'thermal wraps', slathering your body in a mask, then cocooning you in a reflective thermal blanket, to help retain body heat and ensure you gain the greatest benefit from moisturising or de-toxifying ingredients. Hot towels work, but they'll need thorough washing afterwards. A more efficient way to keep the body heat in (and the mess) is to invest in a mountaineer's 'space' blanket (see DIRECTORY for mail order from sports and hiking shops). (You can also keep this hypothermia-beater in the car as snowdrift insurance between at-home spa sessions.) If you have enough space on the bathroom floor, make a pillow for your head and pad the

flooring with towels, unless it's plushly carpeted. Then lay out the space blanket, sit in the middle of it, apply your body mask and wrap the space blanket around you. It will keep you amazingly warm.

For your D-I-Y seaweed wrap, simply soak dried seaweed (such as large sheets of kombu, available at health food stores) in water, then scoop the slippery gel onto your skin. As an alternative to seaweed, mix your own custom-blended deep-cleansing clay body mask: take some clay or Fuller's Earth (available at health food stores and chemists), add enough water to make a paste, then add a few drops of essential oil into the mix. Try mixing three drops each of orange and lemon, or lavender and sandalwood, or patchouli and rose. Slap it on all over with your hands, wrap yourself in the blanket and lie down, with your head on a folded towel, for 20 minutes. Shower thoroughly, moisturise and relax again…

This is a good time to try a little brow grooming, the professional way (see *Brow Beat*, page 61, for the secrets of perfect tweezing).

Sunday p.m.

Get out in the fresh air, whether walking or gardening.

Sunday Night

In the last decade, firm evidence has emerged to back up what aromatherapists have long understood: that scented oils have tangible effects on the nervous and immune systems; they kick-start or calm, help overcome fatigue or beckon sleep. (See *Aromatherapy For You*, page 198.) So before you go to bed, give yourself an aromatherapy massage, with a blend of super sleep-inducing oils that will deeply relax you. (If two of you are spending a spa weekend together, it's now the turn of the person who gave last night's massage to lie back and relax.)

Excellent oils for insomnia and sleep problems, or just to help you drift off, are valerian, marjoram, chamomile Roman, clary sage, lemon and sandalwood. Make a blend using a total of five drops of one or more of these oils, added to one teaspoon of carrier/base oil. (The most effective are sesame, almond or jojoba oils.) Pour a little of the blended oils into your palm to warm them between your hands. Then, using long, slow strokes, massage from feet upwards, always moving towards the heart. Allow the oils to sink in thoroughly, then it's time for bed. For once, you'll start the week perfectly poised to cope with anything life can throw at you.

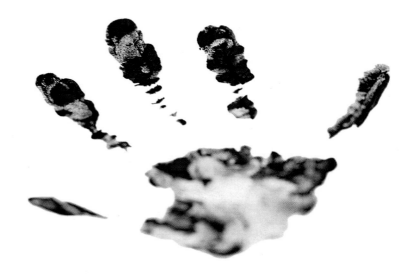

SKIN SMOOTHERS

Exfoliant creams, mitts or loofahs slough away dead skin cells to reveal fresher, brighter skin underneath. They also make moisturisers penetrate more efficiently. Skin is generally tougher on the body than the face, but, with the exception of the hard skin on feet and ankles, you should still treat it with respect. So don't be brutal, and, if you do buy an exfoliant cream, always make sure it has gentle, rounded particles which won't scratch the skin. (See *Here's the Scrub*, page 77.)

MUD SLINGING

The kind of mud used in body and face treatments is not the same as the mud you used to play in as a child. These muds and clays are dug from deep in the earth, or taken from the sea bed, and contain skin-enhancing ingredients. They come in a rainbow of colours: yellow, white, red, green, black and brown. Sources include Italy's Montecatini thermal springs, Morocco (for rhassoul mud), the Black Sea and the Dead Sea. Mud from the Dead Sea contains mineral salts that are ten times more concentrated than those in sea water and scientists have declared it to be extremely therapeutic. It has been found to help certain forms of eczema and psoriasis, which is why companies such as Ahava (see DIRECTORY) are now incorporating it into D-I-Y body treatments.

Mud's healing properties have been recognised for centuries, but it is rapidly becoming a fashionable beauty ingredient, incorporated into skin creams and salon treatments. Mud acts almost like a vacuum cleaner on the skin's surface, drawing out surface debris such as excess sebum, dead cells and pollution, which can then be rinsed away.

Mud treatments are suitable for all skin types, but are particularly beneficial for oily and combination skins. The types of mud you're most likely to find on sale are:

✦ pure, white, powdery kaolin, an excellent cleanser which has an astringent effect, improves circulation and lymphatic flow and is particularly good for normal to oily skins.

✦ Fuller's Earth, a soft, brown clay which is incredibly stimulating and cleansing, and also sloughs off dead skin cells. Good for normal to oily skins.

✦ green clay, a miraculous skin-balancer, which is good for treating acne and for tackling wrinkles. You can find it in some health food stores.

You can enjoy a mud bath at home, mixing Fuller's Earth or green clay with warm water until it's muddy, but not slimy. The first time you take a dip, just stay in for five to ten minutes. Every few days, have another mud bath, increasing the time you spend in it from ten to 20 minutes. (Mud is de-toxifying, so you should take it easy and not overdo it.)

Other muds we love to wallow in include Princess Marcella Borghese Fango-Active Mud, said to be a favourite of **Diana, Princess of Wales**, and Pierre Cattier Argile Mud (see DIRECTORY) and E'SPA's Pink Hair & Scalp Mud, which is a wonderful scalp deep-cleanser. A spa weekend is the perfect time to enjoy a mud treatment, but if you're going to have a full-body mud wrap, find some old towels to drape over a bathroom chair first. It's messy!

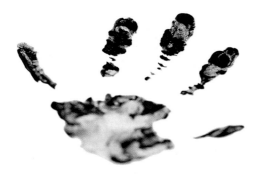

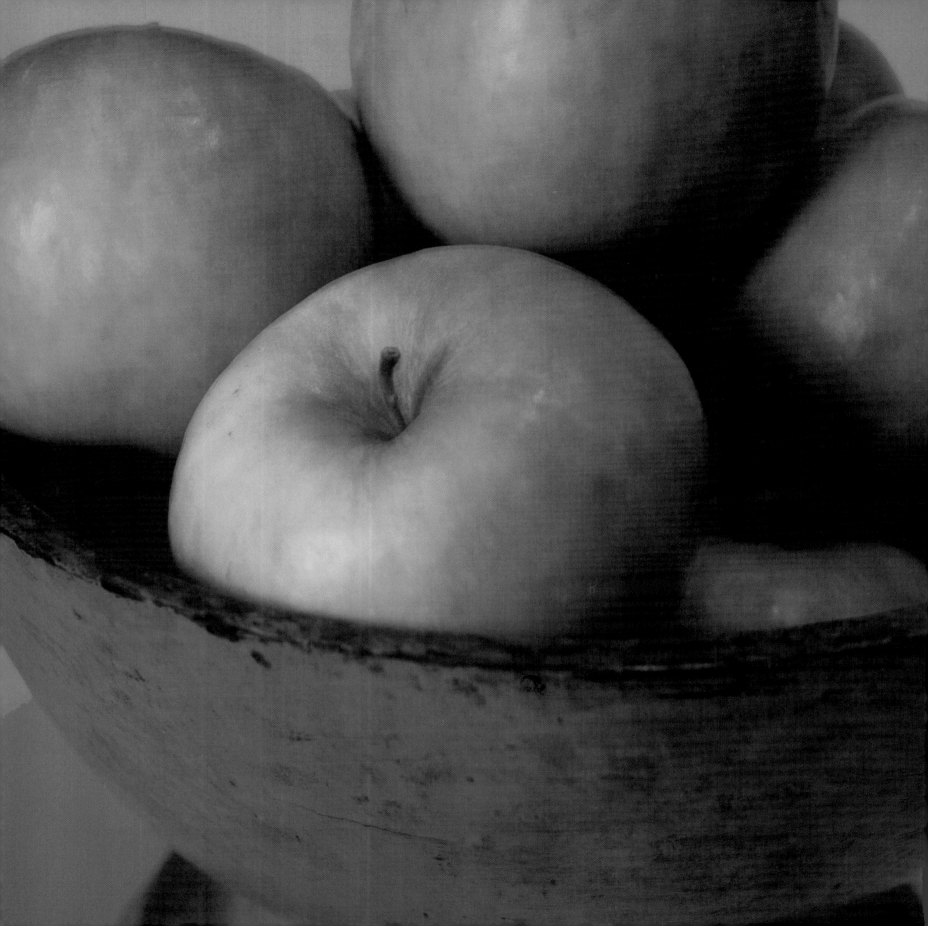

MORE SPA SECRETS

✦ Drink pure spring water, all weekend; naturopaths prescribe it slightly warm or room temperature, not iced.

✦ Spend as much time as you like daydreaming or listening to soft music with your eyes closed.

✦ Preferably don't lie in – it may disturb your body clock for the coming week. But feel free to go to bed as early as you like.

✦ Design your meals around foods with angst-easing properties: apricots, bananas, oranges, papayas, broccoli, carrots, peppers, lentils, wholegrains, pulses and wheatgerm (sprinkle this particular stress-beater on everything you eat over the weekend).

✦ Try starting the day with a 'power shake': ground sunflower and sesame seeds, whizzed in a blender with apple juice, soya milk, some live yoghurt and slices of any fruit that is to hand.

✦ Eat your meals by candlelight.

✦ Discover the joys of seaweed: the iodine-rich sea veggie balances metabolic function and encourages the body to burn fat more efficiently. It helps protect against pollution, too. You'll find dried seaweeds at your health food store. (If you can't stand the rock-poolish taste, the least seaweed-flavoured one is nori, which can also be ground up and used on food as a condiment.)

✦ Buy yourself a big bowl of organic green apples and leave them on the kitchen table. Snack on them whenever you feel like it. Alan Hirsch, M.D., Director of Chicago's Smell and Taste Foundation, has discovered that the scent actually reduces anxiety by increasing the brain's alpha waves, which are directly linked with relaxation.

SEAWEED – IN-DEPTH

You may steer clear of it at the beach, but in future you can expect to encounter a lot more seaweed incorporated into face and body treatments. Seaweed, long used as a thickening agent in everything from ice cream to hand cream, is now taking an active role in a variety of skincare products.

Fans say that seaweed – actually a generic term for more than 20,000 species of algae that grow in the world's oceans – can moisturise, control oil production, fight the ageing effects of pollution on the skin and possibly protect against UV light. What's more, certain parts of the plant can be used in place of animal-derived ingredients, making seaweed a 'politically correct' cosmetic component.

In traditional medicine, seaweed paste is used to treat burns because it can soothe and inhibit bacterial infections. Today, it's most often used as an ingredient in body treatments and bath additives because it helps draw toxins to the surface of the skin.

Skincare treatments using seawater and/or seaweed (known as thalassotherapy) are on offer in many beauty salons and over-the-counter products. Ranges to look out for include Thalgo, E'SPA, Repêchage and Phytomer (see DIRECTORY).

BACK BASICS

When it comes to your back, out of sight can mean out of mind. Because it's frequently neglected, back skin can often be in need of a boost.

If the skin on your back is less than bareable, poor circulation could be the problem, so start with regular skin brushing, with a long-handled brush to make it easier.

If your back is blemished, apply a face mask for oily complexions all over your back.

If your skin is dry and flaky, enlist a friend for a mutual back-scratching session. Start with a home-made salt-and-oil scrub, applied with a loofah or sisal mitt: dip the mitt in olive oil or jojoba oil, then into coarse sea salt, and rub briskly all over shoulders and back. Rinse, then pat dry and apply a rich body lotion or massage oil. Then swap places!

LEARN HOW TO MEDITATE

Meditation can be a short-cut to relaxation, resulting in significant health benefits. When you're calm and relaxed, you look better, too – no furrow-lines or frowns. Research shows that this technique, when practised regularly, can help keep at bay a wide range of complaints, from headaches to asthma, eczema, PMS, hypertension – even heart attacks. The physical effects of meditation are a significant reduction in the metabolic rate, the heart rate and in breathing speed, while circulation improves and muscle tension disappears. Stress ebbs away, leaving us better able to cope with forthcoming activities.

The idea of meditation is to clear the mind – at least temporarily – of extraneous thoughts which sap our energy, by focusing on just a single thought. That's why we suggest learning to meditate during your 'spa retreat' weekend, a time which should be free from interruptions and when you should be quite relaxed in any case.

After only a few minutes, practised meditators can feel more clear-headed and rested. To the novice, however, even attempting to meditate can be stressful. Just as you're trying to empty your mind, it seems to fill instantly with 'To Do' lists. Or your limbs develop Lotus-position-ache. So here is the experts' advice on how to maximise the benefits of meditation, while avoiding the pitfalls.

✦ Choose a quiet spot where you won't be interrupted. Insist, like Greta Garbo, that friends/partners/family leave you alone.
✦ Don't eat or drink for half an hour beforehand. Don't meditate before a meal, either; hunger pangs will put you off.
✦ Turn down the lights or draw the curtains/blinds.
✦ Sit comfortably in an upright position, with your hands resting in your lap. Creaky knees or a painful back will make you fidget. If you still aren't comfortable, lie down – although most meditation teachers prefer the seated position, to avert the danger of *over*-relaxation (i.e. nodding off). The idea is to remain calm but alert.
✦ Imagine every part of your body relaxing: start with your scalp, moving down the body, and feel the tension ebb away from your jaw, neck, shoulders, arms, fingers, stomach, legs, feet and toes.
✦ Prevent stimulating ideas or niggling problems entering your mind by concentrating on one neutral or calmly pleasing thought: the colour blue, a cloudless horizon, a mountain vista.
✦ Let breathing settle into a natural rhythm. Don't try to change the pattern. One highly effective meditation technique is to focus on breathing itself: feel the air as it enters your nostrils, moving down to fill the lungs completely, then slowly exhale. Breathe from the abdomen, not the chest; feel your tummy swell as you inhale. Count slowly as you breathe in and out, taking as long to expel each breath – fully – as you did to inhale.
✦ Whenever a distracting thought breaks in, simply acknowledge it and let it go. American meditation master Ram Dass advises transforming each thought into a cloud and watching it float away in your mind's eye.
✦ When you've finished, slowly open your eyes, stretch and wait a minute or two before standing up, to avoid dizziness.
✦ Start small – two to five minutes, then ten, then as long as you want or can carve out of your schedule. To begin with, establish a regular time each day for meditation. When you become practised you can meditate almost anywhere: on the train, at your desk.

✦ There is no right way or wrong way to meditate. What works for you is the right way. Some experts believe that repeating a phrase (or 'mantra') time and again can lull the mind into a state of meditative bliss. Meditation author Lawrence LeShan suggests looking up two names in a phone book, at random, and combining the first syllable of each to create your own mantra.

GO INTO DE-TOX

A stress-free, quiet weekend is the perfect time to try out a de-toxification regime. If you can manage one or two days without caffeine and alcohol, largely eating fruit and vegetables, you will feel great benefits. However, expelling toxins from an overloaded system can temporarily induce headaches or other aches and pains, dizziness and a degree of lassitude. To combat this, drink as much pure water as possible (2 to 5 litres daily), submerge yourself in warm baths, and rest. If you drink a lot of caffeine during the week – say, more than four cups of coffee a day – it will make a 'de-tox' headache more likely. (Tea drinkers may not experience such dramatic symptoms, but be alert to unpleasant withdrawal side-effects.) To avoid a headache, keep on drinking caffeine but cut right down to one cup in the morning, or switch to decaffeinated. But do ask yourself what all that caffeine is doing to your system the rest of the time...

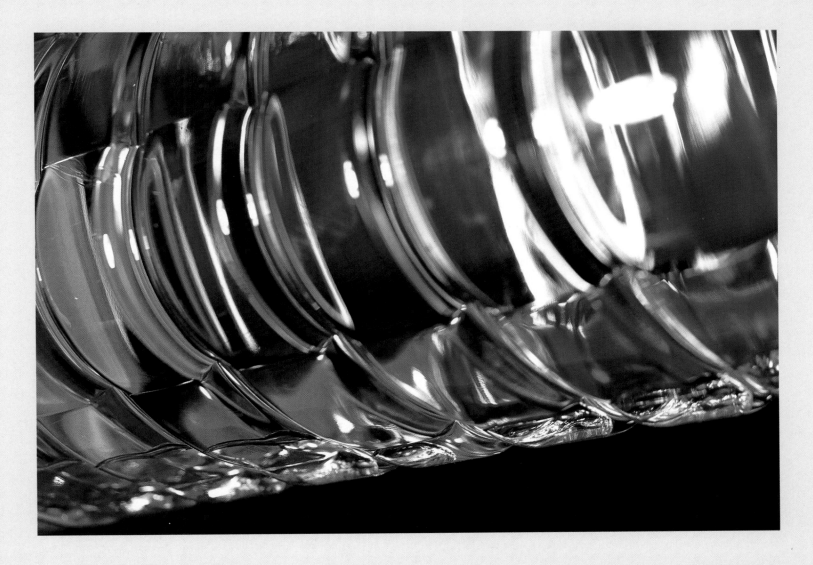

In her book *Food Combining in 30 Days*, Kathryn Marsden details an easy two-day de-tox plan.

✦ Breakfast on as much fruit as you like: kiwi, apples, pears, grapes, mango, papaya, peaches or nectarines, singly or in combination.

✦ After a mid-morning snack of a banana and, if you wish, a cup of weak China tea (more alkaline than Indian), herb tea or pure water, lunch should be a large raw salad, of, for example, dark-leaved lettuce, skinned cucumber and tomato, cauliflower or broccoli, avocado, grated carrot, peppers (any colour), chicory and parsley. Serve with a dressing of extra virgin olive oil and cider vinegar.

✦ At teatime, munch on a handful of sunflower and pumpkin seeds or unblanched almonds, washed down with water or weak herb tea.

✦ For dinner, prepare a large portion of steamed or gently poached vegetables. Choose from a selection of leeks, cauliflower, broccoli, root vegetables, onion, marrow, celeriac, aubergine, peppers, courgette or red cabbage, flavoured with herbs – fresh, if possible.

✦ Before bed, eat a small carton of fresh, plain, additive-free bio-yoghurt, and then relax.

Your whole system will really have benefited from the rest you have given it.

AROMATHERAPY FOR YOU

An aromatherapy massage, with sweet-smelling essential oils, is an irresistible treat, but you can also give yourself the benefit of their subtle powers at home. Leigh Richmond, one of the UK's leading aromatherapists who has created a range of her own blends, has compiled these lists of suggested oils for *The Beauty Bible*.

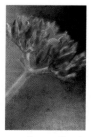

First Aid Kit

These ten oils will help with physical ailments. Keep them in your bathroom and use them either in your bath, or as a burning oil, or massage them in to your skin, diluted in a carrier/base oil; in the case of aches, pains or bruises, use them as a compress diluted in warm water.

These oils should be seen as complementary to conventional medical care. If you have a serious problem, always consult a qualified practitioner. Leigh advises against using them in pregnancy.

Eucalyptus: antiseptic, warms up respiratory system, helps alleviate colds, coughs, flu, congestion, fever, sinusitis and sore throats.

Geranium: most effective in regulating and balancing extremes on both physical and emotional levels, especially PMT, depression and post natal depression (don't use if breastfeeding); can help treat endometriosis.

Ginger: helps treat digestive disorders, spasms, appetite loss or disorders; also effective for colds, flu, muscular aches and pains, rheumatism and arthritis; strengthens immune system.

Juniper: stimulates the circulation, helps to purify and detoxify the blood; stimulates a sluggish liver; brings mental clarity, powerful in diffusing negativity.

Lavender: known as the universal panacea of essential oils, this balances and regulates the nerves; effective in treating depression, insomnia, exhaustion; highly antiseptic, so good for burns, blisters, bruises and bites (in compress form); helps soothe and alleviate pain.

Lemon: highly antiseptic, so helpful in alleviating symptoms of colds and flu; purifies and de-toxifies blood; helps lower blood pressure, stimulates the brain and helps you focus.

Peppermint: powerful decongestant effective in all kinds of nasal colds/stuffiness; calms digestive disorders and nauseous migraines; refreshing, helps clear mental fog.

Pine: alleviates respiratory problems, coughs, colds, flu, eases muscular aches and pains; refreshing, brings mental clarity.

Rosemary: beneficial in sluggish circulation, rheumatism, muscular aches and pains; also hair loss and dandruff; stimulates memory, enlivening mind and sharpening powers of recall.

Tea tree: versatile anti-bacterial and anti-viral oil useful in treating colds, flu, skin conditions and viral infections such as warts, herpes, thrush and candida, and athlete's foot.

First Aid for Stress and Emotional Problems

Essential oils can be very beneficial, effective treatments for emotional problems. Whether these are the result of grief and bereavement, stress at work, or a life-changing decision, the many devotees of essential oils know that they can help you through those 'can't cope, can't sleep' times which affect most of us at some stage.

Chamomile: calms and soothes the nervous system, allaying fear and anxiety; good for phobias, depression, obsessive behavioural patterns and insomnia; ideal for children (in low dosage), and hypersensitive people.

Clary Sage: will help lift the dark clouds of severe depression, bringing lightness and peace; strengthens nerves, so good for anxiety, fears, oversensitivity to other people, paranoia, obsessive behaviour. Use with a grounding oil such as sandalwood, vetyvert or juniper.

Frankincense: very spiritual oil, bringing tranquillity; good for excess and addictions, obsessive behavioural patterns, allaying unexplained fears and phobias; helps promote insight, peace, mental calm. Use with a grounding oil.

Jasmine: uniquely uplifting effect on emotions, aphrodisiac; good for alleviating anxiety, post natal depression and labour pains (apply as compress).

Juniper: good for depression, stops you being over-vulnerable to other people's problems and taking them on board as your own; quells negativity, especially in stressful environments.

Lavender: highly effective against depression, regulates nerves, brings greater clarity and peace of mind; effective against insomnia.

Neroli: gently soothes, calms and allays fears; best used for nervous conditions, anxiety, depression, phobia, shock and insomnia; also good for calming hyperactive or anxious children.

Rose: known as the queen of essential oils, this balances emotional disorders, promotes inner poise and confidence; acts as a gentle opener for repressed painful emotions, especially grief.

Sandalwood: calming, balancing and grounding; ideal for getting problems off your chest; gives impetus to cope with difficult and stressful situations.

Vetyvert: known as the oil of tranquillity, deeply relaxing, beneficial for anxiety, stress and insomnia; helps promote inner calm, poise and confidence; helps you cope in times of major upheaval and grief.

First Aid for Pregnancy

Choose from neroli, frankincense and chamomile, with jasmine and rose (only in the last trimester) in moderation. Massage blends of chamomile and neroli or frankincense and rose onto the stomach to help prevent stretch marks. Use two drops of neroli to five of chamomile or four frankincense and one rose in 10ml of carrier/base oil (almond – unless you have a nut allergy – grapeseed or peach kernel); try adding in the contents of a capsule of vitamin E.

Combine two, three or four of these oils using two drops of each in 10ml of carrier/base oil, (10ml of carrier/base oil is enough for a facial, 20ml a full body massage). Or you could use up to five drops of the oil you feel you need most with a drop each of the other essential oils.

WARNING If you are using clary sage or frankincense, do not drive or use heavy machinery afterwards ✿ Keep essential oils out of the reach of children ✿ Store in a cool, dark place

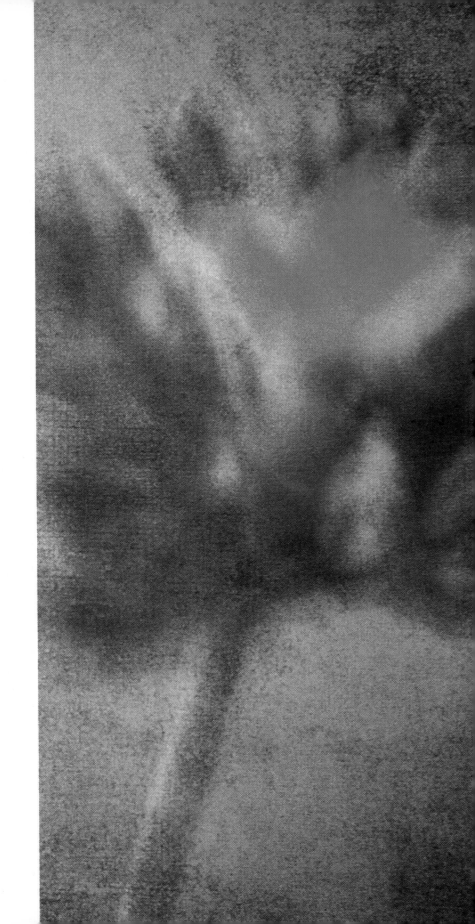

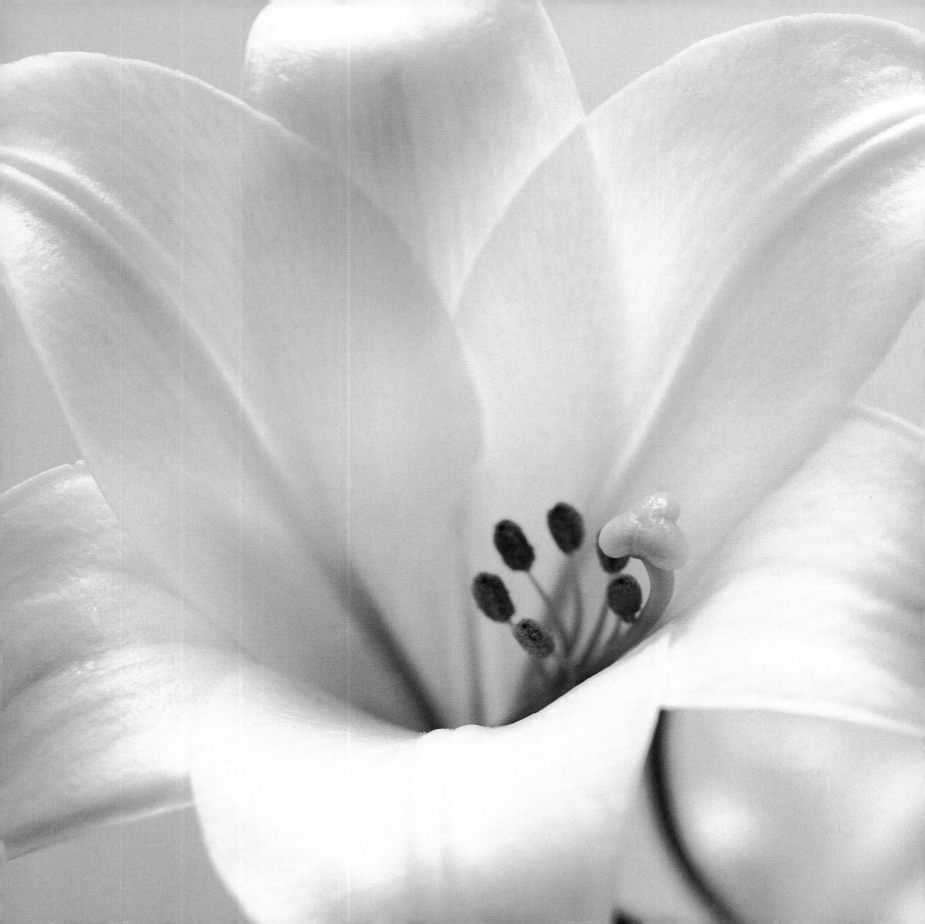

7 Fragrance

This is the era of the 'fragrance wardrobe'. **While some women are faithful for life to an old favourite, many more are discovering the joy of experimenting with scents that match their mood.** But, since perfume is one of the most expensive beauty indulgences, getting it right is essential. Especially since fragrance develops differently on different skin types. Here's our guide to finding your perfect scent – and to making the most of its mood-lifting potential.

HOW TO BUY A FRAGRANCE

Just as a woman's clothes can enhance innate style and have a profound effect on everyone around, so can scent. But it is vital to choose the right one for your personality and your mood. Here's how to waft wisely.

Never be too impulsive when buying a perfume, advises Lorna McKnight, an independent consultant to the perfumery and cosmetics industry and former perfume buyer for Harrods. Always shop in a fragrance hall or store where you can try the scents rather than just buy bottles off the shelf, and preferably somewhere you can get individual advice from a trained perfumery sales assistant.

Before you start spraying fragrance on yourself, ask the assistant to spray the perfumes onto 'blotters' – absorbent strips of blotting paper. This helps you identify which fragrance you might like to try on your skin, and saves you from walking around drenched in something which is more a turn-off than a turn-on. (We've all done that.) You can now sample the scent exactly as professional 'noses' (the fragrance creators) do: hold the blotter at the non-scented end between thumb and forefinger, and place the scented end about two inches below your nostrils. Use your second finger to tap the blotter lightly so that it vibrates; this will help disperse the scent into the air so that you can smell it better. Once you've found a scent you're attracted to, try it on your body.

'You should sample one fragrance at a time,' advises Lorna McKnight, 'and *really* wear it before you make up your mind, rather than spray one on the back of your hand, one on the other, one on your wrist, which is what a lot of women do. You want to know how it develops on *you*, and you can't tell if you're being confused by other scents. Close your eyes, really smell it. Ignore the packaging and the marketing and concentrate on the scent itself. And ideally – to avoid any chance of an expensive mistake – go back and repeat the exercise a couple of times before you buy it.' (Scent-strips in magazines are a good clue as to whether a fragrance is a hate-at-first-sniff or a 'maybe'. But never buy on the basis of these alone. You must find out how fragrance reacts on your own skin.)

The top note – a perfume's first impression – lasts just fifteen or so minutes. So, more important than whether you take to the initial smell is how you feel about the middle notes (lasting up to an hour) and bottom notes (which linger for several hours). Scents smell different on each of us; skin, make-up and diet are all an influence, which is why you should never buy a fragrance just because you love it on your best friend or on the scent-strip. Fragrances alter on your skin as your cycle progresses, too – and according to the time of year. Just as you don't feel like eating heavy food or drinking red wine in summer, there are scents appropriate to different seasons. Good reasons, therefore, to build up a personalised perfume 'wardrobe' to match your moods. And the weather...

How to Pick the Perfect Perfume – For You

The sheer number of fragrances out there – dozens of old faithfuls and non-stop new versions – is nose-boggling. With more than 100 scents launched each year, how are we ever to find our perfect match?

Identifying which ones say 'me' could take countless time-consuming trips to the fragrance counter. And scent-speak descriptions don't help anyone outside the beauty business much, either, with descriptions such as 'aldehydic', 'floral', 'green', and so on. Little wonder we stick to the ones we know – or make repeated expensive perfume errors, which gather dust on our dressing tables.

Fragrance 'Portraits'

But there is, in fact, a fascinating short-cut which can point you in the direction of scents you're likely to love: fragrance 'portraits' – designed (like scent itself) to go straight for your emotions. This helps you 'see', rather than guess, which scents suit you.

It couldn't be simpler. Which group of pictures on the following pages are you instinctively drawn to? Let the list which accompanies your chosen collage of images be your starting point next time you visit a fragrance counter.

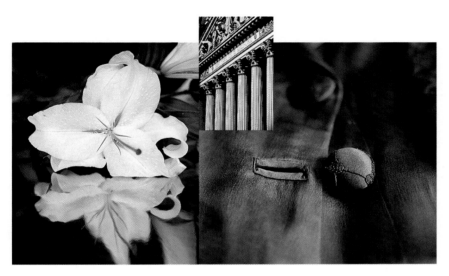

1.

These scents are rich, but also soft and subtle. They're like bottled essence-of-elegance:

Hermès *24 Faubourg*   Lancôme *Poême*
Cartier *So Pretty*   Van Cleef & Arpels *First*
Chanel *No. 5*   Rochas *Madame Rochas*
Lanvin *Arpège*   Worth *Je Reviens*
YSL *Y*

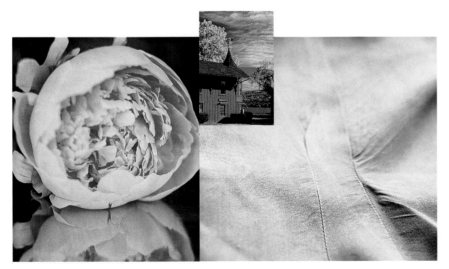

2.

Outdoorsy, innocent, breath-of-fresh-air scents that you should find irresistible:

Estée Lauder *Pleasures*   Guerlain *Jardins de Bagatelle*
Calvin Klein *cKOne*   Giorgio Armani *Acqua di Giò*
Cacharel *Anaïs Anaïs*   Salvador Dali *Eau de Dali*
Nina Ricci *L'Air du Temps* YSL *Paris*
Chanel *Cristalle*   Chanel *Allure*

You may be attracted to more than one set of photos, which is fine; your choice may vary with your mood.
But this approach to choosing a scent still eliminates much time-wasting and wrist-sniffing.

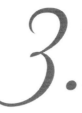

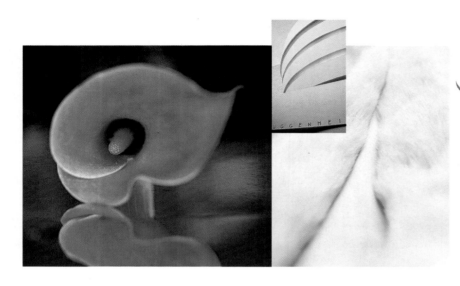

3.

Scents with sensuality, these love-them-or-hate-them fragrances evoke passionate responses:

Boucheron *Jaïpur*   Salvador Dali *Eau de Dali*
Chanel *Coco*   Estée Lauder *Youth Dew*
YSL *Opium*   Cacharel *Loulou*
Donna Karan *Donna Karan*   Lancôme *Magie Noire*
Calvin Klein *Obsession*   Jean Patou *1000*

4.

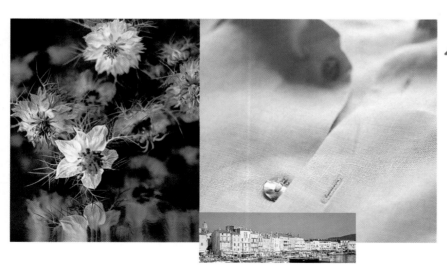

These fragrances have a casual, natural mood – stylish and easy to wear:

Halcyon Days   Rochas *Femme de Rochas*
Chanel *No. 22*   *4711*
Coriandre   Prescriptives *Calyx*
Giorgio *Red*   Paco Rabanne *Calandre*
YSL *Rive Gauche*   *Comme des Garçons*

Just why are these at-a-glance perfume portraits so effective? According to perfume expert Dr Luca Turin, 'Scent is actually about much more than our sense of smell; it brings together all the senses.'

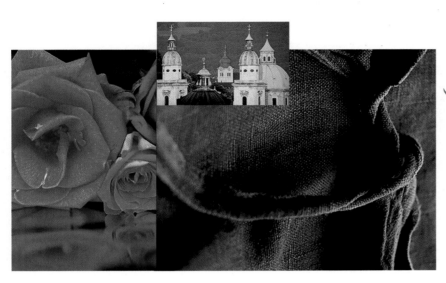

5.

Upbeat scents for the woman who wears her confidence on her sleeve:

Carolina Herrera *Flore*   Giorgio *Giorgio*
Antonia's Flowers   Estée Lauder *Beautiful*
Tiffany *Trueste*   Roger & Gallet *Pour Femme*

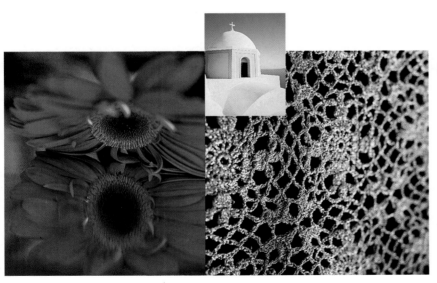

6.

A mix of soft flowers, sweet spices and fruitiness, for fashion-lovers:

Chopard *Casmîr*   Nikos *Sculpture*
Christian Dior *Dolce Vita*   Kenzo *Kashaya*
Guerlain *Un Aire de Samsara*   Gucci *Accenti*
Caron *Nocturnes*

We've found this method foolproof on virtually all the women we know, and we hope you will too.

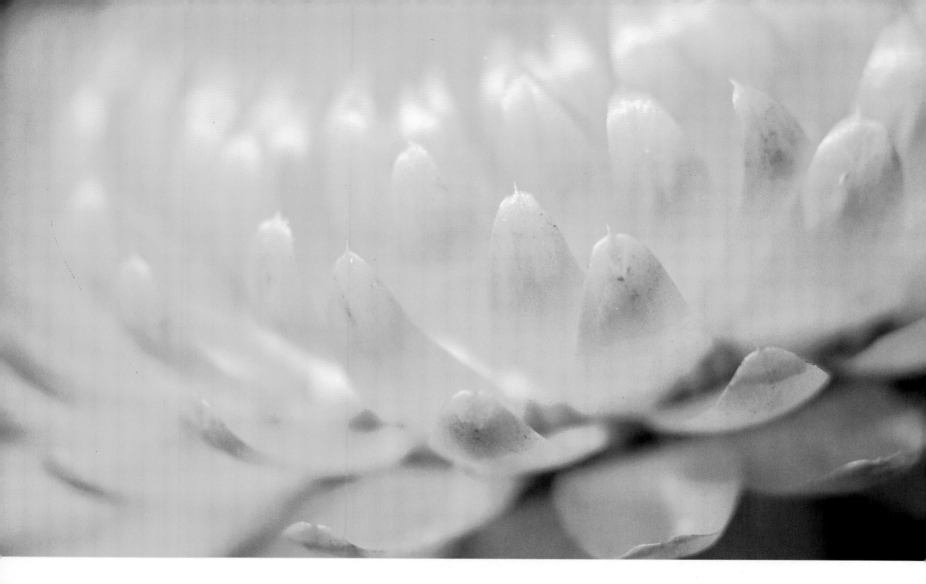

Your Body's Scent-Spots

Next time you spritz on a scent, consider skipping behind the ears. Scientists have located no less than 16 pulse-points on the body, including the temples, crook of the elbows, wrists, (between) your bosom, either side of the pubic bone, the back of your knees and the front of your ankles. If you do apply scent to your neck, dab it either side of the throat about eight centimetres (three inches) *below* your ear. There's another reason you might want to set your scent-sights a little lower: fragrance floats up on your body heat, so scenting below the waist will weave a head-to-toe aura for hours. Freshly washed hair is also a good fragrance carrier, as are clothes made of natural fabrics; try spraying under hems and collars. You could also spray or dab scent on a ribbon and tie it around your hair or wrist.

Too Little – Or Too Much?

We can't go through life asking everyone, 'How do I smell?'. But your own nose does start tuning out your scent after the first few minutes and, barring a deliberate sniff, stops picking it up completely after about 15–30 minutes. So the across-the-board rule of thumb is that whatever you can smell, others can smell more.

The strength of scent you wear controls the distance it can be smelled from, and how long it lasts. If the fragrance is alcohol-based (cologne, eau de parfum, eau de toilette), it will plummet sharply at first, then level off. But oil- or cream-based perfumes – for instance, body creams or bath oil, worn as perfume – taper off more gradually. If you 'layer' your fragrance (see opposite) you will achieve more lingering results.

> **Cologne** typically lasts one to four hours.
> **Eau de toilette/eau de parfum** usually lasts four to six hours.
> **Body lotion** or **body cream** lasts from three to eight hours.
> **Perfume** usually lasts from three to eight hours.
> You can also spray scent on clothes, where it's long-lasting – but harder to remove.

Deciphering Perfume-Speak

Top notes are the initial smells which hit you when you open the bottle and spray it onto your skin. They last for a very short time.
Middle, heart or soul notes describe the smells which evolve after about ten minutes exposure to oxygen and the skin.
Base notes are the smells which slowly develop to hold the whole fragrance together and which will linger at the end of the day. Never buy a fragrance unless you like the base notes; these are the ones which you – and everyone around you – will have to live with.

Layer Upon Layer

Most women apply perfume too lavishly on the pulse-points in the hope of making their fragrance last longer. This just makes the fragrance overpowering for the first few hours, before it fades away. By using complementary bath and body products, the fragrance is literally 'layered' on the skin: as the body heats and cools during the day each product 'comes alive', so ensuring a subtle, delicate aura which lasts consistently throughout the day or evening. The principle is this: start with a body shampoo/foam bath/bath oil/soap. Then use the *matching* body cream or lotion, with optional dusting powder or talc on top, and, a little later, apply just a light touch of perfume, eau de parfum or eau de toilette. As a ritual, it's truly the last word in pampering self-indulgence.

TRIED & TESTED

FRAGRANCED BODY LOTIONS

Bear in mind that these are all designer fragrances – with price tags to match, so they are real luxuries. However, our testers were really impressed with the following, giving very high marks indeed for scent, velvet quality, smoothness of application, softening ability and enduring improvements in skin texture.

Top Five Treats

Hermès Calèche Body Cream
COMMENTS: 'softened skin and smells beautiful', 'fragrance lasted all day and I had many compliments at work'.

Clarins Eau Dynamisante Moisturising Body Lotion
COMMENTS: 'skin felt smooth and nourished with a definite improvement on elbows, which became much softer', 'lovely lemony, fresh smell'.

Issey Miyake L'Eau d'Issey Crème Parfumée Pour Le Corps
COMMENTS: 'skin felt lovely, sensuous, soft and silky', 'particularly good on heels and knees', 'easily absorbed and skin felt great'.

Caron Fleur de Rocaille
COMMENTS: 'quite a cooling and summery scent', 'felt and smelt so good', 'rich and creamy, like a mousse'.

Calvin Klein Escape Body Cream
COMMENTS: 'loved it to bits', 'skin-calming with a very smooth and creamy texture'.

WHO WEARS WHAT?

Michelle Pfeiffer wears Donna Karan's *Donna Karan New York* perfume, 'Because it's sexy, intimate and sensual – but not so upfront that you feel it's wearing you.' She's also a fan of Giorgio Armani's *Acqua di Giò* – as is **Faye Dunaway**.

Model **India Hicks**: 'I bought Yves Saint Laurent's *Champagne* because I loved the witty packaging. Then I found it reminded me of every celebration I'd ever been to.'

Naomi Campbell likes to have a wardrobe of fragrances. Top of the list: *Diorissimo* and *Route du Thé* (see DIRECTORY), the signature scent of New York department store Barney's.

The Princess of Wales, **Anouk Aimée** and **Jacqueline Bisset** love Lanvin's *Arpège*, the ultra-sophisticated French classic.

The Prince of Wales favours Geo F. Trumper's *Extract of Limes* toiletries, from the Royal barber. (**Diana** likes the zingy scent, too; she keeps a supply of their Bath & Shower gel.)

Supermodel **Carla Bruni** likes *Shalimar* by Guerlain. 'I'm very classic when it comes to perfume. When I wear fragrance, I tend to choose the old French ones.'

Princess Michael of Kent: 'I have a range of scents which I vary according to my mood, the season and the occasion – but I always return to *L'Air du Temps*, by Nina Ricci.'

Madonna likes to wear Paco Rabanne's ultra-sophisticated *XS*.

The Queen's signature scent? *Joy*, by Jean Patou, renowned as the costliest fragrance in the world. (Other *Joy*-lovers: **Joan Rivers**, **Barbara Taylor Bradford**, the late **Ella Fitzgerald** and the late **Jackie Onassis**.)

Kylie Minogue likes *Nocturnes* by Caron.

Catherine Deneuve drops into Parisian perfume mecca Octée to stock up on supplies of their No. 2 scent.

First Lady **Hillary Rodham Clinton** likes to wear *Tantra Perfume Diffusion*, from New Age beauty company Aveda. **Cindy Crawford** spritzes herself with Aveda's *Chakra No. II 'Attraction'*, while **The Duchess of York** indulges herself with Aveda's *Tangerine Absolute Essence*.

Annick Goutal's fragrances have notched up dozens of famous fans. What did **Madonna**, **Prince** and the late French premier **François Mitterand** have in common? Annick Goutal's *Eau d'Hadrien*. **Isabelle Adjani** and supermodel **Stephanie Seymour** go for *Eau de Camille*, while *chanteuse* **Juliette Greco** prefers Annick Goutal's *Tubereuse*.

Bianca Jagger loves Chopard's floriental *Casmîr*.

Who's been carried away by Thierry Mugler's *Angel*? Everyone from **Nicole Kidman** to **Elton John** via **Hillary Clinton** and **Iman**...

Helena Christensen likes *Opium* by YSL and *Chloë* by Lagerfeld. 'They're quite old-fashioned, and I love putting them on with old dresses.' Another big fan of *Chloë* is **Olivia Newton John** – maybe because it's not just a great scent, it's the name of her daughter...

TV presenter **Katie Puckrick**: 'I wear *Ultima II Sheer Scent*. It's a real boy magnet! All the guys breathe in deeply when they catch a whiff of this and want to know more about me! Even the ridiculously cheesy packaging is great – but it's a fairly well-kept secret.'

Melanie Griffith loves *Le Must* by Cartier. 'Ten years ago I smelled it on an actress called Helen Shaver and said, "What's that?" And I've worn it ever since.'

Elle Macpherson's favourite scent? *Vetiver* by Guerlain. 'I like the way male fragrances smell on me.'

Model-turned-designer **Inès de la Fressange**: 'When I was 19, there was a girl at school who I thought was so glamorous. She wore *Chanel No. 19*. I thought that if I wore the same perfume, I would be just as glamorous. That was my first perfume. I tend to change fragrances when I change my life – a new boyfriend, a new apartment. But my favourites are the old French perfumes, like *Shalimar* and *Vol de Nuit* by Guerlain. Another Guerlain fan is **Sophia Loren**, who wears *L'Heure Bleu*.

Actress **Patsy Kensit** loves Chanel's *Cristalle*.

Jane Asher wears *Je Reviens* by Worth. 'It's an old one, but people still stop me and ask what I'm wearing.'

TIPS

☀ If you've sprayed on too much perfume and stepping back into the shower isn't a viable option, dilute the scent by rubbing with a warm, soapy washcloth. But if you tend to be heavy-handed with fragrance, stick with eau de toilette, which isn't as strong as perfume or eau de parfum.

☀ Estée Lauder, one of the *grandes dames* of the beauty world, recommends perfuming yourself by spraying the air, then walking through the fragrant cloud. She also suggests spraying your hair with scent, not just your pulse-points.

☀ High altitudes decrease the longevity of perfume as well as the potency of its aroma. So if you're flying off for a romantic weekend in the mountains, you might apply your fragrance more often – or choose a stronger concentration.

☀ Women have a better sense of smell than men, and it's particularly sharp in the first half of the menstrual cycle.

☀ It's often said that you can't wear more than one scent a day or it'll 'clash'. But Annette Green, of The Fragrance Foundation in New York, says that most fragrances don't linger longer than about three to four hours, so you can wear several in the space of one day if the mood takes you. She's been known to wear up to four in 24 hours.·

☀ Each one of us has an 'odour fingerprint' – the sum total of many factors including heredity, complexion and even diet. Fragrance doesn't last as long on dry skin as on oily skin, and perfume may smell stronger on someone who has just eaten a lot of high-fat or spicy foods.

☀ Avoid wearing your usual fragrance in the sun, unless it's available in a special alcohol-free version. Many scents contain ingredients that trigger an adverse reaction in sunlight, causing rashes with itching or prickliness, or turn the skin brown. (You could apply it to your clothes, instead.)

☀ Never apply perfume straight after bathing; warm water causes pores to dilate, temporarily leaving skin more sensitive to any product applied to it; the alcohol in perfume can sting or burn. You can, of course, use a scented body lotion instead.

☀ Science has recently confirmed what we always hoped: women who sprayed themselves with a floral scent twice a day were found to have improved moods and less anxiety and fatigue.

ON OUR (RATHER CROWDED) DRESSING TABLES

SARAH:

Christian Dior Diorissimo

Guerlain Mitsouko and Shalimar

Jean Patou Joy

Chanel Allure

Antonia's Flowers

Lanvin Arpège

Escada Acte 2

Issey Miyake Pour Homme

Cartier So Pretty

Clinique Aromatics

Perfumer's Workshop Tea Rose

Estée Lauder Knowing

L'Artisan Parfumeur La Haïe Fleurie du Hameau

JO:

Guerlain Mitsouko

Chanel Cristalle

YSL Champagne

L'Eau par Kenzo

Lancôme Poême

Shiseido Ambre Sultan (only available from the Shiseido boutique in the Palais Royal, Paris)

An old bottle of Shocking, by Schiaparelli

Cartier So Pretty

Christian Dior Eau Sauvage

Lanvin Arpège

Nina Ricci Deçi-Dela

Chanel No. 19

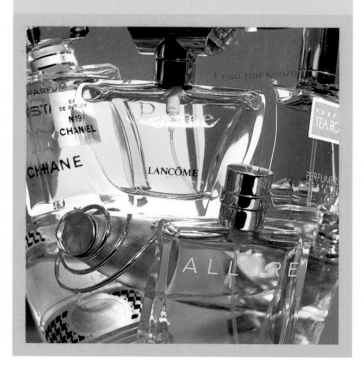

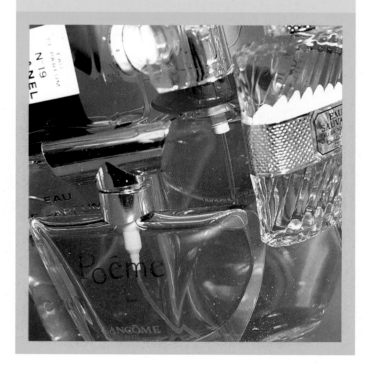

Perfume After-Care

Knowing how to look after your perfume will protect your investment. Air, heat and light are a fragrance's worst enemies. Here's how to exercise some scent sense.

✳ The lifespan of an unopened bottle of fragrance depends on its blend, but usually you can keep it safely for up to three years, as long as it's away from heat and light. Bathrooms aren't the ideal place to store fragrance, because of the temperature fluctuations.

✳ Limit your perfume's exposure to air as much as possible. Once you open the bottle, it will begin to deteriorate – like wine, but not so fast. Experts recommend sticking to one or two scents and using them up quickly; if you like to have a wider choice, always buy the smallest size.

✳ If you do buy larger bottles of fragrance, which are more cost-effective, fill an atomiser with a very small amount of scent at a time, and keep the big bottle in the fridge.

✳ Alternatively, keep the bottle in its box, which limits its exposure to light.

✳ All fragrances have about a year to 18 months of shelf life. If they smell vinegary, go darker or orangey in appearance, or become sticky in texture, they are past their best.

Unisex Scents

Traditionally, men's scents contain masculine notes such as cedar, clary sage, tarragon, vetiver, leather, tobacco and oak moss, in contrast to more flowery notes in women's scents: ylang-ylang, tuberose, jasmine, iris and lily of the valley. But the line between 'his' and 'hers' scents is blurring, as unisex scents become bestsellers (e.g. Calvin Klein cKOne). So if you'd like to share a scent, here are some to try:

Christian Dior Eau Sauvage	Calvin Klein cKOne
Eau de Givenchy	4711
Paco Rabanne Dalimix Paco	Guerlain Jicky
Rochas Eau de Rochas	Eau de Caron
Bulgari Eau Parfumée	Opium Pour Homme Eau de Parfum

The Ten Wonders of the Perfume World

The volume of new and old scents is overwhelming. So how do you discover the truly great scents among the also-rans?

We asked Dr Luca Turin, author of *Parfums Le Guide* (published by Hermès and available in French only), probably the only unbiased guide to scents, to nominate his favourite all-time classics. Some of them are easy to find, others need a little detective work – for some you may need to make a pilgrimage to Paris, still the world's perfume capital. (See DIRECTORY.)

Caron *Royal Bain de Champagne* – 'rarest of all, a laughing perfume'

Caron *Tabac Blond* – 'perfumed darkness'

Chanel *Bois des Iles* – 'mulled ambrosia'

Chanel *Cuir de Russie* – 'devil-may-care luxury'

Guerlain *Après l'Ondée* – 'just miraculous'

Guerlain *Jicky* – 'for large cats of both sexes'

Guerlain *Mitsouko* – 'dramatic, mysterious'

Thierry Mugler *Angel* – 'futuristic, sensual'

Patricia de Nicolaï *New York* – 'the purest form of bottle intellect'

Shiseido *Feminité du Bois* – 'austere but brilliant temptation'

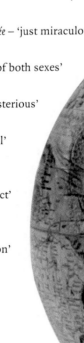

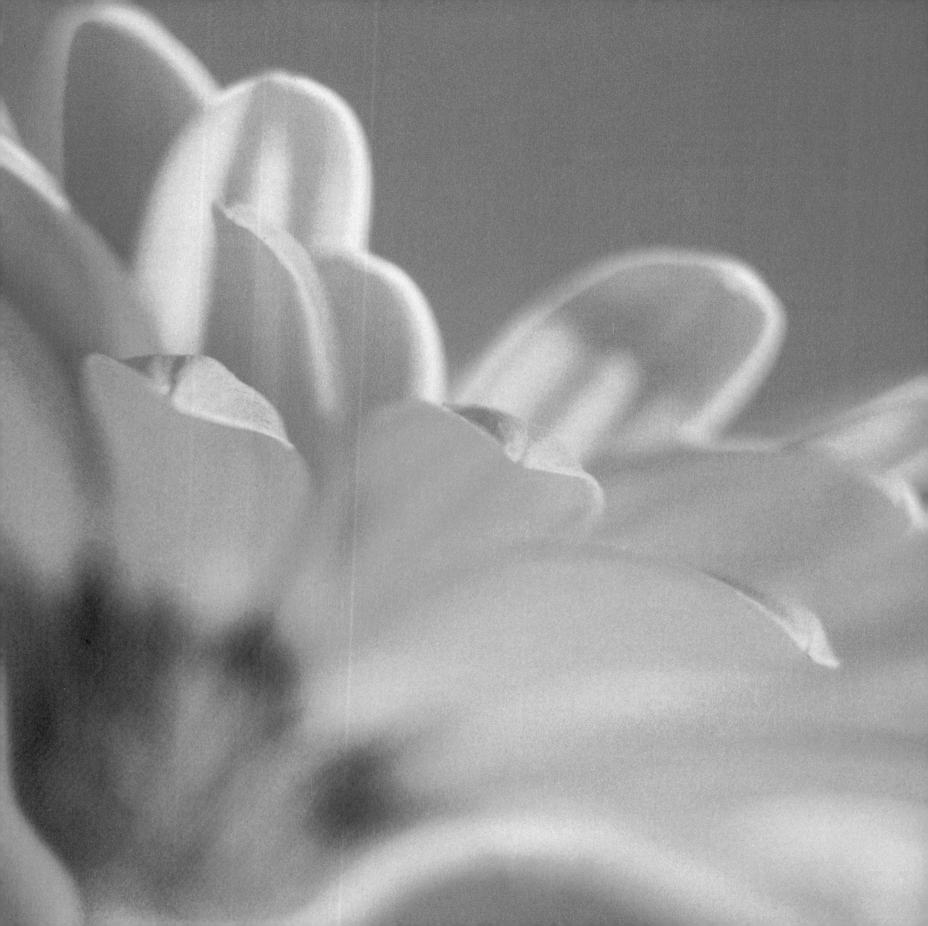

8 Directory

EXPERTS' GUIDES

LONDON GUIDE

The capital of the UK is one of the great beauty and health meccas of the world. Here are our insider secrets – the places we depend on and really like to visit. We hope you will, too.

Beauty Shopping

Dickins & Jones
224 Regent Street,
London W1A 1DB
Tel: 0171 734 7070
Light, bright and spacious, this redesigned Beauty Hall is the only one to have the feel of a New York department store. It offers an exclusive service: a personal shopper who will steer you towards the best skincare and make-up choices for you.

Crabtree & Evelyn
6 Kensington Church Street,
London W8 2PD
Tel: 0171 937 9335
and 134 King's Road,
London SW3 4XB
Tel: 0171 589 6263
A wonderful source of scented presents with very pretty packaging. As well as their range of nostalgic fragrances, they are now introducing effective skincare, footcare and bodycare.

Harrods
87–135 Brompton Road,
London SW1X 7XL
Tel: 0171 730 1234
Harrods' Beauty Hall and Fragrance Hall are an Aladdin's Cave of beauty, skincare, make-up and perfume treasures – flatteringly uplit, acres of marble and an unrivalled air of luxury. Visit the elegant Fifth Floor Hair & Beauty Salon for anything from a Jessica manicure to a full, top-to-toe makeover. They also offer a bridal service.

Liberty
210–220 Regent Street,
London W1R 6AH
Tel: 0171 734 1234
The last privately owned department store in London, Liberty has a real feeling of intimacy, with a small beauty hall which manages to squeeze in a cornucopia of unusual brands, as well as the more traditional names. Great for fragrance.

Lush
7 The Market,
Covent Garden,
London WC2E 8RA
Tel: 0171 379 5423
and 123 King's Road,
London SW3 4PL
Tel: 0171 376 8348
Truly wacky, with soap-by-the-yard if you feel like it! Inexpensive, fun and innovative. You can also buy fresh cosmetics; they are hand-made with natural ingredients so need to be kept in a fridge.

M.A.C. Cosmetics
109 King's Road,
London SW3 4PA
Tel: 0171 349 0601
This Canadian company, recently taken over by Estée Lauder, offers the ultimate in value-for-money fashion cosmetics – which is why its counter is sometimes three-deep in beauty hunters. Saturday tends to be a zoo, so if you can go another time, do.

Neal's Yard Natural Remedies
15 Neal's Yard,
London WC2H 9DP
Tel: 0171 379 7222
and 9 Elgin Crescent,
London W11 2JA
Tel: 0171 727 3998
Started by Romy Fraser when almost nobody outside France had heard of aromatherapy, Neal's Yard has grown like topsy. We love the translucent blue bottles and the delicious products inside them, including Seaweed & Arnica Foaming Bath (for our tired backs). A bonus is the fact that you can buy base creams and add your own blend of essential oils. Make a point of exploring Neal's Yard itself, with its therapy rooms, food shops and herbal dispensary.

Harvey Nichols
109–125 Knightsbridge,
London SW1X 7RJ
Tel: 0171 235 5000
Recently redesigned, the ground floor beauty hall now boasts three private rooms where you can experience a variety of treatments using the ranges on sale. A unique feature is FRED, a fragrance computer which helps you pinpoint the scents you might like.

Space NK Apothecary
Thomas Neal Centre,
41 Earlham Street,
London WC2H 9LD
Tel: 0171 379 7030
If you want the latest international beauty lines, head for Space NK. Proprietor Nicola Kinnaird (NK) sniffs out and secures ranges before anybody else knows they even exist, including LORAC, Stila, François Nars and Poppy lipsticks. A store which virtually has its own fan club.

L'Artisan Parfumeur
17 Cale Street,
London SW3 3QR
Tel: 0171 352 4196
This sells perfumer Jean Laporte's own fragrance creations, many of them flower-based. (The Tuberose is a favourite with women who can't buy Fracas any more.) Also matching scented candles, clever presents and a range of costume jewellery.

Les Senteurs
227 Ebury Street,
London SW1W 8UT
Tel: 0171 730 2322
Fragrance-aholics the world over should add this Pimlico boutique to their global shopping list. Carries a truly unique collection of lesser known perfumes, candles, soaps and other scented products from around the globe.

Santa Maria Novella Pharmacy
117 Walton Street,
London SW3 2BP
Tel: 0171 460 6600
If you can't get to its Renaissance home in Florence, visit this shoebox-sized London outpost of the famous pharmacy in chic Walton Street. We can unreservedly recommend Crema Pedestre for pavement-weary feet.

Screen Face
24 Powis Terrace,
London W11 1JH
Tel: 0171 221 8289
This was a favourite with international make-up artists, models and film stars long before the recent invasion of M.A.C. and Bobbi Brown. It's open to non-pros, too: piled floor-to-ceiling with exclusive ranges you won't find elsewhere, hundreds of shades of all types of make-up, plus sponge bags, brushes and other tools of the trade.

Selfridges
400 Oxford Street,
London W1A 1AB
Tel: 0171 629 1234
The beauty hall in this famous Oxford Street landmark is at last being given a makeover. It's particularly good for fragrances, bath goodies and special 'gift-with-purchase' promotions.

Yves Rocher
7 Gees Court London,
St Christopher's Place,
London W1M 5HQ
Tel: 0171 409 2975
A tiny shop stuffed to bursting with bargain priced, botanically based cosmetics from this French company.

When we feel traditional, we head for this clutch of boutiques offering an old-fashioned selection of delicious scents and exciting bits and bobs:

Czech & Speake
39 Jermyn Street,
London SW1Y 6DN
Tel: 0171 439 0216

Crown Perfumery
35 Park Street,
London W1Y 3HG
Tel: 0171 493 1717

Floris
89 Jermyn Street,
London SW1Y 6JH
Tel: 0171 930 2885

Penhaligon's
41 Wellington Street,
London WC2E 7BN
Tel: 0171 836 2150

Natural Health

Ainsworths
36 New Cavendish Street,
London W1M 7LH
Tel: 0171 935 5330
If you need a homoeopathic remedy for anything from hay fever to travel sickness, this friendly pharmacy can meet every need.

All Hallows House Centre for Natural Health
St Dunstan's Church,
Idol Lane,
London EC3R 5DD
Tel: 0171 283 8908
This Christopher Wren church, now a dedicated natural health centre, has proved a life-line for stressed-out/weary businesspeople. Many City companies now have contracts with the centre for use by their employees. Patients, some of whom come especially from abroad, say the place itself is healing – as are the practitioners.

Aromatherapy Associates
68 Maltings Place,
Bagleys Lane,
London SW6 2BY
Tel: 0171 731 8129
A bit out of the way but worth the trip. **The Prince** and **Diana, Princess of Wales'** favourite aromatherapists practise here, and it deserves every word of its reputation. Life-enhancing treatments and marvellous oils to take home.

Hale Clinic
7 Park Crescent,
London W1N 3HE
Tel: 0171 631 0156
In this beautiful, cream-painted Georgian house opposite Regent's Park, you will find the largest choice of alternative and complementary therapies in the UK. It is owned and run by Theresa Hale, a former yoga teacher who will advise on the most appropriate therapy for you. The basement houses the Nutri-Centre, one of our favourite sources for supplements, health foods and health books, with an extremely swift global mail order service.

Life Centre
15 Edge Street,
London W8 7PN
Tel: 0171 221 4602
Brainchild of Louise White, this former chapel offers the best schedule of non-stop, seven-day-a-week yoga classes for all levels of experience, plus a handpicked team of natural health practitioners (from aromatherapy to Shiatsu), operating out of some of the most beautiful treatment rooms you can expect to find anywhere.

Nelsons
73 Duke Street,
London W1M 6BY
Tel: 0171 629 3118
This old-fashioned homoeopathic pharmacy with stained-glass panels first opened in 1860. It makes its own range of homoeopathic remedies and carries a full range of Bach Flower remedies.

The Back Shop
24 New Cavendish Street,
London W1M 7LH
Tel: 0171 935 9120
If you, like us, suffer from back problems, you'll want to know about this store dedicated to back care, stocking everything from chairs to shoes via travel pillows.

The Sanctuary
12 Floral Street,
London WC2E 9DH
Tel: 0171 240 9635
For women only, this pioneering retreat with its own swimming pool now offers a selection of natural therapies plus facials, make-up lessons and beauty treatments. It puts together special day packages for top-to-toe pampering.

Wild Oats
210 Westbourne Grove,
London W11 2RH
Tel: 0171 229 1063
This is a pioneering health food supermarket offering a terrific choice of vitamins and natural beauty products plus a complete range of organic foods. A haven for those on special diets (no sugar, gluten-free etc.). Fashion designer **Rifat Ozbek** moved to Notting Hill especially to be within walking distance.

London Day Spas

Elizabeth Arden Red Door
29 Davies Street,
London W1Y 1FN
Tel: 0171 629 4488
In New York, Elizabeth Arden's Red Door spa is the legendary one-stop beauty pit-stop for the best-groomed women in town. Now London has its own Elizabeth Arden Red Door hair and beauty spa, in a Mayfair townhouse, offering escapist pampering, stress-busting treatments, first-class facials, cut and colour (from Pierre-Charles, who's ex-Harrods), plus professional make-up for special occasions.

The Dorchester Spa
The Dorchester,
Park Lane,
London W1A 2HJ
Tel: 0171 495 7335
In the basement of this legendary hotel you will now find a world-class day spa. This pampering paradise constantly attracts visiting movie stars, from **Nicole Kidman** and **Cher** to **Barbra Streisand** and **Anne Archer**, who particularly like the 'panthermal bath', which sweats out post-travel toxins.

Screen Face
48 Monmouth Street,
London WC2
Tel: 0171 836 3955
This new branch carries all of the Screen Face must-haves – conveniently located on the borders of Covent Garden and Soho.

The Urban Retreat and Aveda Concept Salon
4th Floor, Harvey Nichols,
109–125 Knightsbridge,
London SW1
Tel: 0171 201 8610
The New Age has dawned in Knighsbridge: at this Aveda spa, you can leave shopping madness behind to enjoy their unique aromatherapeutic beauty treatments and stress-busting haircare – or sit on a vibrating pedicure 'throne' to unkink your muscles while your toes are painted. The deliciously healthy food is by Joy, London's top organic caterer.

TOP TEN UK HOTELS WITH SPAS

These days, many women's idea of a perfect getaway means good, light food and a menu of sybaritic beauty treatments. Hotels are responding to demand by rapidly developing their spa facilities available. We asked Susan Harmsworth, spa consultant and creator of the E'SPA range (which we're big fans of), to nominate her top ten UK hotels with spas. Here they are, in the order that she rates them:

❶ **Turnberry Hotel**, Golf Courses and Spa
Turnberry,
Ayrshire,
Scotland KA26 9LT
Tel: 01655 331000

❷ **Lucknam Park Hotel**
Colerne,
Wiltshire SN14 8AZ
Tel: 01225 742777

❸ **Chewton Glen Hotel**, Health & Country Club
New Milton,
Hampshire BH25 6QS
Tel: 01425 275341

❹ **St Andrew's Old Course Hotel**
St Andrew's,
Fife,
Scotland KY16 9SP
Tel: 01334 474371

❺ **Sprowston Manor Hotel**
Sprowston Road,
Norwich,
Norfolk NR7 8RP
Tel: 01603 410871

❻ **Gleneagles Hotel**
Auchterarder,
Perthshire,
Scotland PH3 1NF
Tel: 01765 662231

❼ **The Bath Spa Hotel**
Sydney Road,
Bath,
Avon BA2 6JF
Tel: 01225 444424

❽ **St Pierre Country Club Resort**
Chepstow,
Gwent NP6 6YA
Tel: 01291 625261

❾ **Sopwell House Hotel**
Cottonmill Lane,
St. Alban's,
Hertfordshire LA1 2HQ
Tel: 01727 864477

❿ **The Runnymede Hotel**
Windsor Road,
Egham,
Surrey TW20 0AG
Tel: 01784 436171

Questions to Ask When Booking

The pace at some spas is very laid back and languid, while others offer a dawn till dusk schedule of get-fit-quick activities. Because spa visits are never exactly cheap, it's important that you find one that matches your pace and goals, in order not to waste your time – and money. To ensure you know exactly what to expect before you book a spa break, Susan Harmsworth has put together a list of questions that you should ask if you've never visited the spa before. These should help you make the right choice for you.

1) What exactly is included in the package – e.g. initial consultation, treatments, exercise classes, meals, use of all facilities? If certain elements aren't included, what are the individual costs?

2) Should you book treatments before you arrive or are timings very flexible? If you are advised to pre-book, but are not sure what you want, then block out time with a therapist and decide on actual treatments when you arrive.

3) Are treatments available seven days a week and in the evenings?

4) What facilities do they have – e.g. sauna, steam room, separate facilities for men and women? Do they have exercise classes and a full gym with plenty of cardiovascular equipment?

5) Do they carry out a fitness assessment?

6) Do they offer specific programmes – e.g. for de-toxifying, stress management, weight loss, etc. – or can they put one together for the individual?

7) Can they cope with special dietary needs? Do they offer healthy eating menus? What kind of food – hot or cold – is available at meal times, and is there a choice?

8) Are children allowed in the spa?
9) Is there any special clothing you should bring – e.g. do they supply robe and slippers? Is it casual dress, or do people dress for dinner?

10) Do they allow smoking, and if so, where? (This is relevant both to smokers and non-smokers.)

In addition, ask for a complete information pack before you go and speak directly with the spa regarding treatments and booking, not just the hotel reception. Look carefully at the type and length of treatments, and be aware that all-inclusive treatments can sometimes be of a lesser quality or take a shorter time – so don't necessarily compare all-inclusive treatments with those on the treatment list.

TEN LEADING UK SPAS

Alas, Britain still lags behind in the spa stakes. In the UK, for the most part, the level of luxury and cuisine doesn't measure up to what you'll find in the USA, where the creation of luxurious getaway spas has almost become an art form. UK spas are learning fast, though, and you can find some British retreats which are truly relaxing and pampering. To ensure you choose the right spa for you, do make a point of asking all the questions suggested by spa expert Susan Harmsworth (left).

Cedar Falls Health Farm
Bishops Lydeard,
Taunton,
Somerset
Tel: 01823 433233
This is a small health farm with a relaxed and cosy atmosphere, and log fires in winter. It is set in 40 acres of mature gardens, woodland and fishing lakes alongside the Cedar Falls Golf Course. Alternative treatments are taken very seriously; the Natural Therapy Clinic offers aromatherapy, hypnotherapy, reflexology, kinesiology, iridology, Reiki healing, lymph drainage massage and sports injury treatment. There are more than 50 beauty treatments on offer (Clarins, René Guinot, Thalgo and Ionothermie). The emphasis is on anti-stress and total relaxation.

Champneys Health Resort
Wigginton,
Tring,
Hertfordshire HP23 6HY
Tel: 01442 863351
Champneys is Britain's original, world-famous health farm, renowned for its combination of luxury and professional expertise. It offers everything you could want health-wise and beauty-wise, with a very extensive range of activities and exercise classes, from juggling lessons to yoga via light therapy and Shiatsu, and offers more than 80 beauty treatments (Christian Dior, René Guinot, Decleor). Champneys is set in 170 acres of parkland; perfect for bracing walks. The resort is something of a 'status symbol' venue (leave those tattered sweatpants at home), but popular with couples because of its five-star hotel atmosphere. Offers excellent spa cuisine and top-class, luxurious service – but at prices to match.

Forest Mere
Forest Mere,
Liphook,
Hampshire GU30 7JQ
Tel: 01428 722051
Forest Mere's slightly outdated facilities are currently undergoing major modernisation which should create a state-of-the-art spa. Quiet and relaxed, this lakeside spa is deep in the heart of the Hampshire countryside and the recently introduced hiking programme makes it popular with walkers; it's not ideal for action-seekers but makes the perfect tranquil getaway. There are five types of bedroom (to suit most pockets) and a smart but friendly dining room. It offers a wide range of exercise classes, alternative therapies, relaxation and stress management classes, plus treatments by René Guinot and Clarins. The gym is open from 10–15 hours a day. As only about ten per cent of guests are couples, it is ideal for a solo spa trip.

Grayshott Hall Health & Fitness Retreat
Headley Road
Grayshott,
Nr Hindhead,
Surrey GU26 6JJ
Tel: 01428 604331
Grayshott is affordably luxurious, based in the former country house of Alfred Lord Tennyson, and has 47 acres of gardens. (Ask for a room in the main house rather than the extension.) It provides delicious and plentiful food (no need to starve here), and meals can be served in your room. There is an extensive selection of exercise classes and a well-equipped gym. Therapies and activities on offer include Qi-gong, T'ai Chi, relaxation counselling and assertiveness training;

there are indoor tennis courts and a nine-hole golf course. On the list of 70 treatments you'll find names like René Guinot, Clarins and Sisley. The ratio is 50/50 men and women guests and nobody would feel out of place here on their own. A four-night minimum stay is recommended, to maximise the benefits of the retreat.

Henlow Grange Health Farm
Henlow,
Bedfordshire SG16 6DB
Tel: 01462 811111
Set in a Georgian mansion, Henlow is perfect for spa goers looking for a packed schedule and a wide range of treatments, since there are more than 120 masseurs and therapists working here, offering Clarins, René Guinot, Decleor, Thalgo. In addition to a huge ozone-treated pool, there is a gym with 30 fitness stations; it is open 24 hours a day for the super keen. Henlow Grange is suitable for all levels of fitness, offering everything from aerobics to relaxing yoga. With a down-to-earth, relaxed but bustling atmosphere, it's considered extremely good value for money, but as a result don't expect too many extra frills.

Inglewood Health Hydro
Kintbury,
Berkshire RG17 9SW
Tel: 01488 682022
Set in beautiful countryside, just an hour from London, Inglewood is comfortable rather than deluxe, but offers affordable health and beauty packages with absolutely no pressure to power dress. It is good for alternative therapies including shiatsu massage and yoga, and has more than 40 beauty treatments, many of them more unusual than you tend to find elsewhere – e.g. peat facials, seaweed wraps, etc. Supervised walks and stress management lectures are available, but there is generally a very relaxed atmosphere. A plus is that the nearby Norland Nursery will take in guests' children.

Ragdale Hall Health Hydro
Nr Melton Mowbray,
Leicestershire LE14 3PB
Ragdale Hall offers tailor-made programmes to help each visitor meet his/her goals, whether that's to unwind, be pampered or boost fitness; the gym and pool are open around-the-clock. (There are both indoor and outdoor pools.) Renowned for its menu of beauty treatments, there are more than 70 on offer, including Clarins, Decleor, René Guinot, Kanebo and Ionithermie. A comfortable Victorian pile, Ragdale provides a friendly, professional service. If you want to 'stop the world and get off' for a few days, you could have stress counselling or spend time in the floatation tank.

Shrubland Hall Health Clinic
Coddenham,
Ipswich,
Suffolk IP6 9QH
Tel: 01473 830404
Shrubland Hall is a truly beautiful Palladian building set in 4,500 acres, with a stunning Italian garden and extensive woodlands to explore. (Ask for a room in the main house.) It has an old-fashioned feel – more like health farms of old – and attracts a devoted clientele who return year after year for first-class holistic therapies and a healthy, raw food diet; dietary requirements are taken very seriously. Shrublands is generally quite strict – it is a health clinic, not a sybaritic spa – but there are plenty of beauty treats to make you feel pampered (RoC, Clarins, E'SPA). Don't expect rigorous, energetic exercise: the emphasis is on body conditioning (Pilates, yoga). If you like the quiet life, this is a wonderful place to switch off.

Springs Hydro
Packington,
Nr. Ashby-de-la-Zouch,
Leicestershire LE65 1TG
Tel: 01530 273873
Britain's only purpose-built health resort and pool complex – perfect for mermaids because it features an indoor heated pool, sauna and steam rooms, whirlpool, plunge and splash pools, plus a floatation tank. Popular with mothers and daughters visiting together, and with professional sportsmen, because of the standard of fitness facilities, including aquarobics, aerobics, dance, yoga and relaxation. There are around 100 treatment options, by Clarins, Thalgo, Decleor and René Guinot. The atmosphere is more like a health club than a country house hotel, but Springs offers excellent value for money.

Stobo Castle Health Spa
Peeblesshire,
Scotland EH45 8NY
Tel: 01721 760249
An hour's drive south of Edinburgh, Stobo Castle's brooding Gothic appearance hides a warm, cosy welcome with a country house feel (complete with log fires – sometimes a necessity). A great antidote to the stresses of modern life, Stobo is much more a place to unwind – with daily relaxation classes, for instance – than a get-fit destination. The pool is compact and the gym tiny, but there are acres of countryside to walk briskly across. Alongside the usual treatments – from Thalgo, Ionithermie and Stobo's signature range – you'll find non-surgical facelifts and aromatherapy. Meals focus on the best of local Scottish produce, and meals can be taken in your room – which are well furnished and comfortable.

LEADING SPAS IN THE REST OF THE WORLD

The steamy hot, mineral-rich waters of natural spas have attracted seekers of holistic health from the Romans onwards. Today, spa centres, many with marvellous beauty facilities, are bubbling up all over the world, even in such apparently unlikely spots as Japan and Thailand. We asked Dr Susan Horsewood-Lee, a London-based private doctor who runs the Spa Consultancy and has travelled widely inspecting spas, to recommend her favourite mid-market options in mainland Europe and the Far East.

Austria
Grand Hotel Sauerhof (with Marbert Beauty Farm)
Weilburgstrasse 11-13,
2500 Baden,
Nr Vienna
Tel: (+43) 2252 41 2510
Fax: (+43) 2252 48 047
This spa, with sulphur baths near the Viennese Woods, used to focus solely on rehabilitation treatments and arthritis but has now launched into a wide range of beauty treatments – including ones targeted at slimming and cellulite – and complementary therapies. The stylish, traditional hotel and beautiful countryside make it a perfect summer retreat with sports facilities which include golf and tennis.

France
Hélianthal
Place Maurice Ravel,
64500 St Jean de Luz
Tel: (+33) 59 51 51 51
Fax: (+33) 59 51 51 54
This spa is utterly French, based in a modern hotel in a very beautiful old port town. The food is wonderful, with a dietetic menu arranged by the resident nutritionist. The heavenly pool is behind sliding glass doors at sea level so that, in cooler weather, you can at least still see and hear the sea. The spa is notable for its thalassotherapy – marine and seaweed treatments and mud baths. These are beneficial for many conditions including bad backs (there is a dedicated back clinic), heavy legs (due to poor circulation or lymphoedema) and for slimming. An inspiring place to learn how to look after the rest of your life.

Hungary
Danubius Thermal Hotel
Heviz
Tel: (+36) 83 41 180
Fax: (+36) 83 40 666
Heviz Spa is set in particularly beautiful countryside overlooking the steaming waters of Lake Balaton, a naturally warm lake (32°C in summer) with lily ponds. Hungary has a tradition of using its beneficial mud to relax, rejuvenate and treat aches and pains. This peaceful area used to be the home of state-run sanatoria for rheumatism and now has high-quality, up-to-date hotels with lots of outdoor living on offer, including water sports and sailing.

Indonesia
Javana Spa
Cangkuang,
Sukabumi,
West Java
For info, contact PT Sarana Prima Budaya Raga,
Danitama Plaza Building 1st Floor,
Jln. Sultan Hasanuddin No. 47–48,
Kebayoran Baru,
Jakarta 12120
Tel: (+62) 21 739 0416/ 739 0452/ 739 4943
Fax: (+62) 21 739 7847
This is a retreat for both body and mind. Individual spa programmes combine the best of Western and Eastern philosophies aimed at attaining internal and external balance. The atmosphere is peaceful and meditative and every guest is given a local companion to guide them through each day. The spa is notable for its wonderfully pure, de-toxifying food, hikes to the local waterfalls, mud treatments, and aromatic and traditional massage.

Italy
Grotta Giusti Spa
Via Grotta Giusti,
171-51015 Monsummano Terme,
Tuscany
Tel: (+39) 572 51008
Fax: (+39) 572 51007
This spa consists of a brand new treatment centre based in beautifully revamped caves which is attached to a traditional hotel and spa. This region of Tuscany is famous for its natural hot springs with volcanic mud. The wonderfully pure water emerges at 34°C, so it's marvellous for all sorts of rheumatic disorders and sports injuries. There is a huge repertoire of mud treatments (quite odourless) and a very good beauty section. The anti-cellulite treatment is excellent. Guided therapeutic walks include sessions on especially designed aerobic equipment set in the woods. There are also many sports facilities in the area.

Japan
Ryokan-Kannawa-en (ryokan means hotel)
Kannawa,
Beppu,
Kyushu
Tel: (+977) 66 2111
Fax: (+977) 66 2113
Beppu is a large town with eight separate natural springs, each with different qualities. There is a range of hotels, both traditional – such as Ryokan-Kannawa-en – and modern, plus 75 public bath houses. A fairly rigorous regime is on offer, involving steam baths, hot and cold dips, massage, sand baths – where women dig you into hot sand – and mud baths. The food is wonderful and, for a Westerner, a stay in this fascinating region can end up being as much about sightseeing as health.

Switzerland
Hotel Maison Blanche
39655 Leukerbad
Tel: (+41) 27 62 11 61
Fax: (+41) 27 61 34 74
Leukerbad is a magical small mountain retreat perched 5,000 ft (1,524m) up in the Swiss Alps where three million gallons of steaming water gush daily from the rocks. Of the several hotels and medical treatment centres (noted for sports injuries and all rheumatic problems), the Maison Blanche, although not the most expensive, is the most charming. It has its own thermal pools; the trick in the mornings is to fall out of bed into a swimsuit and straight into a natural jacuzzi outdoors where, warm as toast, you can gaze up at the snow-tipped peaks. Amongst the memorable treatments available are the Romische/Irische (Roman/Irish) baths – a two-hour thermal extravaganza of vapour and water baths with a brush/soap massage and relaxation – and the wonderful Institut Isabella which provides a range of beauty treatments. A place with well-being in the air.

Thailand
Chiva-Som
73/4 Petchkasem Road,
Hua Hin,
Prachuab Khiri Khan 77110
Tel: (+66) 32 536 536
Fax: (+66) 32 511 154
A small oasis of peace and serenity by a lake in a rapidly developing area. The Thai staff are incredibly helpful and immediately you set foot there, stresses and strains float away. The facilities are very good, with separate male and female rooms: the spa's Thai massage has to be the best thing ever. The excellent food (plenty of fresh fruit and vegetables cooked European-style with a Thai

slant) is not presented as a weight loss regime, although little notes of calorie content make you aware of what you're eating. Rooms are beautiful, with suites in separate little bungalows, some overlooking the lake.

Turkey

Kervansaray Thermal Hotel
Çekirge Street,
Çekirge-Bursa
Tel: (+90) 224 233 9300
Fax: (+90) 224 233 9324
Bursa, a beautiful and traditional town with a marvellous covered bazaar, has several hot springs but the best facilities are to be found at the Kervansaray Hotel, which has access to traditional baths and offers five-star accommodation at three-star prices. The naturally hot water has a very high mineral content so it's very good for rheumatism and post-operative recovery, but the notable treatment is the Turkish bath massage. Traditional masseuses, who (like all the staff) are charming, surround the baths and, using local mud, pummel stiff bodies into submission. The food is good but since thinness is not the Turkish style, it is not aimed at weight loss.

TIPS FOR TRIPS: HOW TO LOOK GOOD ON THE GO

Whenever you travel, you pay a beauty toll. Flying, in particular, can be terrible for your appearance, because cabin air is so intensely dry. But we have some sky-high solutions to going places and looking great. What's more, if you follow a few simple tips, you can reach new heights of in-flight relaxation.

Before the Flight

★ Pre-order a diet or vegetarian meal, so you don't have to eat the usual high-fat, high-calorie airline meal.

★ Buy before you fly: Aromatherapeutics and Danièle Ryman both offer kits containing aromatherapy oils specially designed to help you recover from air travel and adjust to new time zones. (See DIRECTORY.)

★ Choose sensible clothes: wear layers of comfortable, natural fabrics and wrinkle-free knits. You can dress them up with a smart blazer and flat shoes. Take your own pair of cotton-rich 'slouch socks' for long-haul flights (which are invariably much more pleasant to wear than the synthetic versions the airline will give you).

★ Try to book an aisle seat, which will allow you to move around more easily without disturbing seat-mates. Also ask which seats offer extra leg room.

★ When you're booking your hotel, find out whether they offer massage, either in your room or in a hotel spa. Massage, particularly using aromatherapy oils, can really help tackle jet lag: it can be uplifting if you need to be awake, relaxing when it's nighttime but your body clock still says it's daytime.

During the Flight

★ Drink loads of water before and during the flight; cabin air is drier than the Sahara, at just six per cent humidity. Avoid alcohol or coffee, which will make you feel even more dehydrated.

★ Remove your make-up when you get on board (or don't put it on in the first place) and slather on plenty of moisturiser instead. (Prescriptives Flight Cream is justifiably legendary.) Put mascara on eyes and apply make-up just before landing.

★ Walk up and down the aisles of the plane as often as you can. When you're standing (for instance, waiting in a queue for the loo), stretch your legs by slowly bending back one knee at a time. Reach back and catch hold of your foot, pulling it towards your body. Hold for a slow count of five, then repeat with the other foot. Also good for legs: Decleor Circulagel, a menthol-scented gel which boosts sluggish circulation.

★ Pressurised cabins can make eyes puff up, so take a gel-formulation treat for tired and puffy eyes (see *Tried & Tested Treats*, page 59). Alternatively, take along chamomile tea bags; ask for hot water, let them steep and cool, then wring them out and place them on your eyes.

★ Planes are filled with 'ambient electricity', which makes for flyaway hair. Smooth hair down with a tiny dab of our favourite hair-sleeker, Kiehl's Silk Groom (see DIRECTORY), which banishes static and restores shine. If you have long hair, pack a 'scrunchie', which can make hair look neat and groomed after a long flight.

★ If you feel scared or nauseous at any time, try Shiatsu: place one hand on your knee, palm up. Rest the fingers of the other hand face down on your palm, placing the thumb just below your wrist. (No need to press hard.) These points are linked with anxiety and travel sickness.

★ Our trick for sleeping well on a long-haul flight, which Ford Models founder **Eileen Ford** also swears by, is to cram a pillow into your hand luggage. It makes any seat instantly comfortable and allows you a much better night's sleep than an airline pillow. And, according to Eileen Ford, 'If you sleep well, you look well.' Alternatively, try an inflatable neck pillow, widely available through mail order catalogues and department stores.

When You Arrive

★ Light therapy is fantastically effective for helping conquer jet lag. We have heard excellent reports of the Hale Clinic's approach (see DIRECTORY), which combines light therapy – exposing the traveller to full-spectrum lighting (equivalent to the light on a spring day) with reflexology. If you can't find a therapist or health centre offering a similar approach simply get out in the daylight and have a walk, which will help to reset your body clock. (If it's dark when you arrive, try to make a point of getting plenty of light the next day.)

★ Designer **Donna Karan** travels with her own food, packing bags of carrots, wholewheat pretzels and fresh fruit – which sure beats airline stodge. She also takes along slices of lemon, which she drops into hot water. 'And I take a gramme of vitamin C every hour, to stop water retention.'

★ Spritz water on your face to keep it moisturised: models swear by Evian or Vichy sprays. **Helena Christensen**'s favourite is Remo Facial Mist, which she picks up from Sydney's most fashionable store of the same name.

★ **Calvin Klein** is so keen on Prescriptives Flight Cream that he once bought up the entire stock of this in-flight skin rehydrator from a New York department store.

★ Make-up artist **Mary Greenwell** has mastered the art of looking glamorous when she flies. 'If you're wearing cashmere – the best texture to travel in – you'll always look glamorous. I don't go anywhere without my cashmere socks and sweater.'

DIRECTORY

USEFUL ADDRESSES

All products mentioned in this book are available to overseas readers via The Overseas Posting Company, a one-stop shopping service for overseas customers. Contact them at:

The Overseas Posting Company
74 Denmark Road,
London SW19 4PQ
Tel/fax: +44 (0) 181 944 7719
(24 hours)

ALTERNATIVE AND COMPLEMENTARY THERAPIES

Acupuncture
Governing body:
British Acupuncture Council
Park House,
206–208 Latimer Road,
London W10 6RE
Tel: 0181 964 0222
List of local practitioners available free of charge. For a copy of the complete register send sae and cheque/postal order for £3.50.

Alexander Technique
Alexander Technique International (ATI)
142 Thorpdale Road,
London N4 3BS
Tel: 0171 281 7639
Send A5 sae for list of 200 teachers.

Alexander Teaching Network (ATN)
PO Box 53,
Kendal,
Cumbria LA9 4UP
Send sae for register of 80 teachers.

The Society of Teachers of the Alexander Technique (STAT)
20 London House,
266 Fulham Road,
London SW10 9EL
Tel: 0171 351 0828
Send sae for list of 550 teachers.

Allergies
British Society for Allergy and Environmental Medicine with **The British Society of Nutritional Medicine**
PO Box 28,
Totton,
Southampton SO40 2ZA

Allergy Care
Pollards Yard,
Wood Street,
Taunton,
Somerset TA1 1UP
Tel: 01823 325023
Suppliers of specialist foods, supplements and dietary aids. Also food allergy testing service.

The Allergy Shop Ltd
PO Box 196,
Haywards Heath,
West Sussex RH16 3YF
Tel: 01444 414290

Anthroposophical Medicine
Anthroposophical Medical Association
For list of 25 practitioners send sae to:
Anthroposophical Medical Movement,
c/o Park Attwood Clinic,
Trimpley,
Bewdley,
Worcestershire DY12 1RE

Applied Kinesiology
To find nearest practitioner, send sae and £1 in stamps to:
The Association for Systemic Kinesiology
39 Browns Road,
Surbiton,
Surrey KT5 8ST
Tel: 0181 399 3215

or, for list of their 200 practitioners, send sae to:
Kinesiology Federation
PO Box 7891,
Wimbledon,
London SW19 1ZB
Tel: 0181 545 0255

Aromatherapy
Umbrella Organisation with 4,500 practitioners:
Aromatherapy Organisations Council
For info and names of practitioners in your area send A5 sae to:
The Secretary,
3 Latymer Close,
Braybrooke,
Market Harborough,
Leicester LE16 8LN
Tel/fax: 01858 434242

or, for register of practitioners, send sae with cheque/postal order for £2 to:
International Society of Professional Aromatherapists
ISPA House,
82 Ashby Road,
Hinckley,
Leicestershire LE10 1SN
Tel: 01455 637987

or send sae plus £2 to:
International Federation of Aromatherapists
Stamford House,
2–4 Chiswick High Road,
London W4 1TH
Tel: 0181 742 2605

The Tisserand Institute
runs a 'Discovering Aromatherapy' course at:
65 Church Road,
Hove,
East Sussex BN3 2BD
Tel: 01273 206640

Leigh Richmond
The Life Centre, 15 Edge Street,
London W8
Tel: 0171 221 4602

For stockists of essential oils, send A5 sae to:
Aromatherapy Trade Council
PO Box 52,
Market Harborough,
Leicestershire LE16 8ZX
Tel: 01858 434 242

For details of nearest stockists of blended oils, and mail order:
Aromatherapy Associates Ltd
68 Maltings Place,
Bagleys Lane,
London SW6 2BY
Tel: 0171 371 9878

Autogenic Training
For groups outside Greater London, send sae to:
The British Association for Autogenic Training & Therapy
100 Harley Street,
London WJN 1AF

For groups in the London area, send sae to:
Autogenic Training Centre
100 Harley Street,
London W1N 1AF

Biodynamic Psychotherapy
Gerda Boyesen Centre
For info on their network of practitioners, write to:
Acacia House, Centre Avenue,
Acton Park,
London W3 7JX
Tel: 0181 743 2437

Bioenergetic Medicine
Institute of Bioenergetic Medicine
103 North Road,
Parkstone, Poole,
Dorset BH14 0LU
Tel: 01202 733762

Wimbledon Clinic of Natural Medicine
1 Evelyn Road
London SW19 8NU
Tel: 0181 543 5477

Biomagnetic Therapy
The British Biomagnetic Association
For info and local practitioners send sae to:
The Williams Clinic,
31 St Marychurch Road,
Torquay,
Devon TQ1 3JF
Tel: 01803 293346

Chinese Herbal Medicine
For register of 190 practitioners, send A5 envelope and cheque/postal order for £2 to:
Register of Chinese Herbal Medicine (RCHM)
PO Box 400,
Wembley,
Middx HAG 9NZ
Tel: 0181 904 1357

Chiropody & Podiatry
For details of nearest practitioner, send sae to:
Society of Chiropodists and Podiatrists
53 Welbeck Street,
London W1M 7HE
Tel: 0171 486 3381

Chiropractic
The British Chiropractic Association
Equity House, 29 Whitley Street,
Reading,
Berkshire RG2 0EG
For details of nearest practitioner:
Tel: 01734 757557

or send sae to:
British Association for Applied Chiropractic
The Old Post Office,
Cherry Street,
Stratton Audley, Nr Bicester,
Oxfordshire OX6 9BA
Tel: 01869 277111

For info and directory of practitioners, send £1.50 and a 50p stamp to:
McTimoney Chiropractic Association
21 High Street,
Eynsham,
Oxfordshire OX8 1HE

Colonic Irrigation
For nearest practitioner, send sae to:
Colonic International Association
16 Englands Lane,
London NW3 4TT
Tel/fax: 0171 483 1595

Colour Therapy
For list of practitioners, send sae to:
Hygeia College of Colour Therapy
Brook House,
Avening,
Tetbury,
Gloucestershire GL8 8NS
Tel: 01453 832150

Counselling
Send A4 sae to:
British Association for Counselling (BAC)
1 Regent Place,
Rugby CV21 2PJ
Tel: 01788 578328

Cranial Osteopathy
For register of members, send sae to:
The Secretary,
Cranial Osteopathic Association (CrOA)
478 Baker Street,
Enfield,
Middlesex EN1 3QS
Tel: 0181 367 5561

Craniosacral Therapy Association
For info/practitioners, send sae to:
27 Old Gloucester Street,
London WC1N 3XX

Crystal Therapy
For nearest practitioner, send A5 sae to:
Affiliation of Crystal Healing Organisations
46 Lower Green Road,
Esher,
Surrey KT10 8HD
Tel: 0181 398 7252

The School of Electro-Crystal Therapy
117 Long Drive,
South Ruislip,
Middlesex
Tel: 0181 841 1716 for courses in ECT and details of your nearest practitioner.

Feng Shu
For more info, telephone their International Network on:
0171 935 8935
or contact:
Community Health Foundation
The East West Centre,
188 Old Street,
London EC1V 9FR
Tel: 0171 251 4076

Floatation
For list of floatation centres, contact:
Float Tank Association
PO Box 11024,
London SW4 7ZF
Tel: 0171 627 4962

Flower Remedies
Dr Edward Bach Centre
Mount Vernon,
Sotwell, Wallingford,
Oxfordshire OX10 0PZ
Tel: 01491 834678
Send sae for list of practitioners.

For info and mail order of Bach Flower Remedies:
A. Nelson & Co Ltd
73 Duke Street,
London W1M 6BY
Tel: 0171 495 2404

The Flower and Gem Remedy Association
For leaflet and price list of their mail order, contact:
Suite 1, Castle Farm,
Clifton Road,
Deddington,
Oxfordshire OX15 0TP
Tel: 01869 337349

The Nutri-Centre at The Hale Clinic
7 Park Crescent,
London W1N 3HE
Tel: 0171 436 5122

Findhorn Flower Essences
Mail order catalogue from:
Phoenix Community Stores,
The Apothecary,
The Park,
Findhorn Bay, Forres,
Morayshire IV36 0TZ
Tel: 01309 691044
Fax: 01309 690933

Healing Herbs Flower Remedies
PO Box 65,
Hereford,
Herefordshire HR2 0UW
Tel: 01873 890218

Bailey Flower Essences
7–8 Nelson Road,
Ilkley,
West Yorkshire LS29 8HN
Tel: 01943 432012

Healing
College of Healing
for register of 250 practitioners write to:
Runnings Park,
Croft Bank, West Malvern,
Worcestershire WR14 4DU
Tel: 01684 566450

National Federation of Spiritual Healers
For details of nearest practitioner, tel: 0891 616080 between 9am – 5pm (calls charged at 49p per minute) or write to:
Old Manor Farm Studio,
Church Street,
Sunbury-on-Thames,
Middlesex TW16 6RG

Herbalists
Send sae to:
General Council and Register of Consultant Herbalists
Grosvenor House, 40 Sea Way,
Middleton-on-Sea,
West Sussex PO22 7BA

Homoeopathy
To find your nearest practitioner, send sae to:
Society of Homoeopaths
2 Artizan Road,
Northampton NN1 4HU
Tel: 01604 21400

or send large sae to:
The UK Homoeopathic Medical Association
6 Livingstone Road,
Gravesend,
Kent DA12 5DZ
Tel: 01474 560336

or, to find a doctor who is also a homoeopath, send sae to:
Faculty of Homoeopathy
Hahnemann House,
2 Powis Place,
Great Ormond Street,
London WC1N 3HT
Tel: 0171 837 9469

Hydrotherapy
For nearest practitioner, contact:
The British College of Naturopathy and Osteopathy
6 Netherhall Gardens,
London NW3 5RR
Tel: 0171 435 7830

Hypnotherapy
For nearest practitioner, send sae to:
Central Register of Advanced Hypnotherapists
28 Finsbury Park Road,
London N4 2JX
Tel: 0171 359 6991

or send sae to:
The National Register of Hypnotherapists & Psychotherapists
12 Cross Street,
Nelson,
Lancashire BB9 7EN
Tel: 01282 699378

For leaflet and nearest practitioner write to:
UK College for Complementary Healthcare Studies
St Charles Hospital,
Exmoor Street,
London W10 6DZ
Tel: 0181 964 1205

Iridology
For advice and nearest qualified practitioner, send sae to:
Guild of Naturopathic Iridologists
95 Grosvenor Road,
London SW1V 3LF
Tel: 0171 834 3579

For list of practitioners, send sae to:
Society of Iridologists
998 Wimborne Road,
Bournemouth BH9 2DE
Tel: 01202 518078

Light Therapy
SAD Association
PO Box 989,
Steyning PN44 3H6
Tel: 01903 814942

SAD Lightbox Company
Unit 1, Riverside Business Centre,
Victoria Street,
High Wycombe HP11 2LT
Tel: 01494 526051

Manual Lymphatic Drainage
For nearest practitioner, send sae to:
MLD UK
8 Wittenham Lane,
Dorchester on Thames,
Oxfordshire OX10 7JW

Martial Arts – T'ai Chi
For national list of instructors, send sae to:
T'ai Chi Union for Gt Britain
69 Kilpatrick Gardens,
Clarkston,
Glasgow G76 7RF

Massage
For list of local practitioners representing Eastern and Western massage, send large sae to:
British Massage Therapy Council
Greenbank House,
65a Adelphi Street,
Preston PR1 7BH
Tel: 01772 881063

Clare Maxwell-Hudson is one of Britain's most respected massage teachers. For details of her massage courses, write to:
Clare Maxwell-Hudson School of Massage
PO Box 457,
London NW2
Tel: 0181 450 6494
Clare has also written many books on the subject, including
The Complete Book of Massage
(Dorling Kindersley, £9.99)

Leigh Richmond
The Life Centre,
15 Edge Street,
London W8
Tel: 0171 221 4602

Medical Herbalism
National Institute of Medical Herbalists
For register of 310 practitioners send large sae and 29p stamp to:
56 Longbrook Street,
Exeter,
Devon EX4 6AH
Tel: 01392 426022

Meditation
Transcendental Meditation
For details of your nearest teaching centre, tel: 0800 269303

Naturopathy
General Council & Register of Naturopaths, NAD MRN
Goswell House,
2 Goswell Road,
Street,
Somerset BA16 0JG
Tel: 01458 840072
Send cheque/postal order for £2.50 and sae for register of 213 practitioners.

British College of Naturopathy and Osteopathy
6 Netherhall Gardens,
London NW3 5RR
Tel: 0171 435 7830 for personal consultations.

Nutritional Therapy
Institute of Optimum Nutrition
Blades Court, Deodar Road,
London SW15 2NU
Tel: 0181 877 9993
for in-depth health check including hair analysis.

Osteopathy
For nearest practitioner, send sae to:
Osteopathic Information Service
PO Box 2074,
Reading,
Berkshire RG1 4YR
Tel: 01734 512051

Polarity Therapy
For nearest practitioner, send A4 sae plus £1.50 to:
UK Polarity Therapy Association (BCMA/ICM affiliated)
Monomark House,
27 Old Gloucester Street,
London WC1N 3XX
Tel: 01483 417714

Psychotherapy
For info, write with sae or tel:
UK Council for Psychotherapy
167–169 Gt Portland Street,
London W1N 5FB
Tel: 0171 436 3002

The British Association of Psychotherapists
37 Mapesbury Road,
London NW2 4HJ
Tel: 0181 452 9823

The Guild of Psychotherapists
19b Thornton Hill,
London SW19 4HU
Tel: 0181 947 0730

Reflexology
The British Reflexology Association
Monks Orchard,
Whitbourne,
Worcestershire WK6 5RB
Tel: 018868 21207

Shiatsu
The Shiatsu Society
Tel: 01483 860771 for nearest practitioner, or send sae for list of their graduates to:
British School of Shiatsu
6 Erskine Road,
London NW3 3AJ
Tel: 0171 483 3776

Stress Management
International Stress Management Association (UK)
Southbank University, LPSS,
103 Borough Road,
London SE1 0AA
Write for nearest practitioner.

Stress Reduction Techniques
For details of how to order tapes and books, send sae to:
British Holistic Medical Association
Royal Shrewsbury Hospital South,
Shrewsbury SY3 8XF
Tel: 01743 261155
Fax: 01743 353637

Yoga
The British Wheel of Yoga
1 Hamilton Place,
Boston Road,
Sleaford, Lincolnshire
Tel: 01529 306851

Umbrella Organisations
Institute for Complementary Medicine
PO Box 194,
London SE15 1QZ
For info send sae and three first-class stamps.

Council for Complementary and Alternative Medicine
179 Gloucester Place,
London NW1 6DX

For info on standards, send sae and cheque/postal order for £1.50.
The British Complementary Medicine Association
9 Soar Lane
Leicester LE3 5DE
Tel: 0116 242 5406

The British Council of Complementary Medicine
works for public education, sets standards and discipline.

The British Register of Complementary Practitioners
(linked to **The British Council**)
For info send sae with three first class stamps to:
PO Box 194,
London SE16 1QZ

British Homoeopathic Association
27a Devonshire Street
London W1N 1RJ
Tel: 0171 935 2163

British Homoeopathic Dental Association
For register of 150 practitioners, send sae to:
12 Wellington Road,
Watford,
Hertfordshire WD1 1QW

British Reflexology Association
Monks Orchard
Whitbourne
Worcester WK6 5RB
018868 21207

BEAUTY SALONS

Harrods Hair & Beauty
5th Floor, Harrods Ltd,
87–135 Brompton Road,
London SW1X 7XL
Tel: 0171 581 2021

Clarins Gold Salons
Clarins offer probably the widest range of facials and body treatments of any cosmetics company. They have a nationwide network of salons, and these are the *crème de la crème*. (If there isn't one near you featured on this list, tel: 0171 629 2979 to locate one.)

CENTRAL LONDON
Bambos
428 Muswell Hill Broadway,
London N10
Tel: 0181 883 5723

Beauty Plus
The Cannons Sports Club,
Cousins Lane,
London EC4
Tel: 0171 621 0579

Chrysalis
59–61 Turnham Green Terrace
London W4
Tel: 0181 995 7360/994 6427

Winchmores Health & Beauty Clinic
3 Wades Hill,
London N21
Tel: 0181 8827909

EAST ANGLIA
Top-To-Toe
27 Hill Street,
Wisbech,
Cambridgeshire
Tel: 01945 584272

Beauty Profile
21 Paradise Road,
Downham Market,
Norfolk
Tel: 01366 385917

Trudi's Beauty Centre
6 St Andrews Hill,
Norwich, Norfolk
Tel: 01603 613153

HOME COUNTIES &
CHANNEL ISLANDS
Anita's Hair & Beauty
The Old Bakery,
Basingstoke Road,
Spencers Wood,
Nr Reading,
Berkshire
Tel: 01734 885955

Forresters Beauty Salon
203a Halls Road,
Tilehurst, Reading,
Berkshire
Tel: 01734 455223

The Cutting Company
69 High Street,
Woburn Sands,
Buckinghamshire
Tel: 01908 585251

The Elusive Butterfly
At Ambers of Amersham
The Millstream, London Road,
Old Amersham,
Buckinghamshire
Tel: 01494 434646

Les Mains D'Or Salon de Beauté Ltd
31 Connaught Avenue,
Frinton-on-Sea,
Essex
Tel: 01255 677479

The Beauty Studio
31 Hutton Road,
Shenfield,
Essex
Tel: 01277 230330

Scentsations Parfumerie
68 Bedford Place,
Southampton,
Hampshire
Tel: 01703 230333

The Elusive Butterfly
3 Lower Road,
Chorleywood,
Hertfordshire
Tel: 01923 284161

Bromley Health Lido
The Beauty Clinic,
Bath Road,
Off Southlands,
Bromley,
Kent
Tel: 0181 466 8040

Ambers Beauty Studio
40 Long Chaulden,
Hemel Hempstead,
Hertfordshire
Tel: 01442 248002

Bodyshapers
4 Temple Court,
St John,
Jersey
Tel: 01534 862884

Fridolin's Beauty Clinic
27 High Street,
Pinner,
Middlesex
Tel: 0181 8682443

Totally You
Station Road North,
Egham, Surrey
Tel: 01784 432345

Inches of Oxted
38 Station Road West,
Oxted, Surrey
Tel: 01883 722555

The Still Room
St Andrews Mews,
St Andrews Lane,
Lewes,
East Sussex
Tel: 01273 479660

Circe
Kings Court,
170 High Street,
Uckfield,
East Sussex
Tel: 01825 766476

Q Hair & Beauty
37 North Street,
Chichester,
West Sussex
Tel: 01243 781585

Richard John Hair & Beauty
1 The Arcade,
Worthing,
West Sussex
Tel: 01903 230375

MIDLANDS
Ashleigh Beauty Clinic
26 Stoneygate Road,
Leicester
Tel: 0116 2707948

Jackie Walker Hair & Beauty Centre
21–23 Biggin Street,
Loughborough,
Leicestershire
Tel: 01509 266262

Richardsons of George Row Beauty
The Courtyard,
George Row,
Northampton,
Northamptonshire
Tel: 01604 259259

Chantilly
23 High Street,
Stone,
Staffordshire
Tel: 01785 814627

Belle Sante
11 Guys Place East,
Leamington Spa,
Warwickshire
Tel: 01926 337113

Mr Nicholas
15–19 High Street,
Tettenhall,
West Midlands
Tel: 01902 756519

NORTH EAST
Cameo Health & Beauty Studio
8 High Street,
St Martins,
Stamford,
Lincolnshire
Tel: 01780 52725

One Hundred & One The Beauty Studio
101 Walkergate, Beverley,
East Yorkshire
Tel: 01482 865074

Beau Visage
19 Hill Street,
Corbridge,
Northumberland
Tel: 01434 633011

Complexions
19a High Street,
Arnold,
Nottinghamshire
Tel: 0115 9208144

Pretty Woman
625 Roundhay Road,
Oakwood,
Leeds,
West Yorkshire
Tel: 0113 2492733

House of Beauty
The Manse Chambers,
18 Pitt Street,
Barnsley,
South Yorkshire
Tel: 01226 296646

Je Ne Sais Quoi
10 Terminus Road,
Millhouses,
Sheffield,
South Yorkshire
Tel: 0114 2621921

The Beauty Rooms
22 Gills Yard,
Wakefield,
West Yorkshire
Tel: 01924 291547

NORTH WEST
Essentials
317/319 Hale Road,
Hale Barns,
Altrincham,
Cheshire
Tel: 0161 9804401

Braeside Beauty Centre
138 Chester Road,
Northwich,
Cheshire
Tel: 01606 75358

Skin Deep
Unit 2, Feather Development,
High Street,
Tarporley,
Cheshire
Tel: 01829 733900

Options Beauty Centre
18 Cairo Street,
Warrington,
Cheshire
Tel: 01925 234692

Options Beauty Centre
36 Derby Street West,
Ormskirk,
Lancashire
Tel: 01695 570588

Salon Classique
20 Breck Road,
Poulton-le-Fylde,
Lancashire
Tel: 01253 892555

Salon Classique
46 Wood Street,
St Annes,
Lancashire
Tel: 01253 725714

SOUTH WEST
Jennifer Luckham Beauty Clinic
32 Monmouth Street,
Bath,
Avon
Tel: 01225 428741

Westbury Health & Beauty Clinic
25 Canford Lane,
Westbury-on-Trym,
Bristol,
Avon
Tel: 0117 9768001

The County Salon
6 Lower Lemon Street,
Truro,
Cornwall
Tel: 01872 70090

The Beauty Spot
The Coach House,
2a Bull Lane,
Winchcombe,
Gloucestershire
Tel: 01242 604017

Lifestyle Health & Beauty
Priory Coach House,
Hankerton,
Malmesbury,
Wiltshire
Tel: 01666 577636

WALES
Vogue Health & Beauty Salon
22 Hill Street,
Haverfordwest,
Pembrokeshire
Tel: 01437 767913

Vogue Health & Beauty Salon
Bridge House,
Swan Square,
Haverfordwest,
Pembrokeshire
Tel: 01437 762544

Skin Deep
10 High Street,
Rhuddlan,
Clwyd
Tel: 01745 590693

SCOTLAND
Beauty Box
18 Newmarket Street,
Ayr
Tel: 01292 263492

KLM Beauty Studio
24 Thunderton Place,
Elgin Moray
Tel: 01343 551140

Beauty Base
8 Creswell Lane,
Glasgow
Tel: 0141 3345031

Beauty Essentials
The Dalmahoy Golf & Country
Club,
Edinburgh
Tel: 0131 335 3992

Charlie Taylor Hair & Beauty
20/28 South Methven Street,
Perth
Tel: 01738 441711

Decleor Gold Salons

Decleor is a skincare range from
France based on the powers of
aromatherapy and phytotherapy.
Many of Decleor's face and body
treatments begin with a back
diagnostic massage which also
relaxes you completely.

CENTRAL LONDON
207 Health & Beauty
207 Worple Road,
London SW20 8QY
Tel: 0181 946 6444
Contact: Anita Brady

The Body Clinic
32 The Market Place,
Falloden Way
London NW11 6JJ
Tel: 0181 458 9412
Contact: K McDonagh

Burlingtons Hair Cutters
166–168 Clerkenwell Road,
London EC1R 5DE
Tel: 0171 833 4506
Contact: Angie Lenci

Christine Beauty Salon
489 Lordship Lane,
London SE22 8JY
Tel: 0181 693 8528
Contact: Christine Vella

The City Beauty Clinic
26 Widegate Street,
London E1 7HP
Tel: 0171 247 8500
Contact: Fiona Sadek

Claudia Aston
24 North Road,
London NW11
Tel: 0181 954 5652
Contact: Antonella Noto

Daniel Bryant H & B Care
131 Station Road,
London E4
Tel: 0181 559 4800
Contact: Daniel Bryant

Dolphin Square Trust Ltd
Chichester Street,
London SW1
Tel: 0171 798 8685
Contact: Angie

Et Quo
50 Cross Street,
London N1 2BA
Tel: 0171 704 2982
Contact: Angela Broh

Face It Beauty Salon
17 High Gate, High Street,
London N6 5JJ
Tel: 0171 431 3510
Contact: Donna Gershinson

The Feel Good Factor
Last But Not Least Unit,
Asda Superstore,
151 East Ferry Road,
London E14 3BT
Tel: 0171 537 1114
Contact: Ann Craddock

Good Looks Health & Beauty
22 Blackheath Village,
London SE3
Tel: 0181 852 0651
Contact: Evelyn

Mystique Health & Beauty Centre
77 The New Broadway,
London W5 5AL
Tel: 0181 840 4435
Contact: Shabneez

The Retreat at Headmasters
32–34 The Ridgeway,
London SW19 4TQ
Tel: 0181 947 0506
Contact: Liza

Ritz Health & Beauty Salon
43 Heath Street,
London NW3
Tel: 0171 431 5208
Contact: Mr V Patel

Riverside Club
Dukes Meadows,
London W4
Tel: 0181 994 9496
Contact: Fiona Brackenbury

Total Look
281 Fulham Road,
London SW10 9QA
Tel: 0171 351 1123
Contact: Mrs Koritsas

Village Affair
The Harbour Club,
95 High Street,
London SW19 5EG
Tel: 0171 371 7744

Worthingtons
12 Charlotte Place,
London W1P 2AP
Tel: 0171 631 1370
Contact: Jane Worthington

HOME COUNTIES
Altered Images
69 London Road,
Sevenoaks,
Kent TN13 1AX
Tel: 01732 456 151
Contact: Madeleine Taylor

Amanda Beauty Therapist
16 High Street,
Botley, Southampton,
Hampshire SO23 2EA
Tel: 01489 789 589
Contact: Amanda Holt

Antoniou Hair Fashion
60 High Street,
Maidstone,
Kent ME14 1JL
Tel: 01622 690 998
Contact: Nikki Creelman

Apollo Health & Beauty
51 Thorpe Road,
Peterborough,
Cambridgeshire DE3 6AN
Tel: 01733 63983
Contact: Maggie Perkins

BJ's Hair & Beauty Salon
34 Station Road East,
Oxted,
Surrey RH8 0PG
Tel: 01883 714072
Contact: Sally

Beauty Business
65 Western Road,
Hove,
East Sussex BN3 2JQ
Tel: 01273 822 476
Suzanne Goldstone

The Beauty Rooms
15 The Broadway,
Beaconsfield,
Buckinghamshire HP9 2PD
Tel: 01494 672 211
Maria Ray

Beauty Secrets
10b Market Square,
Pump Alley,
Horsham,
West Sussex RH12 1EU
Tel: 01403 240 489
Contact: Beryl Martin

The Beauty Spot
122 London Road,
Knebworth,
Hertfordshire
Tel: 01438 812114
Contact: Mrs Kenny

The Beauty Studio
211a Three Bridges Road
Three Bridges,
Crawley
West Sussex RH10 1LG
Tel: 01293 522 491
Contact: Christine Collyer

Beauty Within
High Street,
Cuckfield,
West Sussex RH17 5JX
Tel: 01444 459 277
Contact: Helen Marshall

Bennissimo Beauty Salon
27 Maldon Road,
Witham,
Essex CM2 2AA
Tel: 01376 502 303
Contact: Carol Ann Lunnon

Bodyline
9 Batholomew Street,
Newbury,
Berkshire RG14 5DY
Tel: 01635 550 262
Contact: Kerry

Body Matters
10 Nightingale Corner,
Little Chalfont,
Buckinghamshire
Tel:01494 765000
Contact: Kate Edwards

Bonnie Cook Beauty Salon
30 Red Lion Street,
Richmond,
Surrey TW9 1RW
Tel: 0181 332 6630
Contact: Bonnie Cook

Bourne Beautiful
3 Cheam Road,
Ewell Road,
Ewell Village,
Surrey KT17 1SP
Tel: 0181 786 7121
Contact: Nicola Webb

Broadways Health & Leisure
2a Devonshire Road,
Bexleyheath,
Kent DA6 8DS
Tel: 0181 304 4909
Contact: Julia Clarke

Cedars Health & Beauty Suite
Richmond Hill,
Richmond,
Surrey TW10 6RW
Tel: 0181 940 2247
Contact: Suzanne Summers

Cherry Trees Beauty Clinic
High Grange,
Cherry Tree Lane,
Hemel Hempstead,
Hertfordshire HP2 7HS
Tel: 01753 867003
Contact: Lesley

Cloud Nine
14 Oxford Road East,
Windsor,
Berkshire SL4 1EF
Tel: 01753 867003
Contact: Helen Thacker

Cottesmore Beauty Salon
Cottesmore Club,
Buchan Hill, Crawley
West Sussex RH11 9AT
Tel: 01293 520 321
Contact: Sandra Cook

The Dolls House
Church Road,
Penn,
Buckinghamshire HP10 8LN
Tel: 01494 812 411
Contact: Linda Kent

Essence Health & Beauty
Lower Ground Floor,
3 Collier Row Road,
Romford,
Essex RM5 3NP
Tel: 01708 737611
Contact: Wendy Stallworthy

Eternal Youth
79–81 High Street,
Waltham Cross,
Hertfordshire EN8 7AF
Tel: 01992 701 110
Contact: Lynn Bowers

Face Facts
1st Floor, 4 High Street,
Chesham,
Buckinghamshire HP5 1EP
Tel: 01494 775412
Contact: Sara Paul

Falltricks Beauty Salon
146 Balgores Lane,
Gidea Park,
Essex RM2 6BP
Tel: 01708 735195
Contact: Leigh Applebee

Figure Shapers
95 Western Road,
Hove,
East Sussex BN3 1FA
Tel: 01273 728467

French at 48
48 Queens Road,
Buckhurst Hill,
Essex IG9 5BY
Tel: 0181 504 6600
Contact: Paula French

Hadley Spa
4 Heddon Court Parade,
Cockfoster Road,
Cockfosters,
Hertfordshire EN4 0DB
Tel: 0181 449 0236
Contact: Mrs Joseph

Head Quarters
Stockley Park Arena Ltd,
Stockley Park, Uxbridge,
Middlesex UB11 1AA
Tel: 0181 813 6842
Contact: Hugh Morgan

Health & Harmony
1494 London Road,
Leigh On Sea,
Essex SS9 2UR
Tel: 01702 471 797
Contact: Jennifer

The Hunting Beauty Clinic
55 St Lukes Road,
Maidenhead,
Berkshire SL6 7DN
Tel: 01628 22261

Images Beauty Rooms
7a Downham Road,
Ramsden Heath
Billericay Essex
Tel: 01268 711577
Contact: Tracey Jane Nicholls

Inches Away
1–3 Rectory Road,
Beckenham,
Kent BR3 1HL
Tel: 0181 663 6110

Jasmines Beauty Salon
12 Gildredge Road,
Eastborne,
East Sussex BN21 4RL
Tel: 01323 726 997
Contact: Nicola Vaughan

La Peche Salon
2 Chestnut House,
High Street,
Crowthorne
Berkshire RG11 7AD
Tel: 01344 778540

The Leisure Club
Selsdon Park Hotel,
Addington Road,
Sanderstead,
Surrey CR2 8YA
Tel: 0181 657 8811
Contact: Lena Christou

Lena White Nails & Beauty
34 Watford Road,
Northwood,
Middlesex HA6 2AT
Tel: 0181 868 2811
Contact: Lena White

Maria Elena Health & Beauty
8 Tudor Parade,
Rickmansworth,
Hertfordshire WD3 4DF
Tel: 01923 896117
Contact: Maria Alexandrou

Micheala Giles
62 Chestnut Avenue,
Billericay,
Essex CM12 9JG
Tel: 01277 622096

Milo Hawkins
116 Oaklands Drive,
Weybridge,
Surrey KT13 9OB
Tel: 01932 851850

Neroli
192 Hutton Road,
Shenfield,
Essex CM15 8NR
Tel: 01277 232300
Contact: Eileen Holmes

New Verity's
25–27 Weyhill,
Haslemere,
Surrey GU27 1DA
Tel: 01428 642 100

L'Orchidee
48 Charter Place,
Watford,
Hertfordshire WD1 2RR
Tel: 01923 249 412
Contact: Carol Andrea

Panache
11 Brook Lane,
Warsash, Southampton,
Hampshire SO31 9FH
Tel: 01705 550 562
Contact: Penny Coe

Raffles Beauty Studio
23 Denmark Street,
Wokingham,
Berkshire RG11 2AY
Tel: 01734 788 111
Contact: Helen Smith

Riverside Club
Ducks Hill Road,
Northwood,
Middlesex HA6 2DR
Tel: 01923 840840
Contact: Emma Dixon

The Riverside Club
Hanibal Way,
Off Stafford Road,
Croydon
Surrey CR0 4RW
Tel: 0181 681 1331
Contact: Sarah Ford

San Souci Beauty
9 Holmesdale Road,
Reigate,
Surrey RH2 0BA
Tel: 01737 221 219
Contact: Mrs Perry

Sandra Dawn Health & Beauty
179 High Street,
Guildford,
Surrey GU1 3AW
Tel: 01483 506364
Contact: Sandra Dawn

Santina Ltd
115 Station Road,
Burchington,
Kent CT7 9RE
Tel: 01843 848223
Contact: L Macgowan

Skin & Tonic Health & Beauty
218 Cobham Road,
Fetcham,
Leatherhead
Surrey KT22 9JQ
Tel: 01372 360285

The Studio Health & Beauty
Northbridge Road,
Berkhamsted,
Hertfordshire HP4 1EH
Tel: 01442 878660
Contact: Penny Eastman

Sunrise Health & Beauty
The Wedding Centre
46 West Street,
Marlow
Buckinghamshire SL7 2NB
Tel: 01628 487719
Contact: Dawn O'Shaughnessy

Supermops
36 Franklin Road,
Hayward Heath,
West Sussex RH16 9DF
Tel: 01444 870800
Contact: Lesley Bridgestock

Utopia Health & Leisure Spa
Rowhill Grange,
Top Dartford Road,
Wilmington,
Kent DA2
Tel: 01322 667433
Contact: Jennifer Gorman

Venus Studio
47 Newlands Road,
Woodford Green,
Essex IG8 0RS
Tel: 0181 508 8257
Contact: Beryl Tibbetts

The White House
2 East Street,
Thame,
Oxfordshire OX9 3JS
Tel: 01844 260 080
Contact: Amanda

EAST ANGLIA
Amanda Jane Beauty
46 Abbeygate Street,
Bury St Edmunds,
Suffolk IP33 1LB
Tel: 01284 764544
Contact: Amanda Jane

Carolyn Hammond
15 Fore Street,
Ipswich,
Suffolk IP4 1JW
Tel: 01473 226900
Contact:

Potters Holiday & Leisure
Hopton On Sea,
Nr Yarmouth,
Norfolk NR31 9DX
Tel: 01502 732306
Contact: Jane Potter

CHANNEL ISLANDS
Emma's Health & Beauty
Le Bourg De Bas,
Forest,
Guernsey GY8 0BE
Tel: 01481 38583
Contact: Emma

The Hotel De France
St Saviours Road,
St Helier,
Jersey JE4 8WZ
Tel: 01534 58144
Contact: Nathalie

Mahogany Health & Beauty
The Hotel De France,
St Saviours Road,
St Helier,
Jersey JE4 8WZ
Tel: 01534 58144

SOUTH WEST
The Beauty Spot
The Coach House, 2a Bull Lane,
Gloucestershire GL54 5HY
Tel: 01242 604 017
Contact: Carmela Rosbottom

The English Rose H & B Salon
29 Church Street,
Calne,
Wiltshire SN11 0HZ
Tel: 01249 821 158
Contact: Tracey Deeming

Visage
St Olaves Close,
Exeter,
Devon EX4 3TP
Tel: 01392 420 601
Contact: Brenda Anvari

WALES
The Aromatherapy Clinic
227 Pantbach Road,
Rhiwbina Village,
Cardiff CF4 6AE
Tel: 01222 521 206

Beauty With Sara
3 Church Street,
Wrexham,
Clywd LL13 8LS
Tel: 01978 357232
Contact: Sara Shoemark

MIDLANDS
Absolute Hair & Beauty
4 Oakfield Shopping Centre,
Rad Valley Road
Copthorne,
Shropshire SY3 8BD
Tel: 01743 351591
Contact: Karen Taylor

The Beauty Clinic
First Floor, The Buttermarket,
Newark,
Nottinghamshire NG24 1BF
Tel: 01636 612 844
Contact: Tracey

The Beauty Mill
Barnsley Road,
New Millerdam,
Wakefield WF2 6QQ
Tel: 01924 259718
Contact: Sonia Edwards

The Beauty Room at Treats
93c Melton Road,
West Bridgeford,
Nottinghamshire NG2 6EN
Tel: 01159 822287
Contact: M Roberts

Charisma
10a Beeches Walk,
Sutton Coldfield,
West Midlands B73 6HN
Tel: 0121 354 9513
Contact: Sheila Short

Christina Louise H & B Centre
14 Francis Street,
Stoneygate,
Leicestershire LE2 2BE
Tel: 01162 704995
Contact: Christina Sykes

Clarendon Beauty Salon
515 Hagley Road,
Smethwick,
Birmingham B66 4AX
Tel: 0121 429 9191
Contact: Helen McElroy

Courtyard Beauty Salon
5 Potters Yard, Potter Street,
Melbourne,
Derbyshire DE73 1DW
Tel: 01332 864 461
Contact: Angela Smithson

Eden Health & Beauty
The Key Health & Fitness,
Bunny Lane,
Keyworth,
Nottinghamshire NG12
Tel: 01159 375216
Contact: Louise

Elegance Beauty
120 Damson Lane,
Solihull,
Birmingham B92 9JS
Tel: 0121 705 9554
Contact: Doreen Collins

Essential Beauty
7/8 The Colanade,
Eastgate Street,
Stafford ST19 9HY
Tel: 01785 257711

Femi Latif
Unit 71, The Shires Walk,
High Street,
Leicester LE10 3JA
Tel: 01162 532393

First Impressions
24–26 Maid Marion Way,
Nottinghamshire NG1 6JS
Tel: 0115 948 3814
Contact: Sue Johal

The Gallery Health & Beauty
Hinckley Island Hotel,
A5 Hinckley,
Leicestershire
Tel: 01455 250809
Contact: Emma Snowden

Hellidon Lakes Hotel
Hellidon,
Daventry,
Northamptonshire NN11 6LN
Tel: 01327 262550
Contact: Jackie Nicoll

Inches Health & Beauty Salon
14 Manor Walk,
Market Harborough,
Leicestershire LE16 9BP
Tel: 01858 463483
Contact: Carol Grant

Jane Green
35 Blackwood Road,
Dosthill,
Tamworth,
Staffordshire B77 1JW
Tel: 01827 283076

Lygon Arms Country Club
Lygon Arms,
Broadway,
Worcestershire WR12 7DU
Tel: 01386 854421
Contact: Ruth Butler

The Ross Health & Beauty Centre
The Mews,
Church Street,
Ross On Wye,
Herefordshire HR9 6HN
Tel: 01989 564579
Contact: Lynn Snow

Salamanda
892a Woodbrough Road,
Mapperly Plains,
Nottinghamshire NG3 5QR
Tel: 0115 985 665
Contact: Louise Langford

Shapers
9 Guild Street,
Stratford Upon Avon,
Warwickshire B49 6NA
Tel: 01789 299 300
Contact: Sally Gabb

West End Beauty Clinic
6 Chad Road,
Edgbaston,
Birmingham B15 3EN
Tel: 0121 4521060
Contact: Marilyn Hodgkinson

NORTH EAST
Alwoodley Beauty Salon
6 The Avenue,
Alwoodley,
Leeds,
West Yorkshire LS17 9BN
Tel: 0113 261 3374
Contact: Lisa Gordon

Beauty By Christine Clarke
428a Ecclesall Road,
Sheffield,
South Yorkshire S11 8DR
Tel: 01742 682 140
Contact: Christine Clarke

The Beauty Clinic
104a King Street,
Cottingham,
Humberside HU16 5QE
Tel: 01482 875 329
Contact: Miss McKee

The Beauty Spot
Listerdale Shopping Parade,
Rotherham,
South Yorkshire S65 3JA
Tel: 01709 542 605
Contact: A Rounding

Beauty Works
710 Abbeydale Road,
Abbeydale,
Sheffield S7 2BL
Tel: 01142 500210
Contact: Ann Marie Needle

Bedale Beauty
Unit 6,
19 North End,
Bedale,
North Yorkshire DL8 1AF
Tel: 01677 426 557
Contact: Donna Stothard

Belmont Hair & Beauty
86a High Street,
Carrville,
County Durham DH1 1BE
Tel: 0191 386 8859
Contact: Ms Rayna Bowden

Bridge Pharmacy Ltd
Bramhall Beauty Salon,
6 Woodford Road,
Bramhall,
Stockport SK7 1JJ
Tel: 0161 439 2117
Contact: Mrs Whiteley

Classic Beauty
82a Street Lane,
Roundhay,
Leeds
West Yorkshire LS8 2AL
Tel: 01532 369 994
Tracey Large

Cloud Nine
9 Londress Lane,
Beverley,
Humberside HU17 8HA
Tel: 01753 867003
Contact: Nicky Rowbottom

Fine Fettle Beauty Salon
64 Featherbank Lane,
Horseforth,
Leeds LS18 4NW
Tel: 01132 581601
Contact: Vanessa Archer

Grantham Beauty Clinic
13 Vine Street,
Grantham,
Lincolnshire NG31 6RQ
Tel: 01476 61090
Contact: Mrs G Emery

The Gym
30 Something Ventnor Way,
Ossett,
Wakefield
West Yorkshire WF5 8JT
Tel: 01924 262639
Contact: Sam Cullingworth

House of Lindsey
1a Swan Street,
Bawtry,
Doncaster
South Yorkshire DN10 6JQ
Tel: 01302 719 549
Contact: Doreen Bramley

Into Beauty
8 High Street,
Hatfield,
Doncaster
South Yorkshire DN7 6RY
Tel: 01302 351528
Contact: Andrea Larder

Ivy Court Leisure
84 Park View,
Whitley Bay,
Tyne & Wear NE26 2TH
Tel: 0191 281 5237
Contact: Charles Buchanan

Janet Metcalfe
4 Hawksworth Street,
Ilkley,
West Yorkshire LS29 9DU
Tel: 01943 602 133

The Jesmond Clinic
68 Clayton Park Square,
Jesmond,
Newcastle Upon Tyne NE2 4DP
Tel: 0191 281 8775
Contact: Alison Laws

Newcastle Beauty Clinic
2nd Floor,
52 Northumberland Street,
Newcastle Upon Tyne NE1 7DF
Tel: 0191 232 0411
Contact: Susan Howey

Pink Orchid Health & Beauty Salon
5 Alston Road,
Bessacar, Doncaster
South Yorkshire DN4 7HA
Tel: 01302 370 913
Contact: Ruth Waring

Profile
Wellington House,
Cold Bath Road,
Harrogate,
North Yorkshire HG2 ONA
Tel: 01423 507707
Contact: Sally Ramsden

Ponteland Beauty Clinic
Collingwood House,
Meadowfield,
Ponteland,
Newcastle Upon Tyne NE20 9SD
Tel: 01661 822 831
Contact: Charles Buchanan

Ten Out Of Ten Health & Beauty
10 Chapel Street,
Hull,
North Humberside HU1 3PA
Tel: 01482 225 189
Contact: Malcolm Gold

The Works Body & Skin Care Clinic
Tall Trees Academy,
Green Lane,
Yarm,
Cleveland TS15 9FF
Tel: 01642 785440
Contact: Ms Andrea Gillson

NORTH WEST
Beauty With Sara
42 Lower Bridge Street,
Chester,
Cheshire CH1 1RS
Tel: 01244 348483
Contact: Sara Shoemark

Bliss Health & Beauty
Gibbon Bridge Hotel,
Forest Of Bowland,
Lancashire PR3 2TQ
Tel: 01995 61069
Contact: Julia Collinson

Brooklands Health Farm
Calderhouse Lane,
Garstang,
Lancashire PR3 I2E
Tel: 01995 605 162
Contact: Judith Brown

Contours Health & Beauty Centre
42 Revidge Road,
Blackburn,
Lancashire BB2 6JD
Tel: 01254 690 373
Contact: Lesley Barrow

Face & Figure
33 Station Road,
Holmes Chapel,
Cheshire CW4 8AA
Tel: 01477 537192
Contact: Julia Robinson

Karen Taylor Beauty & Skincare
81 Victoria Road East,
Thornton Cleveleys,
Near Blackpool
Lancashire SY5 5BU
Tel: 01253 883094

Lowood Beauty Clinique
Low Wood Hotel,
Windermere,
Cumbria LA23 1LP
Tel: 015394 33338

Neston Natural Health & Beauty
13 Parkgate Road,
Neston,
South Wirral,
Cheshire L64 9XF
Tel: 0151 353 0093
Contact: Jackie Hill

Springs Health & Beauty Clinic
Wrightingtons Country Club,
Moss Lane,
Wigan,
Lancashire 9PB
Tel: 01204 597111
Contact: Andrea Peters

Springs Limited
75 London Road,
Stockton Heath,
Warrington,
Cheshire WA4 6LE
Tel: 01925 262738
Contact: Andrea Peters

Zoes Dalmney Salon
Dalmeny Hotel,
19–30 South Promenade,
Street Annes On Sea,
Lancashire
Tel: 01253 712236
Contact: Zoe Webb

SCOTLAND
AMR Beauty Therapy
25 Clarence Drive,
Hyndland,
Glasgow G12 9QN
Tel: 0141 3395954
Contact: Angela Risk

Cameo Health & Beauty Salon
160/162 Union Street,
Aberdeen AB10 1QT
Tel: 01224 639 982
Contact: Carol Hay or Nicola Nelson

Dom Migele
7–9 Tolbooth Street,
Kircaldy,
Fife KY1 1RW
Tel: 01592 203116
Contact: Frances Panetta

Face Facts Beauty Salon Ltd
1169 Pollockshaws Road,
Shawlands,
Glasgow G41 3NG
Tel: 0141 639 669
Contact: Fiona

Fantasia Beauty Salon
Kings Mill Hotel,
Damfield Road,
Inverness IV2 3LP
Tel: 01463 243 244
Contact: Shirley Tracey

Impressions
4 Earl Grey Street,
Mauchline,
Ayrshire KA5 5AD
Tel: 01290 550 016
Contact: Angela Holland

Iskoka
11 Albyn Terrace,
Aberdeen AB1 1YP
Tel: 01224 641 9000
Contact: Mr M Macneil

Looking Good Skin H & B Clinic
45 Kilbowie Road,
Clydebank G81 1BE
Tel: 01836 786232
Contact: J Briscoe or JA Guyan

Susanne Slimming & Beauty Clinic
51 Cumberland Street,
Edinbrurgh EH3 6RA
Susanne Baird

Sutherland Hair & Beauty
24 High Street,
Newport On Tay,
Fife DD6 8AD
Tel: 01382 541551
Contact: Marion Sutherland

Time Out
51 Holburn Road,
Aberdeen AB1 6EY
Tel: 01224 212 888
Contact: Jill Webster

Totally You Ltd
22 Queens Court,
Sandgate, Ayr,
Ayrshire KA7 1LE
Tel: 01292 619 300
Contact: Tom Stevenson

Top E'SPA Salons
E'SPA is an aromatherapy-based
top-to-toe treatment range which
works on mind, body and spirit. If
you've never had an aromatherapy
massage before, with their menu of
treatments, E'SPA salons are a great
place to start.

CENTRAL LONDON
Caci Clinic
11 Heath Street,
London NW3 6TP
Tel: 0171 431 1033

Catherine England Beauty
Hotel Inter-Continental,
One Hamilton Place,
Hyde Park Corner,
London W1V 3QG
Tel: 0171 409 3131

Espree Leisure Ltd
3 Tudor Street,
London EC4Y OAH
Tel: 0171 867 1222

Joy Weston
142 Notting Hill Gate
London W11 3QG
Tel: 0171 2294141

Village Affair
95 High Street,
Wimbledon Village,
London SW19 5EG
Tel: 0181 946 6222

Michaeljohn
25 Albermarle Street,
London W1X 4LH
Tel: 0171 491 4401

Equilibrium
150 Chiswick High Road,
London W4 1PR
Tel: 0181 742 7701

EAST ANGLIA
Sprowston Manor Hotel
Sprowston Road,
Norwich,
Norfolk NR7 8RP
Tel: 01603 410871

Clarice House Health & Leisure
Bromford Road,
Ipswich,
Suffolk IP8 4AZ
Tel: 01473 463262

Shrubland Hall Health Clinic
Coddenham, Ipswich,
Suffolk IP6 9QH
Tel: 01473 830404

HOME COUNTIES &
CHANNEL ISLANDS
Royal Berkshire Racquet Club
9 Mile Ride,
Bracknell,
Berkshire RG12 4PB
Tel: 01344 869066

Hera Health & Beauty Salon
1 & 2 Broomfield Hall Building,
London Road,
Sunningdale,
Berkshire
Tel: 01344 28282

Lanes Beauty Salon
12 The Highway,
Beaconsfield,
Buckinghamshire HP9 2QQ
Tel: 01494 675050

Bubbles Beauty Salon
26 High Road,
Benfleet,
Essex SS7 5LH
Tel: 01268 795324

Five Lakes Hotel, Golf & Country Club
Colchester Road,
Whitehouse Hill,
Tolleshunt Knights,
Maldon,
Essex CM9 8HX
Tel: 01621 868888

Neroli Beauty Salon
192 Hutton Road,
Shenfield,
Essex CM15 8NR
Tel: 01277 232300

Chewton Glen
The Hotel, Health and Country Club,
New Milton,
Hampshire BH25 6QS
Tel: 01425 275341

Pinnacle St Albans
Cell Barnes Lane,
St Albans,
Hertfordshire AL4 OAN
Tel: 01727 869081

Sopwell House Hotel
Cottonmill Lane,
St Albans,
Hertfordshire AL1 2HQ
Tel: 01727 864477

Kirsten Sand Beauty Salon
Centre Point,
Red Houses,
St Brelade,
Jersey
Tel: 01534 47313

Capel Grange Barn
Badsell Road,
Five Oak Green,
Tonbridge,
Kent
Tel: 01892 833312

Elizabeth Rose
67 High Street,
Tenterden,
Kent TN30 6BD
Tel: 01580 763815

The Runnymede Hotel
Windsor Road,
Egham,
Surrey TW20 0AG
Tel: 01784 436171

Priory Health & Leisure Club
Nutfield Priory,
Nutfield,
Redhill,
Surrey RH1 4EN
Tel: 01737 823510

The Luxury Gap
2 Hillcroft,
Shepherds Hill,
Haslemere,
Surrey GU27 2JL
Tel: 01428 645300

The Treatment Room
15 New Road,
Brighton,
East Sussex BN1 1UF
Tel: 01273 738886

MIDLANDS
Warwickshire Racquet Club
Abbey Road,
Whiteley
Coventry
Warwickshire CV3 4BJ
Tel: 01203 306650

Complexions
19a High Street,
Arnold,
Nottingham,
Nottinghamshire NG14 6AQ
Tel: 01159 920 8144

Village Nottingham
Chilwell Meadows,
Brailsford Way,
Chilwell,
Nottingham
Tel: 01159 464422

First Impressions
24–26 Maid Marian Way,
Nottingham NG1 6JS
Tel: 01159 483814

Salon Professional
22 Lawton Road,
Alsager,
Stoke on Trent,
Staffordshire SG7 2AF
Tel: 01270 882288

Hoar Cross Hall Health Resort
Hoar Cross,
Yoxall,
Nr Burton-on-Trent,
Staffordshire
Tel: 01283 575671

Obsessions
5 Castledyke,
Lichfield,
Staffordshire WS13 6HR
Tel: 01543 254137

Body Sense
Walton Hall,
Walton,
Nr Wellesbourne,
Warwickshire
Tel: 01789 842424

Esporta Health & Fitness
Festival Heights,
Greyhound Way,
Stoke-on-Trent,
Warwickshire ST1 5N2.
Tel: 01782 210210

Caci Clinic
Nicholls Place,
353 Warwick Road,
Dovehouse Parade,
Solihull,
West Midlands
Tel: 0121 706 4420

NORTH EAST
One Hundred and One
The Beauty Studio,
101 Walkergate,
Beverley,
North Humberside
Tel: 01482 865074

The Academy
Oakdale Place,
Harrogate,
North Yorkshire HG1 2LA
Tel: 01423 524052

Peaches & Cream
10a Wesley Street,
Morley,
Leeds,
West Yorkshire LS29 9ED
Tel: 01132 380035

NORTH WEST & ISLE OF MAN
Body Beautiful
46a Chestergate,
Macclesfield,
Cheshire SK11 6BA
Tel: 01625 612312

Options Beauty Salon
18 Cairo Street,
Warrington,
Cheshire WA1 1EH .
Tel: 01925 234692

Mary Haworth Beauty Salon
11 Warrington Street,
Ashton-under-Lyne,
Stockport,
Cheshire
Tel: 01613 304073

Enhance Nail & Beauty Studio
36 Bramhall Lane South,
Bramhall,
Stockport,
Cheshire
Tel: 0161 439 1460

Mount Murray Hair & Beauty
Mount Murray Hotel and Country
Club,
Santon,
Isle of Man
Tel: 01624 661111

Options Beauty Salon
36 Derby Street West
Ormskirk
Lancashire, L39 3NH .
Tel: 01695 570588

Sybaris Beauty Salon
321 The Green,
Eccleston,
Nr Chorley,
Lancashire
Tel: 01257 451651

Secrets Beauty Salon
130 Manchester Road,
Southport,
Merseyside PR9 9BH
Tel: 01704 546339

Village Bromborough
Pool Lane,
Bromborough,
Wirral,
Merseyside
Tel: 0151 643 1616

SOUTH WEST
Laurels Beauty Salon
Bath Spa Hotel,
Bath,
Avon BA2 6JF
Tel: 01225 444424

Esporta
Hunts Brand Road,
Stoke Gifford,
Bristol,
Avon BS12 6HN.
Tel: 0117 974 9747

The Westbury H & B Clinic
25 Canford Lane
Westbury-on-Trym
Bristol,
Avon BS9 3DQ.
Tel: 0117 976 8001

The Dorset Racquets Club
Cabot Lane,
Poole,
Dorset BH17 7BX.
Tel: 01202 642600

Linghams Health Spa
1 Queen's Circus,
Montpellier,
Cheltenham,
Gloucestershire
Tel: 01242 256191

Michaeljohn
c/o Ragdale Spa,
Bishopstrow House,
Warminster,
Wiltshire
Tel: 01985 212512

SCOTLAND
Mary Jeffrey Beauty Salon
Assembly Street
Dumfries, DG1 2RU.
Tel: 01387 269349

Beauty Base
8 Cresswell Lane
Off Byres Rd
Hillhead
Glasgow, G12 8AA.
Tel: 0141 334 5031

Salon X1
11 Park Avenue,
Dunfermline,
Fife KY12 7HX
Tel: 01383 735431

A. L. Beauty Clinic
1 Orchard Street,
Motherwell,
Lanacshire ML1 3HU
Tel: 01698 261565

Elle Beauty Salon
36 Hunter Street,
Kirkcaldy,
Fife,
Tel: 01592 642733

St Andrews Old Course Hotel
St Andrews,
Fife KY16 9SP
Tel: 01334 474371

Gleneagles Hotel
Gleneagles Spa,
Auchterarder,
Perthshire PH3 1NF
Tel: 01764 662231

WALES
Springs Health & Beauty Studio
Old Stable Yard,
Llanrhaeadr, Nr Denbigh,
Clwyd
Tel: 01745 890478

NORTHERN IRELAND
Sanctuary Beauty
4 Church Lane,
Belfast BT1 4QN
Tel: 01232 319288

Patricia Clarke Beauty Salon
86 Antrim Street,
Lisburn,
Co. Antrim BT28 1AU
Tel: 01846 678667

Top Essanelle Salons
Essanelle Salons offer a full range
of beauty treatments.

CENTRAL LONDON
Army & Navy
1st Floor,
101 Victoria Street,
London SW1E 6QX
Tel: 0171 834 1234
Products: Guinot

Barkers
2nd Floor,
63 Kensington High Street,
London W8 5SE
Tel: 0171 937 5149
Products: Guinot, CACI

D H Evans
2nd Floor,
318 Oxford Street,
London W1A 1DE
Tel: 0171 629 1368
Products: Guinot, Decleor,
Designer Nails

Debenhams
1st Floor,
334–348 Oxford Street,
London W1A 1EF
Tel: 0171 580 2471
Products: Mary Cohr, Decleor,
CACI, Ionithermie

Dickins & Jones
4th Floor, 224 Regent Street,
London W1A 1DB
Tel: 0171 734 8326
Products: Guinot, Decleor, Thalgo,
Jessica, CACI, Elizabeth Arden

HOME COUNTIES
Dickins & Jones
1st Floor,
28 Acorn Walk,
Milton Keynes,
Buckinghamshire MK9 3DJ
Tel: 01908 607604
Products: Guinot, Decleor, Jessica,
CACI, Designer Nails

Owen Owen
3rd Floor,
The Exchange Shopping Precinct,
High Road,
Ilford,
Essex IG1 1RR
Tel: 0181 478 9731
Products: Guinot, Mary Cohr

Clements
1st Floor,
The Parade,
Watford,
Hertfordshire WD1 1LX
Tel: 01923 238043
Products: Guinot

Fenwick
1st Floor,
Brent Cross Shopping Centre,
London NW4 3FN
Tel: 0181 202 0323
Products: Guinot, Decleor, Jessica,
Aromazone

Army & Navy
3rd Floor,
Park Street,
Camberley,
Surrey GU15 3PG
Tel: 01276 681446
Products: Guinot, Jessica,
Christian Dior (make-up)

Army & Navy
4th Floor,
105–111 High Street,
Guildford,
Surrey GU1 3DU
Tel: 01483 38598
Products: Guinot

Dickins & Jones
3rd Floor,
George Street,
Richmond,
Surrey TW9 1HA
Tel: 0181 948 2303
Products: Guinot, Jessica

Army & Navy
1st Floor,
St Georges House,
West Street,
Chichester,
West Sussex PO19 1QG
Tel: 01243 786551
Products: Guinot

EAST ANGLIA
Owen Owen
2nd Floor,
The Buttermarket Centre,
Ipswich IP1 1DU
Tel: 01473 286 455
Products: Guinot

SOUTH WEST
Jollys
Upper 1st Floor,
13 Milsom Street,
Bath,
Avon
Tel: 01225 335308
Products: Decleor, Jessica, CACI

MIDLANDS
Rackhams
6th Floor,
35 Temple Row,
Birmingham B2 5JS
Tel: 0121 236 8806
Products: Decleor, Thalgo, Jessica,
CACI, Designer Nails

Rackhams
1st Floor,
The Parade,
Leamington Spa,
Warwickshire CV32 4DA
Tel: 01926 339 211
Products: Guinot, Decleor, Jessica,
CACI

Beatties
1st Floor,
71–80 Victoria Street,
Wolverhampton,
West Midlands WV1 3PQ
Tel: 01902 20409
Products: Guinot, Jessica, CACI

Denners
2nd Floor,
25 High Street,
Yeovil BA20 1RU
Tel: 01935 444444
Products: Guinot, Jessica, CACI

NORTH EAST
Binns
1st Floor, 7 High Row,
Darlington,
County Durham DL3 7QE
Tel: 01325 486876
Products: Guinot, Jessica, Light
Concept, G5

Fenwick
1st Floor,
39 Northumberland Street,
Newcastle NE99 1AR
Tel: 0191 232 0802
Products: Guinot, Decleor, Thalgo,
Jessica, CACI, G5

Binns
3rd Floor, 37 Linthorpe Road,
Middlesborough,
County Durham TS1 5AD
Tel: 01642 223157
Products: Guinot, Jessica, Light
Concept, G5

Binns
1st Floor, 226-231 High Street,
Lincoln LN2 1AY
Tel: 01522 560611
Products: Guinot, Light Concept,
Designer Nails

House of Fraser
2nd Floor, High Street,
Sheffield,
South Yorkshire S1 1QH
Tel: 0114 276 9797
Products: Guinot, Jessica,
Designer Nails

Browns
1st Floor, Daveygate Corner,
York,
Yorkshire YO1 2QT
Tel: 01904 623003
Products: Guinot, Light Concept

NORTH WEST
Browns
3rd Floor, 34–40 Eastgate Row,
Chester CH1 3SB
Tel: 01244 322965
Products: Mary Cohr, Decleor,
Jessica, CACI

Kendals
2nd Floor,
PO BOX 60,
Deansgate,
Manchester M60 3AU
Tel: 0161 832 5298
Products: Guinot, Decleor, Thalgo,
Jessica, Designer Nails, CACI,
Christian Dior

SCOTLAND
Jenners
5th Floor,
48 Princes Street,
Edinburgh EH2 2YJ
Tel: 0131 225 9645
Products: Guinot, Decleor, Jessica,
Designer Nails, CACI, Elizabeth
Arden (make-up)

Frasers
2nd Floor,
21–59 Buchanan Street,
Glasgow, G1 3HR
Tel: 0141 221 2380
Products: Guinot, Decleor, Jessica,
CACI, Givenchy* (*make-up)

Regis Salons
Regis Salons offer a full range of
hair and beauty treatments.

CENTRAL LONDON
Fenwick
63 New Bond Street,
London W1A 3BS
Tel: 0171 629 3765
Products: Guinot, MD Formulations,
Jessica, CACI, Ionithermie, G5

Selfridges
5th Floor,
400 Oxford Street,
London W1A 1AB
Tel: 0171 318 3350/1/2
Products: Guinot, Matis, MD
Formulations, Jessica, CACI,
Ionithermie

Selfridges Spa
5th Floor,
400 Oxford Street,
London W1A 1AB
Tel: 0171 318 3389
Products: Thalgo, CACI, Ionithermie

HOME COUNTIES
Allders
High Street
Bromley
Kent BR1 1HJ
Products: Guiniot, Elemis,
MD Formulations

Allders
North End,
Croydon,
Surrey CR9 1SB
Tel: 0181 667 1741
Products: Guinot, CACI, MD
Formulations, B-Line, OPI, G5, Art
Deco (make-up)

Dingles
Royal Parade
Plymouth
Devon PL1 1DY
Tel: 01752 604106
Products: Guinot

House of Fraser
Lakeside Development,
West Thurrock,
Grays,
Essex RM16 1ZJ
Tel: 01708 891055
Products: Guinot, OPI, Art Deco
(make-up)

Fenwick
101 Royal Victoria Place,
Tunbridge Wells,
Kent
Tel: 01892 549088
Products: Guinot, Ionithermie

Lewis's
27 The Westgate,
Oxford OX1 1LP
Tel: 01865 246237
Products: Guinot, OPI, CACI, Art
Deco

SOUTH WEST
Dingles
45–46 Queens Road,
Bristol BS8 1RG
Tel: 0117 921 5301
Products: Guinot, MD Formulations,
OPI, Ionithermie, Art Deco (make-
up)

WALES
Howells
14 St Mary's Street,
Cardiff,
South Glamorgan CF1 1TT
Tel: 01222 390645
Products: Guinot, OPI, CACI, Art
Deco (make-up)

NORTH-EAST
Allders
The Headrow
Leeds
Yorkshire LS1 1JX
Tel: 0113 2448274
Products: Guinot

NORTH WEST
Lewis's
40 Ranelagh Street,
Liverpool L1 1JX
Tel: 0151 709 8268
Products: Guinot, Ionithermie, Art
Deco

Lewis's
Market Street,
Manchester M60 1TX
Tel: 0161 236 0761
Products: Guinot, CACI

SCOTLAND
Debenhams
97 Argyle Street,
Glasgow G2 8AR
Tel: 0141 204 1036
Products: Guinot, Elemis

Esslemont & McIntosh
25 Union Street,
Aberdeen AB9 8TL
Tel: 01224 647983
Products: Guinot

Steiner Salons
Steiner Salons offer a full range of
hair and beauty treatments.

CENTRAL LONDON
Steiner Beauty
25A Lowndes Street,
London SW1
Tel: 0171 235 3154
Products: Elemis, Guinot, Phytomer
Ultratone

HOME COUNTIES
Steiner Hair & Beauty
Brent Cross Shopping Centre,
London NW4 1YP
Tel: 0181 202 4222
Products: Elemis, La Therapie,
Jessica, Ionithermie

MIDLANDS
Steiner Hair & Beauty
25 Corporation Street,
Birmingham B2 4LF
Tel: 0121 643 7242
Products: Elemis, La Therapie,
Ionithermie

NORTH EAST
Steiner Hair & Beauty
Unit 11/11A Albion Arcade
Bond Street Shopping Centre
Leeds LS1 5BR
Tel: 0113 2433299
Products: Guinot, Elemis

NORTH WEST
Steiner Hair & Beauty
Hoopers,
Alderley Road, Wilmslow,
Cheshire SK9 1PB
Tel: 01625 527469
Products: Elemis, La Therapie

BEAUTY BOOKSHELF

The Allergy Handbook
by Dr Keith Mumby
(Thorsons, £5.99)

Beating Stress at Work (£5.99) and
*Guide to Complementary Medicine and
Therapies* (£6.99),
both by Anne Woodham and
published by the Health Education
Authority.

*The Book of Vitamins and Healthfood
Supplements*
by Rita Greer and Dr Robert
Woodward
(Souvenir Press, £7.99)

The Cellulite Solution
by Dr Elizabeth Dancey
(Coronet Books, £4.99)

*The Complete Guide to Food Allergy &
Intolerance*
by Dr Jonathan Brostoff and Linda
Gamlin
(Bloomsbury Books – rumoured to
be going out of print, but worth
trying to track down secondhand as
it's the definitive handbook)

*A Consumer's Dictionary of Cosmetic
Ingredients*
(Crown, $12, US only)

The Cosmetic Ingredients Decoder
(Dynamo House, £5.99)
From good health food stores – also
available by mail from Wild Oats,
210 Westbourne Grove, London W11
2RH; send a cheque, plus an A5 sae
to the above address.

Creative Visualisation
by Shakti Gawain
(New World Library, £7.99)

*The Doctor's Vitamin and Mineral
Encyclopedia*
by Dr Sheldon Saul Hendler
(Simon & Schuster, US only, $13)

Eating Your Heart Out
by Julia Buckroyd
(Optima, £6.99)

The Encyclopedia of Flower Remedies
by Amanda Cochrane and Clare
Harvey
(Thorsons)

Fear of Food
by Genevieve Blais
(Women's Health, £5.99)

Food Combining in 30 Days
by Kathryn Marsden
(Thorsons, £4.99)

It's Not What You Eat, It's Why You Eat It
by Beechy Colclough
(Vermilion, £8.99)

No Sweat Fitness
by Tania Alexander
(Mainstream, £5.99)

Nutritional Medicine
by Dr Stephen Davies and Dr Alan Stewart
(Pan, £9.99)

The Psychology of Happiness
by Professor Michael Argyle
(Routledge, £9.99)

The Quick Guide to Beating Cellulite
by Liz Earle
(Boxtree, £3.99)

Restful Sleep
by Deepak Chopra
(Ryder, £7.99)

Thin Thighs for Life
by Dr Karen Burke
(Hamlyn, £9.99)

Thorsons Complete Guide to Vitamins and Minerals
by Leonard Mervyn
(Thorsons, £5.99)

Your Personal Trainer
by Anne Goodsell
(Boxtree, £12.99)

BEAUTY MUSIC SHELF

The Fitness Professionals
UEL,
Longbridge Road,
Dagenham,
Essex RM8 2AS
Tel: 0181 849 3567

BEAUTY VIDEO SHELF

Mr Motivator's MOT Workout
(Polygram, £12.99)

Perfect Curves
(Mind & Muscle, £12.99)
Tel: 0171 240 9861 to order.

Shape Up and Slim Down
(EMAP Invision, £12.99)

T'ai Chi, Alexander Technique, Stress Management
VG Productions
93c Priory Road,
London N8 8LY
For their catalogue,
tel: 0181 341 3556

Yoga for Beginners
by Maxine Tobias and John Patrick Sullivan
(£10.50)

CAMOUFLAGE MAKE-UP

British Association of Skin Camouflage (BASC)
send large sae to:
c/o Mrs Jane Goulding,
25 Blackhorse Drive,
Silkstone Common,
Barnsley,
South Yorkshire S75 4SD
Tel: 01226 790744

British Red Cross
The Therapeutic Beauty Care Service Department,
9 Grosvenor Crescent,
London SW1X 7EJ
Tel: 0171 235 5454

Changing Faces
1–2 Junction Mews
London W2 1PH
Tel: 0171 706 4232
Offers counselling for people with facial disfigurement including social skills, building confidence and advice on camouflage make-up.

Chelsea & Westminster Hospital Dermatology Unit
c/o Lady Adamson
369 Fulham Road,
London SW10 9NH
Tel: 0181 746 8167

Disfigurement Guidance Centre
c/o Mrs Doreen Trust, MBE,
PO Box 7,
Cupar,
Fife KY15 4PF
24-hour helpline: 0898 881905

Samples of the **Veil** range for face and body, with details of how to apply, are available for £2 (cheque or postal order) from:
1 & 2 Junction Mews,
London W2 1PN
Tel: 0171 706 4232

CELLULITE

Cellulène by Carilène,
Madecassol by Laroche Naveron and BODI
Available by mail order from:
Beauty by Post
50A High Street,
Poole,
Dorset BH15 1BT
Tel: 01249 819160

Cellulite scrubber by Opal London
Available by mail order from:
Norfolk Lavender Ltd
Caley Mill,
Heacham,
Kings Lynn
Norfolk PE31 7JE
Tel: 01485 570384 for catalogue.

CELLULITE THERAPIES

Ionithermie
For nearest salon and general info contact:
Ionithermie Ltd
9–11 Alma Road,
Windsor,
Berkshire SL4 3HU
Tel: 01753 833900

Mesotherapy
Dr Elisabeth Dancey
55 Wimpole Street,
London W1M 7DF
Tel: 0171 224 1330

COSMETICS AND SKINCARE

Aesop
Personal shoppers/mail order from:
Space NK,
41 Earlham Street,
London WC2H 9LD
Tel: 0171 636 2523

Anne Marie Börlind
For mail order and stockists:
Simply Nature,
Burwash Common,
East Sussex TN19 7LX
01435 882880

Australian Bodycare
For mail order and stockists:
Bodycare House,
15b Church Road,
Southborough,
Tunbridge Wells,
Kent TN4 0RX
Tel: 01892 511 296
(for teatree oil products)

Aveda
Distributors:
A.V.D. Cosmetics Ltd
75/77 Margaret Street,
London W1N 7HB
Tel: 0171 636 7911
Fax: 0171 636 6914

Aveda Brighton Purefumerie
22 East Street,
Brighton,
East Sussex
Tel: 01273 720203

Avon
To contact a local representative,
tel: 0800 663664

Beauty Through Herbs
1 St John's Square,
Thurso KW14 7AN
Tel: 01847 895584

Beauty Without Cruelty
For nearest stockist/mail order:
37 Avebury Avenue,
Tonbridge,
Kent TN9 1TL
Tel: 01732 365291

Beauty Look magnifying mirror
Available through make-up artist
Stephen Glass
Face Facts,
73 Wigmore Street,
London W1H 9LH
Tel: 0171 486 8287

Benefit Cosmetics
On sale at Space NK (see *Aesop*) and Harrods, Knightsbridge in person or by mail order.
Credit card phone line: 0800 730123

Bioforce
This natural health company is now producing ultra-gentle skincare based on violas. For stockists and mail order details, contact:
Bioforce (UK) Ltd,
Olympic Business Park,
Dundonald,
Ayrshire KA2 9BE
Tel: 01563 851177

Blackmore's
For stockists and mail order, contact:
The House of Blackmore,
37 Rothschild Road,
Chiswick,
London W4 5HT
Tel: 0181 987 8640

Bobbi Brown Essentials
On sale at Harrods, Knightsbridge
in person or by mail order.
Credit card phone line: 0800 730123
Also available at selected House of
Fraser stores.

The Body Shop by Mail
Hawthorn Road,
Wick,
Littlehampton,
West Sussex BN17 7LR
Tel: 01903 733888

Burt's Beeswax Lip Balm
Available in person or by mail order
from:
Natural Fact,
192 King's Road,
Chelsea,
London SW3 5XP
Tel: 0171 352 4283

Cellex-C
Available from:
Cellex-C Cosmaceutical Centre
12a Piccadilly Arcade,
London SW1
or, for mail order, call:
0345 402 214

Cosmetics à la Carte
For mail order:
102 Avro House,
Havelock Terrace,
London SW8 4AS
Tel: 0171 622 2318

Crabtree & Evelyn
Customer Services Department,
Freepost,
36 Milton Park,
Abingdon,
Oxfordshire OX14 4BR
Tel: 01235 862244

Dr Hauschka
For details of mail order and
stockists of this all-natural, bio-
dynamic skincare range, contact:
Elysia Natural Skin Care,
Haselor,
College Road,
Bromsgrove,
Worcestershire B60 2NF
Tel: 01527 832863

Efasit
Exclusive to Boots the Chemist

E'SPA
Available in 200 outlets around UK.
For details of nearest stockist and
mail order, telephone their hotline:
01483 454444

Fashion Fair
For nearest stockist,
Tel: 0171 581 5149

Flori Roberts
For nearest stockist,
Tel: 01279 421555.
Also available at
Selfridges,
400 Oxford Street,
London W1
Tel: 0171 318 3720 for mail order.

François Nars
Personal shoppers/mail order from:
Space NK
Tel: 0171 636 2523

Gatineau
For details from appointed Gatineau
salons, and by mail order:
Tel: 01753 620 881

Green & Pleasant
Stockists of many natural ranges of
cosmetics – visit them at:
129 Church Road,
London SW13 9HR
Tel: 0181 563 2349 for mail order.

Helena Rubinstein
Customer care line
For info on all products and mail
order:
Tel: 01732 741000

Hobé Aroma Cosmetics
Natural skincare
PO Box 3760,
London NW3 4YQ
Tel: 0171 483 0469 for mail order

I Coloniali
For stockists and mail order:
Tel: 0181 286 6688

Inchwrap
Finders International Ltd
Orchard House
Winchet Hill
Goudhurst
Kent TN17 1JY
Tel: 01580 211055

Jeanine Lobell's Stila
Personal shoppers/mail order from:
Space NK,
41 Earlham Street,
London WC2
Tel: 0171 379 7000

Joshua Galvin
Exclusive to Superdrug.
Jurlique
For stockists and mail order:
Tel: 0181 995 3948

Juvena
Exclusive to Harrods, who will mail
order:
Tel: 0171 734 1234, ex. 2287

KC Oils
Excellent blended aromatherapy oils
for bathing and massage, in
beautiful bottles. Mail order from:
KC Oils for Shensé,
6 Porton Court,
Portsmouth Road,
Surbiton KT6 4HY
Tel: 0181 399 2934

Kiehl's
See listing under *Hair*

Liz Earle skincare range
Mail order from:
PO Box 7832,
London SW15 6YA
or from QVC, The TV Shopping
Channel.

Lorac Range
created by Carol Shaw
Personal shoppers/mail order from:
Space NK,
41 Earlham Street,
London WC2H 9LP
Tel: 0171 379 7030

M.A.C. (Make-up Arts Cosmetics)
Available from:
109 King's Road,
London SW3 4PA
Tel: 0171 349 0601
also at:
Harvey Nichols,
Knightsbridge.
They also have a limited re-ordering
service by mail at the King's Road
shop.

Maggie Hunt's Make-up Brushes
Order from:
Lion Brush Ltd,
Planet Place,
Killingworth,
Newcastle-upon-Tyne
NE122 0RZ

Mary Kohr
For details of appointed salons:
Tel: 01344 873 123

Nu-Skin
For details of stockists:
Tel: 01494 443 484

Nutri-Metics International
For details of stockists:
Tel: 01908 262 020

Origins
Available from Harrods and major
branches of House of Fraser. For
mail order:
Tel: 0171 730 1234, ext.3371

Philosophy
Available from Harrods, Liberty and
Space NK. For mail order:
Tel:0171 636 2523

Rochas
For info. on all products and mail
order:
Tel: 01902 422 311, ext. 3595

Department Store Mail Order

Harrods Ltd
Grant Way,
off Syon Lane,
Isleworth,
Middlesex TW7 5QD
Credit card phone line: 0800 730123

or contact the relevant department
in the store:
Harrods Ltd
87–135 Brompton Road,
Knightsbridge,
London SW1X 7XL
Tel: 0171 730 1234

Harvey Nichols
109–125 Knightsbridge,
London SW1X 7RJ
Tel: 0171 235 5000 and speak to
relevant department.

Liberty Mail Order Department
Regent Street,
London W1R 6AH
Tel: 0171 734 1234

Muji
26 Great Marlborough Street,
London W1V 1HL
Tel: 0171 494 1197

Selfridges
400 Oxford Street,
London W1A 1AB
Tel: 0171 629 1234 and speak to
relevant department.

Space NK
41 Earlham Street,
London WC2H 9LD
Tel: 0171 636 2523

Make-Up Lessons and Artists
Chanel In-Store Travelling Beauty Schools
Tel: 0171 493 3836 for further info.

Clarins 'Mirror Image Consultation'
Tel: 0171 629 2979 for details.

Clinique
Make-up lessons over the counter.
Tel: 0171 409 6951 for local counters.

Colourings at The Body Shop
Offer 30-minute make-overs.
Contact your local branch of The
Body Shop for an appointment.

Cosmetics à la Carte
Home visits from make-up artists or
lessons at their own studio.
Tel: 0171 622 2318 for details.

Estée Lauder
'Colour on Camera' is a travelling
service by which a trained make-up
artist will give you a lesson while
filming the new look for you.
Tel: 0171 409 6917 for details.
Consultations also available at Estée
Lauder counters. Advisable to book.

The Glauca Rossi School of Make-up
10 Sutherland Avenue,
London W9 2HQ
Tel: 0171 289 7485
Fax: 0171 286 0073

Helena Rubinstein
Travelling make-up artists regularly
visit their counters to give lessons.
Tel: 0171 730 1234, ext 5995, for
details of artists in your area.

Joan Price Face Place
33 Cadogan Street,
Chelsea,
London SW3 2PP
Tel: 0171 589 9062

Kanebo 'Beauty School'
Occasional in-store event.
Tel: 01635 46362 for details.

Lancôme
Lessons tailored to individual
requirements at their private
'studios'.
Tel: 0171 629 8867 for details.

The London Esthetique
75/77 Margaret Street,
London W1N 7HB
Tel: 0171 636 1893
Fax: 0171 636 6914

The Make-up Workshop
Watkins Farm,
Peaceful Lane,
Holwell,
Dorset DT9 5LW
Tel: 01963 23037
Contact: Amanda Jackson-Sytner

Prescriptives
'On Location' workshops move
from store to store.
Tel: 0171 409 6937 for details.

**Princess Marcella Borghese Colour
Wardrobe**
Tel: 0171 629 1699 for details.

Stephen Glass at Face Facts
73 Wigmore Street,
Saint Christopher's Place,
London W1H 9LH
Tel: 0171 486 8287
Fax: 0171 436 0098

Shiseido
Over-the-counter lessons and
occasional workshops.
Tel: 0171 792 1575 for details.

Martha Hill
Order line: 01780 450259

Neal's Yard Remedies
For nearest stockist,
tel: 0171 498 1686
For mail order:
5 Golden Cross,
Cornmarket Street,
Oxford OX1 3EU
Tel: 01865 245436

Philip B (Berkowitz)
Botanical hair & treatment range
Mail order in the UK from:
Space NK,
41 Earlham Street,
London WC2H 9LD
Tel: 0171 379 7030

Rachel Perry natural products
Mail order from:
Nutri-Centre,
7 Park Crescent,
London W1N 3HE
Tel: 0171 436 5122

Screen Face
24 Powis Terrace,
London W11 1JH
Tel: 0171 221 8289
Fax: 0171 792 9357

The Sher System
30 New Bond Street,
London W1Y 4HD
Tel: 0171 499 4022

Shiseido
Available in large department stores
throughout the UK.

Shu Uemura
On sale at Harvey Nichols, London,
in person or by mail order.
Tel: 0171 235 2375

Also on sale at:
Liberty, Regent Street, London
and Space NK, Covent Garden,
London.
For details of make-up parties and
general enquiries contact Head
Office at:
Unit 7, The Quadrangle,
49 Atalanta Street,
London SW6 6TU
Tel: 0171 386 0996

St Ives
St Ives Customer Services,
Alberto Culver Co,
Alberto Road,
Swansea SA6 8RG
Tel: 01792 700118

**Tweezerman's eyelash curlers
and tweezers**
Distributors:
AVD Cosmetics Ltd,
75/77 Margaret Street,
London W1N 7HB
Tel: 0171 636 7911
Fax: 0171 636 6914

Urtekram
For details of this natural and
organic Danish skincare and
haircare range, tel: Barbara Coles on
0171 229 7545
or write to:
269 Portobello Road,
London W11 1LR

Vichy Skin Diagnostics
For an appointment, contact:
Fenwicks, Brent Cross
Tel: 0181 202 0262

Weleda (UK) Ltd
For stockists/mail order:
Heanor Road,
Ilkeston,
Derbyshire DE7 8DR
Tel: 0115 944 8200

Yves Rocher
664 Victoria Road,
South Ruislip,
Middlesex HA4 0NY
Mail order natural skincare.
Tel: 0181 845 1222

COSMETIC SURGERY & COSMETIC DENTISTRY

**British Association of Aesthetic
Plastic Surgeons**
35–43 Lincoln's Inn Fields,
London WC2A 3PN
Tel: 0171 405 2234
Send large first-class sae for list of
accredited cosmetic plastic surgeons.

**British Association of
Dermatologists**
19 Fitzroy Square,
London W1P 5HQ
Tel: 0171 383 0266

**British Association of Plastic
Surgeons**
The Royal College of Surgeons,
35 Lincoln's Inn Fields,
London WC2A 3PN
Tel: 0171 831 5161

British Dental Association
64 Wimpole Street,
London W1M 8AL
Tel: 0171 935 3963

**British Academy of Aesthetic
Dentists**
Suite 152,
84 Marylebone High Street,
London W1M 3DE
Tel: 0171 636 9933
Will send list of qualified dentists in
UK specialising in restorative work
with an aesthetic bias, also details of
reciprocal organisations in rest of
Europe and US.

Stanley Kay
Harley Street Dental Theatre,
Apt 6, 103/105 Harley Street,
London W1N HHD
Tel: 0171 486 1059

Venus Forum
c/o Royal Society of Medicine,
1 Wimpole Street,
London W1M 8AE
Tel: 0171 290 2987

Top Facial Cosmetic Surgeons
Dev Basra
111 Harley Street,
London W1N 1DG
Tel: 0171 486 8055

John Bowen
Flat 1,
30 Harley Street,
London W1N 1AB
Tel: 0171 636 0955

John Celin
34 Hans Road,
London SW3 1RW
Tel: 0171 225 0179

Douglas Harrison
Flat 33,
Harmont House,
20 Harley Street,
London W1N 1AA
Tel: 0171 935 6184

Barry Jones
14a Upper Wimpole Street,
London W1M 7TB
Tel: 0171 935 1938

Basim Matti and Freddie Nicolle
Flat 2, 30 Harley Street,
London W1N 1AB
Tel: 0171 637 9595

Magdi Saad
The Princess Margaret Hospital,
Osborne Road,
Windsor,
Berkshire SL4 3SJ
Tel: 01753 851753

Charles Volkers
29 Hans Place,
London SW1X 0JY
Tel: 0171 584 7435

Norman Waterhouse
55 Harley Street,
London W1N 1DD
0171 637 9684

COSMETO-DERMATOLOGIST

Dr Nicholas Lowe
15 Harley Street,
London W1N 1DA
Tel: 0171 636 7792

DERMATOLOGISTS

British Association of Dermatologists
19 Fitzroy Square,
London W1P 5HQ
Tel: 0171 383 0266

ELECTROLYSIS

British Association of Electrolysists
8 Chaul End Road,
Caddington,
Bedfordshire LU1 4AS
Tel: 01582 487743

EXERCISE

To find a good teacher, look for established qualifications – RSA (Royal Society of Arts), sports science degrees, ACE (American Council of Exercise) and EFIC are all well respected.

To find nearest exercise class or personal trainer, send sae, stating which information you need, to:

The Exercise Association of England
Unit 4,
Angel Gate,
City Road,
London EC1V 2PT

or, for one-to-one training, write to:
The Association of Personal Trainers
Suite 2,
8 Bedford Court,
London WC2E 9OV
Tel: 0171 836 1102
Fax: 0171 379 5552

or send sae to:
The National Register of Personal Fitness Trainers
Thornton House,
Thornton Road,
London SW19 4NG
Tel: 0181 944 6688

Dance
For list of instructors in your area, send large sae, stating which type of dance you are interested in, to:
Imperial Society of Teachers of Dancing (ISTD)
Imperial House,
22–26 Paul Street,
London EC2A 4QE
Tel: 0171 377 1577

Danceworks
Offers a wide choice of dance lessons at:
16 Balderton Street,
London W1Y 1TF
Tel: 0171 629 6183

Exercise Equipment
Energy Express
36 Beech Lane,
Kislingbury,
Northamptonshire NN7 4AL
For price list and order form,
Tel: 01604 832843
They stock hand, wrist and ankle weights and resistance bands.

Medau – the Art of Energy
Available by mail order from:
Lucy Jackson,
23 Springfield Road,
St Johns Wood,
London NW8 0QJ
Tel: 0171 624 3580

The Physical Company
Cherry Cottage,
Hedsor Road,
Bourne End,
Bucks SL8 5DH
Tel: 01628 520208
For mail order of PT Cross Trainer.

Reebok Step and Kettler Trampette
can be obtained from Olympus Sports.
Tel: 0116 265 2484 for stockists.

EYES

David Clulow
For details of your nearest branch, contact:
Jenny de Couteau,
The Optika Clulow Group,
Equitable House,
Lyon Road,
Harrow,
Middlesex HA1 2EW
Tel: 0181 863 8111

Cutler & Gross
16 Knightsbridge Green,
London SW1
Tel: 0171 823 8445
Fashion frames for prescription lenses.

Dollond & Aitchison
For details of your nearest branch, contact:
1323 Coventry Road,
Yardley,
Birmingham B25 8LP
Tel: 0121 706 6133

FACIALS

See also *Beauty Salons*

Clarins
For nearest salon contact:
4 Queen Street,
London W1X 8ND
Tel: 0171 629 2979

For nearest salon contact:
59A Connaught Street,
London W2 2BB
Tel: 0171 262 0403

Dr Hauschka
Details of local therapists and outlets and mail order from:
Elysia Natural Skin Care,
Haselor, College Road,
Bromsgrove,
Worcestershire B60 2NF
Tel/fax: 01527 832863

Elemis
at Harrods and Selfridges, London and 120 beauty salons across the UK.
For details and mail order contact:
57–65 The Broadway,
Stanmore,
Middlesex HA7 4DU
Tel: 0181 954 8033

Janet Filderman
15 Wyndham Place,
London W1
Tel: 0171 262 7034

Eve Lom
Salon:
Tel: 0171 935 9988
Mail order from:
3 Westmead Corner,
Carshalton,
Surrey
Tel: 0181 661 7991

Jo Malone
Shop: 154 Walton Street,
London SW3 2JL
Tel: 0171 581 1101
Mail order: 0171 720 0202

Repêchage
For nearest salon write/tel:
5 Hugh Business Park,
Bacup Road,
Waterfoot,
Rossendal,
Lancashire BB4 7BX
Tel: 01706 211058

Thalgo
For nationwide outlets and mail order contact:
Elgin House,
51 Mill Harbour,
Docklands,
London E14 9TD
Tel: 0171 512 0872

FRAGRANCE

Annick Goutal
For mail order of her perfumes contact:
Les Senteurs,
227 Ebury Street,
London SW1W 8UT
Tel: 0171 730 2322
Les Senteurs' catalogue costs £3, redeemable against your first purchase; they also provide samples of fragrances at £1 each.

L'Artisan Parfumeur
will send their fragrance La Haïe Fleurie du Hameau by mail order from:
17 Cale Street,
London SW3 3QR
Tel: 0171 352 4196

Barney's Route du Thé
Mail order in the UK from:
Space NK,
41 Earlham Street,
London WC2
Tel: 0171 379 7030

Caron
Royal Bain de Champagne and
Tabac Blond available at their
counter or from Harrods mail order.
Credit card phoneline:
0800 730123

Chanel
Bois des Iles and Cuir de Russie
available exclusively through Chanel
fashion boutiques internationally.
London boutiques are at:
26 Bond Street,
London W1
Tel: 0171 493 5040
and
31 Sloane Street,
London SW1
Tel: 0171 235 6631

Chopard's Casmir
Available from selected Boots and
department stores.

Donna Karan's New York
Available from Harvey Nichols,
Harrods, Selfridges and selected
House of Fraser stores.
Also from Harrods mail order.
Credit card phoneline: 0800 730123

Geo F. Trumper
Extract of Limes Toiletries – for mail
order contact them at:
166 Fairbridge Road,
London N19 3HT
Tel: 0171 263 1721
Fax: 0171 281 9337
Their catalogue is free of charge.

Guerlain
Jicky and Mitsouko widely available
nationwide; Après l'Ondée
exclusively at their counter or from
Harrods mail order.
Credit card phoneline: 0800 730123

Halcyon Days
Shop: 14 Brook Street,
London W1
Tel: 0171 629 8811
Mail order: 0800 515925

Patricia de Nicolaï
For mail order of Patricia de Nicolaï
fragrances, including New York,
contact:
Les Senteurs,
(see *Annick Goutal*)

Perfumer's Workshop
Tea Rose is available from Harrods.

Shiseido
Feminité du Bois is widely available.
Or, if in Paris, visit their wonderful
boutique at:

Les Salons du Palais Royal,
Jardins du Palais Royal,
142 Galerie de Valois,
25 Rue de Valois,
75001 Paris
Tel: + 33 (1) 49 27 09 09
Fax: + 33 (1) 49 27 92 912

Thierry Mugler
Angel – widely available.

Perfumes by Mail Order

Anitra Earle Perfume Detective
21 East Chestnut Street,
Chicago,
Illinois 60611,
USA

L'Artisan Parfumeur
17 Cale Street,
London SW3 3QR
Tel: 0171 352 4196

The Crown Perfumery Co Ltd
35 Park Street,
Mayfair,
London W1Y 4HL
Freephone: 0800 220284 (UK only)
International tel: 0171 493 1717

Czech & Speake
244–254 Cambridge Heath Road,
London E2 9DA
Tel: 0181 980 4567

Floris Ltd
89 Jermyn Street,
London SW1Y 6JH
Tel: 0171 930 2885

Jo Malone Sent-a-Scent
Warriner Gardens,
London SW11 4XW
Tel: 0171 720 0202

Penhaligon's Ltd
Crusader Estate,
167 Hermitage Road,
London N4 1LZ
Freephone: 0800 716108 (UK only)
International tel: 0181 880 2050

Scent Direct Fragrances Worldwide
A gift delivery service offering 150
of the world's favourite fragrances,
beautifully packaged and shipped
anywhere in the world. For
details/to order, write to:
Scent Direct,
Bell Vale Lane,
Haslemere,
Surrey GU27 3DJ
Tel: 01428 654575

Les Senteurs
227 Ebury Street,
London SW1W 8UT
Tel: 0171 730 2322

HAIR

Top Hairdressers in the UK
Always check prices when booking
an appointment.

CENTRAL LONDON
Antenna
27a Kensington Church Street,
London W8
Tel: 0171 938 1866

Burlingtons
41 Paddington Street,
London W1
Tel: 0171 935 0140

**The Steven Carey Hair and Beauty
Salon**
112 Mount Street,
London W1
Tel: 0171 495 5353

Nicky Clarke
130 Mount Street,
London W1
Tel: 0171 491 4700

Cobella Hair and Beauty
52 Shepherd Market,
London W1
Tel: 0171 409 0606/0552

Neville Daniel Hair and Beauty
25a Basil Street,
London SW3
Tel: 0171 245 6151

Edmonds
5 Pont Street,
London SW1
Tel: 0171 589 5958

John Frieda
4 Aldford Street,
London W1
Tel: 0171 491 0840

Daniel Galvin
42–44 George Street,
London W1
Tel: 0171 486 9661

The Hair Shop
53 St Martin's Lane,
London WC2
Tel: 0171 242 3737/836 5241

Jo Hansford
19 Mount Street,
London W1
Tel: 0171 495 7774

Harrods Hair and Beauty Salon
Knightsbridge,
London SW1
Tel: 0171 584 8881/581 2021

Daniel Hersheson
45 Conduit Street,
London W1
Tel: 0171 434 1747

Andrew Jose
1 Charlotte Street,
London W1
Tel: 0171 323 4679

Le Léon
2a Ladbroke Grove,
London W11
Tel: 0171 792 9122

MacGregor and McLaughlin
327 King's Road,
London SW3
Tel: 0171 352 9291

Mahogany
17 St George Street,
London W1
Tel: 0171 629 3121
(also Oxford tel: 01865
248143/52494/790245,
Bath tel: 01225 466967)

Mane Line
22 Weighhouse Street,
London W1
Tel: 0171 493 4952/3

Martin Maxey
12 Motcomb Street,
London SW1
Tel: 0171 245 0008

Denise McAdam
14 Hay Hill,
London W1
Tel: 0171 499 8079/493 2461

Michaeljohn
25 Albemarle Street,
London W1
Tel: 0171 629 6969

Paul Nath
224 Shaftesbury Ave,
London WC2
Tel: 0171 836 7152/240 0311

Neville Hair and Beauty
5 Pont Street,
London SW1
Tel: 0171 235 3654

NFB
4 Lumley Street,
London W1
Tel: 0171 499 7831/408 2419

Parsons Skött
243 Westbourne Grove,
London W11
Tel: 0171 243 0939

Vidal Sassoon
60 South Molton Street,
London W1
Tel: 0171 491 8848

Shipton, Leighton & Lowe
18 New Cavendish Street,
London W1
Tel: 0171 487 4048

Trevor Sorbie
10 Russell Street,
London WC2
Tel: 0171 379 6901/240 3816

Toni and Guy
10–12 Davies Street,
London W1
Tel: 0171 629 8348

Gary Wallis
6/7 Lowndes Court,
Carnaby Street,
London W1
Tel: 0171 734 9086/494 1062

Windle
41 Shorts Gardens,
London WC2
Tel: 0171 497 2393

James Worrall
6 Camden Road,
London NW1
Tel: 0171 284 3707

Worthingtons
34 Great Queen Street,
London WC2
Tel: 0171 831 5303

Zah
59 George Street,
London W1
Tel: 0171 935 4441

EAST ANGLIA
Scruffs
76 Mill Road,
Cambridge
Tel: 01223 67672

Level One
14 Highview Parade,
Woodford Avenue,
Gant's Hill,
Essex
Tel: 0181 550 7073

Falltricks
146 Balgores Lane,
Gidea Park,
Essex
Tel: 01708 731753

W1 Hair Design
6 Clements Road,
Ilford,
Essex
Tel: 0181 478 3852

Laurens d'Auray
721 London Road,
Westcliff-on-Sea,
Essex
Tel: 01702 344626

John Oliver Haircutters
13 Red Lion Street,
Norwich
Tel: 01603 627620

HOME COUNTIES
Haringtons
39 Queen Street,
Maidenhead,
Berkshire
Tel: 01628 36747

Forresters
227 Shinfield Road,
Reading,
Berkshire
Tel: 01734 872860

Montage
28 George V Place,
Thames Ave,
Windsor,
Berkshire
Tel: 01753 832 132

Hair Exchange
Exchange House,
458 Midsummer Boulevard,
Central Milton Keynes,
Buckinghamshire
Tel: 01908 230133

Blushes
76 Westgate Street,
Gloucester
Tel: 01452 528342

Storm Hairdressing
10–11a Bedford Place,
Southampton, Hampshire
Tel: 01703 237414

Guy Kremer
Stonemasons Court,
67 Parchment Street,
Winchester,
Hampshire
Tel: 01962 860149/840785

Jon Pereira-Santos at **Toni & Guy,**
Winchester
2 St George's Street,
Winchester,
Hampshire SO23 8BG
Tel: 01962 840422

Unermans
112 Cockfosters Road,
Cockfosters, Hertfordshire
Tel: 0181 449 8444

Greys Hair & Body Shop
62 Spencer Street,
St Albans,
Hertfordshire
Tel: 01727 838909

Altered Image
77 High Street,
Tring
Hertfordshire
Tel: 01442 822609

Altered Image
19 Temple Street,
Birmingham
Tel: 0121 643 1919

Martin Gold
30 The Broadway,
Stanmore,
Middx
Tel: 0181 954 0084

John of Chobham
21 High Street,
Chobham,
Surrey
Tel: 01276 857249

John Carne
270–272 High Street,
Guildford,
Surrey
Tel: 01483 506402/572420

Graduates
2 High Street,
Purley,
Surrey
Tel: 0181 668 8855

The Business Two
7 Grove Road,
Sutton,
Surrey
Tel: 0181 642 4433/643 6785

R J Hair & Beauty
129 Queen's Road,
Brighton,
East Sussex
Tel: 01273 202564

MIDLANDS
Obsession
5 Castle Dyke, Wade Street,
Lichfield,
Staffordsshire
Tel: 01543 254137

Charles Russell
9 Chads Square,
Hawthorn Road,
Edgbaston, Birmingham
Tel: 0121 454 8927/0293

Suyo Hair
71 High Street,
Harborne,
Birmingham
Tel: 0121 427 3229

Giannini
103 Coventry Street,
Kidderminster,
Worcs
Tel: 01562 66411
also at Stourbridge,
Tel: 01384 390720;
Hagley, Tel: 01562 882447;
Birmingham, Tel: 0121 633 0111

Barrows Hairdressing Company
124 High Street,
Pershore,
Worcestershire
Tel: 01386 561275

Julie Drew Hairdressing
8 Mealcheapen Street,
Worcester,
Worcestershire
Tel: 01905 23996

NORTH EAST
Stephen Russell
108 High Street,
Yarm,
Cleveland
Tel: 01642 788461

Mark Scott Hair Design
1st Floor,
6 St Peter's Church Yard,
Derby
Tel: 01332 340538

Bob's Hair Company
20–24 Abbeygate,
Grimsby,
South Humberside
Tel: 01472 362611

Y Salon
97 Clayton Street,
Newcastle,
Tyne & Wear
Tel: 0191 261 0671

The Mark Hill Salon
Hog Lane,
Kirkella, Hull,
Yorkshire
Tel: 01482 656424

Lifestyle Hair & Beauty Centre
48 Jameson Street,
Hull,
Yorkshire
Tel: 01482 225800

NORTH WEST
September Hair Studio
15-17 Queens Street,
Blackpool,
Lancashire
Tel: 01253 28394

Ralph Kleeli Hair
1 Churchbank,
Bolton,
Lancashire
Tel: 01204 361926

Andrew Collinge Hair & Beauty
14 St John's Centre,
Liverpool
Tel: 0151 709 7131

Barbara Daley Hair & Beauty
4 Concourse House,
Lime Street,
Liverpool
Tel: 0151 709 7974

Razor's Edge
1 Royal Exchange Arcade,
Manchester
Tel: 0161 832 7798

also at:
26 Fountain Street,
Manchester
Tel: 0161 832 7747

Ian Henry Hairteam
290 Hoylake Road,
Moreton,
Wirral
Tel: 0151 677 9032

also at:
67 Seaview Road,
Wallasey,
Merseyside
Tel: 0151 639 2862

14 High Street,
Neston,
South Wirral
Tel: 0151 336 8552

141 Ford Road,
Upton,
Wirral
Tel: 0151 606 0011

SOUTH WEST
Marc Sampson Hairdressing
44 Polkyth Road,
St Austell,
Cornwall
Tel: 01726 67012

The Andrew Hill Salon
8 Powderham Road,
Newton Abbot,
Devon
Tel: 01626 65184

Joseph Harling
6 Church Street,
Bradford-on-Avon,
Wiltshire
Tel: 01225 863357

Goldsworthy's Hairdressing
1 Catherine Street,
Swindon,
Wiltshire
Tel: 01793 523817

The Body Beautiful
6 Church Walk,
Trowbridge,
Wiltshire
Tel: 01225 754182

WALES
Ken Picton's Visuals
22–24 Castle Arcade,
Cardiff
Tel: 01222 228688

Andrew Price
6–9 The Mews,
Upper Frog Street,
Tenby,
Dyfed
Tel: 01834 842266

SCOTLAND
Cheynes Hairdressing
46a George Street,
Edinburgh
Tel: 0131 220 0777

also at:
45 York Place,
Edinburgh
Tel: 0131 558 1010

57 South Bridge,
Edinburgh
Tel: 0131 556 0108

3 Drumsheugh Place,
Queensferry Street,
Edinburgh
Tel: 0131 225 2234

Klownz Hair Ltd
1 North West Circus Place,
Edinburgh
Tel: 0131 226 4565

Charlie Miller
13 Stafford Street,
Edinburgh
Tel: 0131 226 5550/1

Paterson SA
129 Lothian Road,
Edinburgh
Tel: 0131 228 5252

Studio One International
17 North Bridge,
Edinburgh
Tel: 0131 557 6968

Dom Migele
7–9 Tolbooth Street,
Kirkcaldy,
Fife
Tel: 01592 203116

Brian Grieve Hairdressing
27 Kirkwynd,
Kirkcaldy,
Fife
Tel: 01592 260516

Alan Edwards Salon
The Briggait,
Bridgegate,
Glasgow
Tel: 0141 552 5232

also at:
56-58 Wilson Street,
Glasgow
Tel: 0141 552 5282

Rita Rusk International
49 West Nile Street,
Glasgow
Tel: 0141 221 1472

John Gillespie Salon
26 St John's Street,
Perth
Tel: 01738 624068

Charlie Taylor Hair & Beauty
20-28 South Methven Street,
Perth
Tel: 01738 633221/633451

N. IRELAND
David Aumonier
1 Little Victoria Street,
Belfast
Tel: 01232 333774

Brave New World
427a Lisburn Road,
Belfast
Tel: 01232 666394

Hair Traffic
58 Wellington Place,
Belfast
Tel: 01232 320837/321150

Keith Kane Hair International
Unit 8,
Town & Country Shopping Centre,
Carryduff,
Belfast
Tel: 01232 813622

The Stafford Salon
45 Queen Street,
Belfast
Tel: 01232 234432

Gatsby International
10a Rathmore Road,
Bangor,
County Down
01247 461244

*List compiled by Jacki Wadeson,
contributing editor to Hair Magazine*

**Hair Products –
Mail Order**
Nicky Clarke Hairomatherapy
Stockists throughout UK including
leading Chemists, Supermarkets
and Department Stores.

La Biosthetique
For details of your nearest salon
contact:
143A Bellevue Road,
Shrewsbury SY3 7NN
Tel: 01743 236246

Kiehl's
UK Mail Order service from Space
NK,
41 Earlham Street,
London WC2
Tel: 0171 379 7030

Philip Kingsley Trichological Clinic
54 Green Street,
London W1Y 3RH
Tel: 0171 629 4004
Larkhall Swiss Laboratories –
hair sample testing to determine
mineral status.
Tel: 0181 874 1130

J.H. Lazartigue
Diagnostic Advisory Hair Centre
20 James Street,
London W1M 5HN
Tel: 0171 629 2250
For mail order including free
diagnostic service, you can also
write or telephone between 10am
and 6pm Mon–Sat.

Lazartigue at Selfridges
Tel: 0171 629 1234

Sam Mcknight
Styling range available from Boots
the Chemists, nationwide.

Molton Brown
Shop: 58 South Molton Street,
London W1Y 1HH
Tel: 0171 499 6474
or by mail order from:
M.B. by Mail,
PO Box 2514,
London NW6 1SR
Tel: 0171 625 6550

Nexxus
For stockists of their products
(including Simply Silver Toning
Shampoo and Clarifying Shampoo
and Treatment):
Unit 2,
Plot 46,
Colville Road,
Acton,
London W3 8BL

Phyto
11 Boundary Passage,
London E2 7JE
For expert advice, mail order and
stockists:
Tel: 0171 613 0265

Redken Laboratories
Contact Sheila Steele for details of
your nearest stockist on:
01908 247253 (direct line) or
01908 247247 (switchboard)

Sebastian
Laminates range
For info, stockists and mail order
Tel: 0345 125545

Schwarzkopf
Aylesbury, Buckinghamshire.
For stockists:
Tel: 01296 314000

Trichologists, Institute of
Send sae for list of members to:
Stockwell Road,
London SW9 9SU

Home Hairdressing

Neville Daniel
Tel: 0171 245 6151

John Frieda
Tel: 0171 491 0840

Daniel Galvin
Tel: 0171 486 8601

Michaeljohn
Tel: 0171 491 4401

Neville
Tel: 0171 235 3654

Charles Worthington
(weddings only)
Tel: 0171 831 5303

Wigs & Hairpieces

Angels & Bermans
119 Shaftesbury Avenue,
London WC2 8AE
Tel: 0171 836 5678
Synthetic wigs with emphasis on
fun.

Banbury Postiche
Little Bourton House,
Southam Road,
Banbury,
Oxfordshire OX16 7SR
Tel: 01295 750606
Wide range of wigs, synthetic fibre.

Trendco
Wigs and hairpieces in modacrylic
fibre. They have some really fun
styles and colours.
For catalogue costing £5,
Tel: 01273 774977

For those who've lost hair through illness
N.B. These wigs tend to be costly.

John Clifton at Mandeville Wigs
12 Upper Mall,
London W6 9TA
Tel: 0181 741 5959
Matched human hair wigs.

Gordon Grieve at Wig Creations
62 Lancaster Mews,
London W2 3QG
Tel: 0171 402 4488
Wigs made of matched human hair.
Fittings at home or hospital if
necessary.

For support and info, contact:
**Hairline International (The Alopecia
Patients Society)**

IMAGE

Federation of Image Consultants
For registry of recommended
consultants countrywide.
Tel: 0956 701018

JET LAG

Daniele Ryman's anti-jet lag packs
available from:
Daniele Ryman Boutique
107b Piccadilly,
London W1
Tel: 0171 753 6708

Aroma Therapeutics Jet Set kit is
available from:
The Barn Business Centre
Great Rissington,
Gloucestershire GL54 2HL
Tel: 01451 822444

Melatonin tablets are available by
mail order from:
Nutrizec
PO Box 3102,
Wokingham,
Berkshire RG41 3YA
Tel: 01734 629120

NAILS

Chelsea Nail Bar
Tel: 0171 225 3889

The Country Club
Tel: 0171 731 4346

Delore
Nail hardener
For nearest stockist,
Tel: Original Additions on:
0181 573 9907

also from:
Amazing Nails
Tel: 0171 355 3634 for
appointments, mail order and
helpline.

The International Nail Association
Call 0171 610 6995 for member
salons and advice.

Jessica
For member salons and advice:
The Natural Nail Company Ltd,
57 Marchmont Street,
London WC1N 1AP
Tel: 0171 713 7793
Fax: 0171 713 7796

Nailtiques
A professional product available
through beauty salons and
hairdressers.
For nearest salon
Tel: 01543 480100.
Fax: 01543 480201

Repair-a-Nail
The Jessica salons (see left) stock
this product.

Super Nail of Los Angeles
Zoom products available in stores
and salons for home use. Try the 15-
minute demonstration of how to use
the products. They also offer
Backscratchers (fibreglass nail
extensions), only available
professionally. For further info
contact their head office at:
101 Crawford Street,
London W1H 1AN
Tel: 0171 723 1163

NON-SURGICAL FACE LIFTS

Amstrad Integra – available from
Boots the chemists.

Bio-Therapeutics
For nearest salon,
Tel: 01926 633020

**CACI (Computer Aided
Cosmetology Instrument)**
For nearest salon contact:
Micromode Medical Ltd,
11 Heath Street,
London NW3 6TP
Tel: 0171 431 1033

Cleo
Available from
Love Ltd,
PO Box 17,
Morley,
Leeds LS27 9EN
Tel: 01132 527744

Dibitron
For nearest salon,
Tel: 0181 202 2264

Eva Fraser's Facial Workout Studio
The Studio,
St Mary Abbots,
Vicarage Gate,
London W8 4HN
Tel: 0171 937 6616/9992

Eva Fraser's book, *Eva Fraser's Facial
Workout*, is published by Penguin
and the video distributed by
Polygram. Both are widely available.

Isolift – available from
Elizabeth Nicoll Products,
PO Box 260,
Bedford MK42 0JW
Tel orders: 01234 365080

Rejuvanessence
Send sae for details of 70
regional facial massage
therapists to:
Belle Vue Lodge,
91 Cheyne Walk,
London SW10 0DQ
Tel: 0171 352 8458

NUTRITION

**Council for Nutrition Education
and Therapy**
For list of local practitioners send
£2 to:
34 Wadham Road,
London SW15 2LR

Diet Breakers,
Barford St Michael,
Banbury,
Oxfordshire OX15 0UA
Send large sae for details.

Eating Disorders Association
Sackville Place,
44 Magdalen Street,
Norwich NR3 1JU
General helpline open
9am–6.30pm, Mon to Fri.
Tel: 01603 621414.
Youth Helpline (18 years &under),
open 4pm–6pm, Mon to Fri.
Tel: 01603 765050
For info and membership details,
write enclosing a large sae.

Overeaters Anonymous
For info, send sae or tel:
PO Box 19,
Stretford,
Manchester M32 9ED
Tel: 0161 762 9348

**Society for the Promotion of
Nutritional Therapy**
PO Box 47,
Heathfield,
East Sussex TN21 8ZX
Tel: 01435 867007
Send sae plus £1 for list of
therapists and info.

**Women's Nutritional Advisory
Service**
PO Box 268,
Lewes,
East Sussex BN7 2QN
Tel: 01273 487366

Supplements
BioCare, Blackmore's, Higher
Nature, Missing Link,
PharmaNord, Quest, Scotia
Pharmaceuticals, Solgar,
Creighton's Naturally. Also a
selection of brands of **Cat's Claw.**
All available for worldwide mail
order (pre-payment by
cheque/credit card) from:
**The Nutri-Centre at The Hale
Clinic**
7 Park Crescent,
London W1N 3HE
Tel: 0171 436 5122

PharmaNord and Quest are also
available at all branches of
Holland & Barrett.

Blackmore's UK Ltd
For nearest stockist/mail order
contact:
37 Rothschild Road,
London W4 5HT
Tel: 0181 987 8640

Co-enzyme Q10
Mail order from:
Nature's Best,
Freepost,
Tunbridge Wells,
Kent TN2 3EQ
Tel: 01892 552117, to order

Foresight
Association for the Promotion of
Pre-Conceptual Care,
28 The Paddock,
Godalming,
Surrey GU7 1XD
Tel: 01483 427839

ORGANIC FOOD

Organic food is becoming more
widely available through health
food stores and major
supermarkets. However, an
increasingly popular way to get
hold of it is via a 'box scheme', in
which seasonal vegetables are
delivered to your door on a
regular basis. To find out details
of your nearest 'Local Food Links'
scheme, or discover more about
how you can support a more
sustainable form of agriculture,
contact:

The Soil Association
Colston Street,
Bristol BS1 5BB
Tel: 0117 929 0661

PERSPIRATION

Mr Renne is consultant surgeon
and expert in micro-surgery to
eliminate excessive perspiration at:
King's College Hospital,
London SE5 9RS
Tel: 0171 346 3017

SEMI-PERMANENT
MAKE-UP

For salon details, contact:
Carole Franck
28 Park Street,
Taunton,
Somerset TA1 4DG
Tel: 01823 271367/421310

SPA PRODUCT
SOURCES

Ahava Mud
Available at Selfridges; for other
stockists write to:
Ahava UK,
PO Box 275,
Cheltenham,
Gloucestershire GL51 5YT
Tel: 01452 864574

The Clay Company
Products available by mail order:
Clay House, Penny Lane,
Liverpool L18 1DG
Tel/Fax: 0151 722 5151

E'SPA
See *Cosmetics & Skin Care*

Mountaineers' Blanket
The Mountain Thermal Blanket is
available from:
Cotswolds,
The Outdoor People
For nearest branch/mail order,
Tel: 01285 643434

Pierre Cattier Argile Mud
For stockists and mail order:
20 Island Farm Avenue,
Molesey Trading Estate,
West Molesey,
Surrey KT8 2UZ
Tel: 0181 979 7261

Spa Tubs
To buy, contact:
Javatub,
3F Brent Mill Estate,
South Brent,
Devon TW10 9YT
Tel: 01364 73909

GLOBAL
DESTINATION
REPORTS

Travelling the globe, whether it's
for business or pleasure, can
leave you in need of an urgent
beauty boost. But it's often well
nigh impossible to know where
to turn for reliable help –
particularly if you don't speak
the language – unless you have a
friend or business contact who
can give you personal
recommendations. We asked
well-groomed women worldwide
to come up with their insider
tips, including hairdressers
(quick wash and dry rather than
a complete restyle), massage
practitioners to ease your
jet-lagged bones and good
manicurists/pedicurists.

Amsterdam
HAIR
Hans Douglas
Grand Hotel Krasnapolsky,
Dam 9-1012 JS
Tel: +31 20 620 554 6095

MANICURE/MASSAGE etc
Clarins Centre de Beauté
at address above
Tel: +31 20 620 26 10/554 60 30

Athens
HAIR
Dino + Gino
Ioannis Metaxa 30,
Glyfada
Tel: +30 1 89 42 026/89 49 182

also at:
52 Panagouli Street,
Glyfada
Tel: +30 1 89 45 972

MANICURE
As above

MASSAGE AND OTHER BEAUTY
TREATMENTS (not hair)
Dino + Gino Beauty Centre
2nd Floor, Ioannou Metaxa 30,
Glyfada
Tel: +30 1 89 45 209/89 47 166/
89 45 209

Berlin
HAIR
Tony & Guy
Kaiser-Friedrichstrasse 1a,
Charlottenburg
Tel: +49 30 341 8545

Vidal Sassoon
Shluterstrasse 38,
Charlottenburg
Tel: +49 30 994 5000

Hanley's
Hackesche Hofe
Mitte
Tel: +49 30 281 3179

MANICURE/PEDICURE
(also reflexology and excellet range
of beauty treatments)
Marie-France
Fasanenstrasse,
Charlottenburg
Tel: +49 30 281 3179

BEAUTY SUPPLIES
KaDWe
Tauentzienstrasse 21
Tel: +49 30 21210
The oldest and best known
department store now has a beauty
salon/cosmetics studio.

Galeries Lafayette
Friedrichstrasse
Tel: +49 30 209 480
The best looking beauty hall in the
hottest street in the former East.

Berlin Cosmetics
Friedrichstrasse 168
Tel: +49 30 201 2220
Old-style cosmetics house with full
consultation service.

Harry Lehmann
Kantstrasse 108
Tel: +49 30 324 3582
Tailor-made fragrances sold by the
gramme.

MASSAGE
Dot Stein (for personal visits)
Tel: +49 30 452 2444

Bombay

Head for the five-star hotels which
all do a decent job with hair and
beauty treatments, particularly
manicure/pedicure. Top
recommendations are:

New Oberoi
Nariman Point
Tel: +91 22 202 57 57

Taj Mahal
Apollo Bunder
Tel: +91 22 202 33 66

Pedicures in India are generally
wonderful. You should also take
time for a head and scalp massage.

Cape Town

HAIR
Linda of London (Hair)
Mount Nelson Hotel,
Orange Street Gardens
Tel +27 21 23 7922/21 24 7817

Carlton Hair International
Shop No.5,
The Place,
Cavendish Square,
Claremont
Tel: +27 21 61 6877

MANICURE/PEDICURE
Linda of London (see above)

Linda van Niekerk, Skincare Clinic
204 Victoria Wharf Centre,
Pier 5,
Waterfront
Tel: +27 21 418 5441/5442

MASSAGE
Linda van Niekerk (see above)

The Chelsea Health & Beauty Clinic
17 Wolfe Street,
Wynberg
Tel: +27 21 797 6754/7066 for a
wide range of natural therapies as
well as beauty treatments (and
there's a hairdresser downstairs)

Geneva

HAIR
Perle
143 Rue de Lausanne,
1202
Tel: +41 22 731 61 81

MANICURE
L'Institute de Beauté Amandine
7 Place du Temple,
1227 Carouge
Tel: +41 22 342 16 16

MASSAGE
Helena Rubinstein
1st floor,
2 Cours de Rive,
1204
Tel: +41 22 311 66 94

Hong Kong

HAIR
Mandarin Hairdressing Salon
Mandarin Oriental Hotel,
Central
Tel: +852 2522 4858
(try for Ronald or Fatima)

MANICURE
Mandarin Hairdressing Salon
Mandarin Oriental Hotel,
Central
Tel: +852 2522 4858
(try for Pat, and, for a special
medical pedicure, Mr So)

MASSAGE
The Beautiful Skin Centre
Shop 344,
Level 3,
Pacific Place
Tel: +852 2506 0928

also at:
B219
Times Square,
1 Matheson Street,
Causeway Bay
Tel: +852 2877 8911

The widest selection of brand-name
cosmetics, aromatherapy oils and
other natural products is available
at:
Seibu Department Store
Pacific Place

Johannesburg

HAIR
Burgundy
Shop 105/106,
1st level,
Sandton Square,
Sandton
Tel: +27 11 884 0192/0193
(and manicure/pedicure)

Carlton Hair Salon
Rosebank Mall,
Cradock Avenue,
Rosebank
Tel: +27 11 788 2914/0113
(and manicure)

MANICURE/PEDICURE
Jill Zander Beauty Clinic
2nd Floor,
Regent Place,
Cradock Avenue,
Rosebank
Tel: +27 11 880 6723
(and full range of beauty treatments)

MASSAGE
**Elaine Brennan Skin & Electrolysis
Clinic**
6 North Park Centre,
3rd Avenue,
Parktown North
Tel: +27 11 788 5213
(and beauty treatments)

Los Angeles

HAIR
Art Luna
8930 Keith Avenue,
West Hollywood
Tel: +1 310 247 1383

Brigitte Danyl or Jamal Hammadi at:
Louis Licari Salon
450 North Cannon Drive,
Beverly Hills
Tel: +1 310 247 0855

Michaeljohn
414 North Camden,
Beverly Hills
Tel: +1 310 278 8333

MANICURE/PEDICURE
Jessica's Nail Clinic
8627 Sunset Boulevard,
West Hollywood
Tel: + 1 310 659 5200

Ole Henritsen
8601 Sunset Boulevard,
West Hollywood
Tel: + 1 310 854 7700

Arcona Studio
5507 Laurel Canyon Boulevard
Tel: +1 818 506 5192

Book your poolside manicure
and pedicure at:
The Peninsula Spa
9882 Little Santa Monica Boulevard,
Beverly Hills
Tel: +1 310 551 2888

MASSAGE
Claudio Tepper at:
The Peninsula Spa
(as above)

Ms Tamara Zalevsky at:
The Health Spa
Regent Beverly Wilshire,
9500 Wilshire Boulevard,
Beverly Hills
Tel: +1 310 275 5200

Madrid

HAIR & MANICURE
Cheska
Velazquez 61
Tel: +34 1 431 6638

Ruphert
Serrano 100
Tel: +34 1 431 0968

Cesar Morales
Marqués de Urquijo 14
Tel: +34 1 559 3576

Borghese
Lagasca 27
Tel: +34 1 576 0058

Llongueras
Ortega y Gasset 23
Tel: +34 1 435 4163

Rachel's
Juan Bravo 12
Tel: +34 1 435 4301

Gente
Hermanos Bequer 4
Tel: +34 1 563 8846

MASSAGE
Llongueras
Lagasca 38
Tel: +34 1 431 7402

Club Abasota
Pradillo 44
Tel: +34 1 519 3450

Edna Cardinale
Claudio Cuello 126
Bajo Derecha
Tel: +34 1 562 3094

BEAUTY TREATMENTS
Centro Estética Carmen Navarro
Nicasio Gallego 4–2
Tel: +34 1 594 4282

COSMETICS
Try **El Corte Inglés** department stores.

Melbourne
HAIR
Adroit Hairdressers
241 Bridge Road,
Richmond,
Melbourne, Vict. 3122
Tel: +61 3 428 1706

MANICURE/PEDICURE
The Hepburn Day Spa Water Shop
100 High Street,
Armidale,
Melbourne, Vict.
Tel: +61 3 9500 2221

MASSAGE
The Hepburn's Spa Resort
Mineral Spring Reserve,
Hepburn Springs, Vict. 3461
Tel: +61 53 48 20 34

Mexico City
HAIR AND BEAUTY TREATMENTS:
Beauty Salon – Hotel Marquis
Paseo de la Reforma,
DF 11500
Tel: +52 5 211 3600

Beauty Salon – Four Seasons Hotel,
Paseo de la Reforma 500,
DF 06600
Tel: +52 5 230 1818

Hotel Spa Ixtapan
(about 100km from Mexico City)
offers a complete range of treatments
Tel: +52 5 264 2613
(also see Santa Fe)

Milan
HAIR & MANICURE/PEDICURE
Aldo Coppola
25 via Manzoni
Tel: +39 2 86 46 21 63
and at:
1 Piazza S. Babila
Tel: +39 2 76 00 40 74
and at:
16 Via Mascheroni
Tel: +39 2 48 00 52 48

The Harbour Club
(the superfitness club beloved of
Diana, Princess of Wales in London)
has opened in Milan at:
Via Cascina Bellaria,
San Siro, 20153
Tel: +39 2 452861

Monaco
HAIR
Jacques Dessange
5 Boulevard des Moulins,
MC 98000
Tel: +377 93 25 01 01

MANICURE
L'Institut des Ongles
Galerie Metropole,
4 avenue de la Madone,
MC 98000
Tel: +377 93 25 77 78

MASSAGE
Les Thermes Marins de Monte Carlo
2 avenue de Monte Carlo,
MC 98000
Tel: +377 92 16 40 40

Moscow
HAIR
Jacques Dessange
Cosmos Hotel,
150 Prospekt Mira
Tel: +007 095 215 0280/215 9780

MANICURE/ PEDICURE/ MASSAGE
Persona Salon
10/13 Sadovo-Triumphalnya,
St Bldng 2
Tel: +007 095 209 0983

Munich
HAIR
Le Coup/Gerhard Meir
23 Theatinerstrasse
Tel: +49 89 22 23 27

Ulrich Graf (uses Aveda)
10 Hans Sachs Strasse
Tel: +49 89 26 70 67

Luitpold Figaro
11 Brienner Strasse
Tel: +49 89 22 09 94

MANICURE/PEDICURE
Janet Sartin Cosmetics
Hotel Bayerischer Hof
5/1 Pranner Strasse
Tel: +49 89 29 63 06

MASSAGE
Janet Sartin Cosmetics
(as above)

New York
HAIR
John Frieda
30, E 76th Street
Tel: +1 212 879 1000

Salon Ishi
70, E 55th Street
Tel: +1 212 888 4744
(ask for the shiatsu shampoo –
while lying horizontal you are given
an incredibly relaxing scalp massage)

MANICURE
Celina Nail & Skincare Salon
348 E 66th Street
Tel: +1 212 737 9500

PEDICURE
Arsi Skincare
Suite 206, 162 West 56th Street
Tel: +1 212 582 5720

MASSAGE
Eastside Massage Therapy Centre
351 E 78th Street
Tel: +1 212 240 2927

New York Wellness Bodywork Centre
80 W 11th St
Tel: +1 212 505 5034

Don't miss having a facial at:
Susan Ciminelli Day Spa
601 Madison Ave
Tel: +1 212 688 5500
This favourite salon of supermodels
like Linda Evangelista also offers
The Ultimate Hour, an amazing
treatment including a facial,
reflexology and seaweed wrap,
squeezed into 60 minutes

DAY SPAS
For recommendations across USA,
the **Day Spa Association** directory
produced by ClubSpa USA lists top
spas. For info,
Tel: +1 201 865 2065

Paris
HAIRDRESSER
Jean-Marc Marcobeal
45 Avenue George V,
75008
Tel: +33 1 47 20 08 81
(Suggested tip 50 FF)

Dominique Peyrot
This roving hairdresser will come to
your hotel
Tel: +33 1 42 28 41 38
Mobile: +33 07 75 81 96

MASSAGE
Institut Guerlain
68 Champs-Elysees,
75001
Tel: +33 1 47 89 71 80
(try the *massage à quatre mains*,
during which you will be lulled into
a state of advanced relaxation by two
therapists at once)

For FACIALS, try:
Jickie Leray
12 Avenue Roosevelt,
75008
Tel: +33 1 42 89 33 85

Prague
HAIR
Hammer SRO
Kadernicky a Kosmeticky Salon,
U Zlate Koruny,
Zelezna 3a
Tel: +42 2 24 21 77 96

MASSAGE
Christian Dior Cosmetic Salon
Paritzska 7
Tel: +42 2 232 73 82

Estée Lauder Shop and Salon
Zelezna 18
Tel: +42 2 24 23 30 23
(opposite the hair salon)

Lancôme Institut de Beauté
Jungmannovo,
Navesii 20
Tel: +42 2 24 21 71 89
(contact: Ludmila Ticha)

Rome

HAIR
Roberto d'Antonio
36 Piazza di Pietra, 00186

also at:
18c Via Guinone Lucina,
Santa Severa
Tel: +39 6 679 3197/6 678 5891
(simple looking, but stars, models
and 'society' flock here)

MANICURE/MASSAGE
(and everything else to do with
beauty and health, including back
and other medical problems):
Prefetti Bellezza
via dei Prefetti
Tel: + 39 6 687 3756

Santa Fe

For the works, go to:
Margarita White
El Palacio de Hierro,
Centro Comercial, DF 11700
Tel: +52 5 257 9200

Singapore

HAIR
Provocative Hair Salon
9 Scotts Road, Pacific Plaza,
Unit 3–11/12
Tel: +65 733 1638

Passion Hair Salon
300 Orchard Road,
The Promenade Unit 02–09
Tel: +65 733 5638

Quest Hair Salon
Raffles City,
Sogo,
Unit 02–34
Tel: +65 388 8949

MANICURE/PEDICURE
Nouvelles Esthetiques
(Clarins products)
6 Raffles Boulevard,
Marina Square,
Unit 03–204
Tel: +65 334 6748

MASSAGE
Renewal Day Spa
Tong Building,
Orchard Road,
Unit 17–02
Tel: +65 738 3521

COSMETICS
Useful stores for cosmetic
supplies include:
C.K. Tangs
Tel: +65 737 5500

Robinson
Tel: +65 733 0888

Seiyu
Tel: +65 223 2222

Metro
Tel: +65 734 3133

Sydney

HAIR
Joh Bailey
Shop 30,
Chifley Plaza,
City
Tel: +61 2 223 7673
(Joh is Sydney's blowdry king and
his salon is handily located in one of
the city's best shopping centres)

MANICURE/PEDICURE
Ali Hamilton Institute
15 Transvaal Avenue,
Double Bay
Tel: +61 2 328 1340/328 1319
(a Sydney institution where the
glitterati go)

Smyth & Fitzgerald
Shop 18,
Ritz Carlton Promenade,
Double Bay
Tel: +61 2 326 1385
(a great one-stop for hairdressing
and all beauty treatments)

MASSAGE
Venestus
31 Oxford Street,
Paddington
Tel: +61 2 361 4014

Zen – The Art of Body Maintenance
116 Darlinghurst Road,
Darlinghurst
Tel: +61 2 361 4200

Tokyo

HAIR, MANICURE & MASSAGE
**Shu Uemura Esthetique & Hair
Styling**
T Place 2F,
4–4–25 Minami Aoyama,
Minato–Ku 107
Tel: +81 3 3486 7578

Many of the large Western hotel
chains offer a good service, but if
you can travel outside Tokyo for a
brief spa getaway, Shu Uemura have
their own thalassotherapy centre:
Shu Uemura Esthetic Salon
Hotel Thalassa Shima,
1826–1 Shirahama,
Uramura-cho,
Toba-shi Mie Pret 517
Tel: +81 599 32 1104
Freephone: 0210 114568

CYBERBEAUTY

One place to check out all the latest beauty happenings is on the Internet. More and more companies are creating 'home pages' on the World Wide Web, which update you on their newest products and share insider beauty tips. In addition, there are discussion groups in which you can exchange beauty information. Some of them will also allow you to mail order products right to your door.

Beware of one problem: if you simply key in the word 'beauty' and do a search, you'll have to sift through hundreds of thousands of locations to find the useful Cyberbeauty sites. To save you, here's a shortlist of our favourites:

AVEDA: http:/ / www.aveda.com
AVON: http:/ / www.avon.com
CLINIQUE: http:/ / www.clinique.com
HAIRNET: http:/ / www.hairnet.com
L'OREAL: http:/ / www.lorealcosmetics.com
MADELEINE'S WORLD OF COSMETICS: http:/ / www.wineasy.se/bjornt/world.html
(which includes an international library of lipstick colours to look at)
REVLON: http:/ / www.revlon.com
SHISEIDO: http:/ / www.toppan.co.jp/shiseido
THE BODY SHOP: http:/ / www.the-body-shop.com
THE GARDEN PHARMACY: http:/ / www.garden.co.uk

**We would love your recommendations for the next edition of *The Beauty Bible*.
Please write to us
c/o Kyle Cathie Ltd, Publishers, 20 Vauxhall Bridge Road
London SW1V 2SA**

INDEX

PHOTOGRAPHIC ACKNOWLEDGEMENTS

CHAPTER 1

page 8   Tr.-Sc., by Claus Wickrath ('Femme'), model Sophia Goth at Elite Los Angeles courtesy of Bobbi Brown

page 12   L.H., mascara courtesy of Bobbi Brown

page 13   L.H. cosmetics courtesy of cosmetics houses shown

page 15   L.H. cosmetics courtesy of cosmetics houses shown

page 16/17 R.H.

page 19   L.H., brush courtesy of Mary Greenwell

page 21   R.P. (top); R.P. (below)

page 22   T.C.L.

page 23   T.C.L.

page 25   D.D.

page 26   L.H., lipstick courtesy of Bobbi Brown

page 27   M.B.

page 28   E.R.

page 29   I.B., by Alfred Gescheidt

page 30/31 L.H.

page 32   E.R.

page 33   D.D.

page 34   I.B.

page 35   D.D.

page 36   L.H., brushes courtesy of Mary Greenwell

page 37   R.F. (x3)

page 38   C.M.

page 39   I.C.L.

page 40   C.M.

page 42/3 D.D.

page 44/5 D.D.

page 46   (top) T.S., by Tamara Reynolds; (below) R.G., courtesy of Warner Bros. courtesy of Senate

page 47   courtesy of Senate

page 49   L.H., scents courtesy of cosmetics houses shown

page 51   D.D.

page 52   E.R.

page 53   I.B., by Michael Gosbee

CHAPTER 2

page 54   T.S., by David Stewart

page 59   C.M.

page 61   D.D.

page 62   R.P. (x4)

page 63   D.D.

page 64   R.H., by Jutta Klee

page 65   L.H., sunglasses courtesy of Sunglass Hut; R.F. (inset)

CHAPTER 3

page 66   Tr.-Sc./Anna/Piccardi

page 71   T.S., by Lori Adamski Peek

page 72   I.B., by Bokelberg

page 73   courtesy of Senate

page 75   L.H.

page 77   L.H.

page 79   Tr.-Sc./Grazia/Carpi

page 81   T.C.L.

page 83   L.H.

page 85   T.C.L.

page 87   M.B., model Carla Williams at Matthews & Powell

page 88   T.C.L.

page 90/91 T.S., by Marc Dolphin

page 92/93 D.D.

page 94   L.H., bottle courtesy of Kay Cooper

page 95   I.C.L.

page 96/97 courtesy of Senate

page 98   T.C.L.

page 101   T.S., by Pete Seaward

page 102   M.B., model Catherine Mceude at Elite New York

page 105   I.B., by Brigitte Lambert

CHAPTER 4

page 106   C.M.

page 111   L.H.

page 113   R.F. (top); R.P. (below x 5)

page 114   T.C.L.

page 115   L.H.

page 116   C.M.

page 118   courtesy of Senate

page 119   D.D.

page 120   L.H.

page 121   A.A.

page 122   courtesy of Nicky Clarke

page 123   courtesy of John Frieda

page 125   by Patrick Demarchelier, courtesy of Sam McKnight

page 126   C.M.

page 127   R.F.

page 130   T.S., by Jerome Tisne

page 131   R.H., by Jutta Klee

page 132   C.M.

page 134   T.S., by Dan Bosler

page 135   C.M.

CHAPTER 5

page 136   T.S., by Nick Dolding

page 144/5 T.S., by D.H. Stewart

page 149   T.S., by Jerome Tisne

CHAPTER 6

page 150   S.P.L., by Clare Park

page 154   I.C.L.

page 155   I.B., by Tomek Sikora

page 156   T.S.

page 158   T.C.L.

page 160/1 D.D.

page 163   L.H.

page 165   L.H.

page 166   T.C.L.

page 168   T.C.L.

page 171   D.D.

page 172   T.C.L.

page 173   T.S., by Ken Scott

page 174   T.S., by Ken Scott

page 177   D.D.

page 179   E.R.

page 181   M.B., model Amanda Wright at Freddies

page 182   D.D.

page 183   D.D.

page 184   I.B., by Andrea Pistoles

page 186   T.C.L.

page 188   I.B. by Simon Wilkinson

page 191   T.S. by Chris Harvey

page 193   L.H.

page 194   L.H.

page 197   L.H.

page 198/9 I.B., by Tomek Sikora

CHAPTER 7

page 200   L.H.

page 205–7 (flowers & material) L.H.

page 205–7 (all buildings) T.S.

page 205   (top) T.S., by Greg Pease; (below) T.S., by Cosmo Condina

Page 206   (top) T.S., by Hiroyuki Matsumoto; (below) T.S., by R Evans

Page 207   (top) T.S., by John Lawrence; (below) T.S., by Hugh Sitton

page 208   I.C.L.

page 211   L.H., scents courtesy of cosmetics houses shown

page 212   L.H., scents courtesy of cosmetics houses shown

page 213   courtesy of Senate

CHAPTER 8

page 214   I.B. by Michael Gosbee

JACKET

(top, left to right)

(i)   M.B., model Nicola Harvey at Select

(ii)   E.R.

(iii)   E.R.

(iv)   M.B.

(bottom, left to right)

(i)   M.B., model Catherine Mceude at Elite New York

(ii)   H.G.

(iii)   E.R.

KEY

The authors and publishers are grateful to the following:

A.A.   Advertising Archive Ltd

C.M.   Christopher Moore Ltd

D.D.   David Downton

E.R.   Erik Russell

H.G.   Hulton Getty

I.B.   The Image Bank

I.C.L.   Images Colour Library

L.H.   Laura Hodgson

M.B.   Maureen Barrymore

R.F.   Rex Features Ltd

R.G.   The Ronald Grant Archive

R.H.   Robert Harding Picture Library

R.P.   Retna Pictures

S.P.L.   The Special Photographers Library

T.C.L.   Telegraph Colour Library

T.S.   Tony Stone Images

Tr.-Sc.   Transworld-Scope